(continued on back)

Managing Attention Disorders in Children

A Guide for Practitioners

SAM GOLDSTEIN, PH.D.
MICHAEL GOLDSTEIN, M.D.

WILEY

A WILEY-INTERSCIENCE PUBLICATION

JOHN WILEY & SONS

New York • Chichester • Brisbane • Toronto • Singapore

This publication is designed to provide accurate and
authoritative information in regard to the subject
matter covered. It is sold with the understanding that
the publisher is not engaged in rendering legal, acccounting,
or other professional service. If legal service or other
expert assistance is required, the services of a competent
professional person should be sought. *From a Declaration
of Principles jointly adopted by a Committee of the
American Bar Association and a Committee of Publishers.*

Library of Congress Cataloging in Publication Data:

Goldstein, Sam.
    Managing attention disorders in children: a guide for
    practitioners / Sam Goldstein, Michael Goldstein.
        p. cm.—(Wiley series on personality processes)
    Bibliography: p.
    ISBN 0-471-61137-9
    1. Attention deficit disorders.   I. Goldstein, Michael.
II. Title. III. Series.
RJ496.A86G65   1989
618.92'8589—dc20   89-9090
                                        CIP

Printed in the United States of America

10 9 8 7 6 5 4 3 2 1

Everyone knows what attention is.
William James, 1890

A proper and effectual remedy for this
wandering of thought, I would be glad to find.
John Locke, 1762

By the time I think about what I am gonna do . . .
I already DID it!
Dennis the Menace
Hank Ketcham, 1988

Series Preface

This series of books is addressed to behavioral scientists interested in the nature of human personality. Its scope should prove pertinent to personality theorists and researchers as well as to clinicians concerned with applying an understanding of personality processes to the amelioration of emotional difficulties in living. To this end, the series provides a scholarly integration of theoretical formulations, empirical data, and practical recommendations.

Six major aspects of studying and learning about human personality can be designated: personality theory, personality structure and dynamics, personality development, personality assessment, personality change, and personality adjustment. In exploring these aspects of personality, the books in the series discuss a number of distinct but related subject areas: the nature and implications of various theories of personality; personality characteristics that account for consistencies and variations in human behavior; the emergence of personality processes in children and adolescents; the use of interviewing and testing procedures to evaluate individual differences in personality, efforts to modify personality styles through psychotherapy, counseling, behavior therapy, and other methods of influence; and patterns of abnormal personality functioning that impair individual competence.

IRVING B. WEINER

University of South Florida
Tampa, Florida

v

Preface

It has long been recognized that problems with attention and arousal constitute the largest single source of referrals to child mental health centers. The cluster of problems, including inattention, overarousal, hyperactivity, impulsivity and difficulty delaying gratification, that is now diagnostically referred to as attention-deficit hyperactivity disorder (ADHD) is probably the most common and one of the most complex disorders of childhood. It affects children's interaction with all areas of their environment. Children with ADHD typically experience difficulty with home and school behavior, peer interaction, academic achievement and psychological adjustment. They are frequently an enigma for their parents and teachers. Their uneven, unpredictable behavior creates stress as well as the erroneous belief that they have problems of motivation and desire, as opposed to physically based inabilities.

Researchers have noted that by the time a child is referred for this set of problems, the clinician is frequently presented with a complex set of difficulties that may be affected by a variety of social and nonsocial factors. Keith Conners (1975a) has observed that evaluation is complicated by the fact that there is no critical diagnostic test for attention problems. There are few exclusionary criteria and no unequivocal, positive developmental markers. ADHD appears to be a disorder distinct from other disorders of childhood because a difference in intensity, persistence and clustering of symptoms rather than the presence or absence or symptoms confirms the diagnosis. Finally, we are now aware that this is not an age-limited disorder but for many in this population presents a set of lifetime problems.

Keith Conners also wrote that this is a disorder marked by contradictions, uncertainty, the unexpected and the bizarre. Over the past 80 years, this cluster of problems has been referred to by at least 30 different descriptive terms. Despite an increasing and enormous volume of research literature, we continue to be uncertain about both the specific cause of these problems and the best course of treatment for these children. The field continues to be plagued by marked differences of opinion as to the cause, definition, evaluation and treatment.

This text is for all practitioners faced with the task of evaluation, guidance and management of attention disorders in children. It is our attempt to offer the practitioner a comprehensive volume providing a research-based understanding of attention disorders, a model for assessment and most importantly, clear, well-defined guidelines for multidisciplinary treatment. The text arises from our years of experience evaluating children with this set of problems, lecturing nationally to parents and professionals and frequent frustration in responding negatively when asked if a text such as this is currently available. Although the text is specifically directed at psychologists and physicians, we believe the breadth and scope of the information provided will prove extremely useful to mental and allied health professionals, educators and parents.

SAM GOLDSTEIN
MICHAEL GOLDSTEIN

Neurology, Learning and Behavior Center
Salt Lake City, Utah
December 1989

Acknowledgments

This work is dedicated to our wives, Janet and Barbara, and our children, Allyson, Ryan, Rachel, Elizabeth and Adam.

We wish to thank Sally Ingalls, Ph.D., for her thoughtful assistance with the manuscript; Elaine Pollock for suggestions in the completion of Chapters 10 and 12; Kathleen Gardner and Sarah Cheminant for organizing and typing the manuscript; Lynn Wilson for library assistance; Connie Cheminant for illustrations in Chapters 1 and 2; and the children and parents we have worked with over the past years, from whom we have learned so much.

S.G.
M.G.

Contents

PART 1

Overview, Background and Etiology

Disorders of attention and arousal are not cured but must be managed throughout childhood. It is for this reason that the practitioner must develop a thorough understanding of the nature, definition and developmental profile of these symptomatic problems if effective treatment is to be initiated. The practitioner must help both parents and other professionals view the world through the eyes of the attention-disordered child.

Chapter 1 is a review of the basic core symptoms of attention disorders and symptom presentation at various developmental ages. The practitioner will be sensitized to the importance of attention, task persistence, reflection and vigilance in everyday living. A number of definitions from various perspectives will be provided. The chapter will provide an analysis explaining the development of secondary adjustment and behavior problems that frequently stem from the core symptoms.

Effective management also presupposes an understanding of etiology. Chapter 2 will provide an overview of brain function and hypothesized brain mechanisms that appear responsible for attention- and arousal-level problems. Theories and research related to specific factors that may affect attention, including heredity, diet, toxins, developmental impairments and injury, will be presented. The data will then be unified into an integrated model of causality.

CHAPTER 1

Attention Disorders

The childhood cognitive and behavioral problems categorized as disorders of attention and hyperactivity present a challenge for the practitioner. These problems constitute the most common chronic behavior disorder (Wender, 1975) and the largest single source of referrals to child mental health centers (Barkley, 1981a). The cluster of problems, including inattention, overarousal, hyperactivity, impulsivity and difficulty with delay of gratification, which diagnostically is now referred to as *Attention-deficit hyperactivity disorder*, or ADHD (APA, 1987), is one of the most complex disorders of childhood. These problems affect children's interaction with all areas of their environment and result in an inability to meet situational demands in an age-appropriate fashion (Routh, 1978). Children with ADHD typically experience difficulty with home, school and community behavior, including peer interaction, academic achievement and general adjustment. They are frequently enigmatic to their parents and teachers. Their uneven, unpredictable behavior creates additional stress and leads to the erroneous belief that these are problems of motivation and desire rather than physically based disabilities.

ADHD problems typically cause significant and pervasive impairment in a child's day-to-day interaction with the environment. The familial, social and academic demands placed on children are primarily determined by the adults in their lives. Restless, inattentive adults can modify their lives so as to minimize the negative impact of these problems. Children cannot do so. Further, these problems appear to have a significant impact on a child's emerging personality and cognitive skills. Although the majority of children appear to outgrow the core symptoms associated with attention deficit (Weiss & Hechtman, 1986; Gittelman, Mannuzza, Shenker & Bonagura, 1985), others do not (Bellak, 1979). It is apparent that years of skill deficit result in a long history of negative interaction with the environment. This in turn becomes a major force on the child's emerging personality (Wender, 1979). A child who experiences years of negative feedback, negative reinforcement and an inability to meet the reasonable demands of family, friends and teachers because of skill deficits will certainly be affected for life. Practitioners must be concerned not only with the core symptoms of this disorder but also with the significant secondary impact they have on both the child and family members.

By the time a child is referred, the practitioner is frequently presented with a complex set of problems that may be affected by a variety of social and nonsocial factors. Evaluation is complicated by the fact that there is no critical diagnostic test for attention problems. There are few exclusionary developmental criteria and no unequivocal, positive developmental markers (Conners, 1975a). Attention deficit appears to be distinct from other disorders of childhood because it is the difference in intensity, persistence and clustering of symptoms rather than the presence or absence of symptoms that confirms the diagnosis (Ross & Ross, 1982). Finally, we are now aware that this is not an age-limited disorder. In some studies, as many as one-third of attention-deficit children present a lifetime set of problems (Gittelman et al., 1985).

Our understanding of attention deficit has been marked by contradictions, uncertainty, the unexpected and, at times, the bizarre (Ross & Ross, 1982). Over the past 80 years, this cluster of problems has been referred to by a multitude of descriptive terms. In the very early 1900s, the disorder was referred to as a *defect in moral control* (Still, 1902). Such terms as *post-encephalitic disorder, hyperkinesis, minimal brain damage, minimal brain dysfunction, Hyperkinetic reaction of childhood, Attention-deficit disorder with and without hyperactivity*, and now *Attention-deficit hyperactivity disorder* are the most familiar to the practitioner. There continues to be disagreement in terminology. It has been argued in the recent literature that perhaps this disorder would be best labeled as a reward-system dysfunction (Haenlein & Caul, 1987), a self-regulatory disorder (Kirby & Grimley, 1986) or a learning disability (McGee & Share, 1988).

ADHD is a disorder that confronts many practitioners, including physicians, psychologists, educators, social workers, speech pathologists and physical therapists. For years each discipline worked in isolation, developing its own set of definitions, ideas for assessment and interventions. This has created problems in communication among disciplines. A psychologist's definition of appropriate attention may be very different from an educator's. Problems persist even within the field of mental health, where there are marked differences of opinion as to the cause, definition, evaluation and best course of treatment. For example, despite an increasing and enormous volume of research literature, the precise definition of this disorder continues to be uncertain. Differing views of the disorder cause different children to be identified as attention disordered in various research studies. This makes it difficult, if not impossible, to compare the outcomes of those studies (Rie, 1980).

Some researchers argue that problems with inattention, hyperactivity and excessive emotionality are cultural phenomena (Block, 1977). They point to various cultures and subcultures as exhibiting a minimal degree of these childhood problems. It is clear, however, that this is a disorder in which the severity of the child's problems results from an interaction of temperamental traits and the demands placed on the child by the environment. An inattentive, impulsive, restless child living somewhere on a tropical island may not gather as many coconuts or catch as many fish as others but may not have significant difficulty meeting the demands of the culture. One hundred years ago in the United States a child with a similar set of problems, struggling at school, would have been asked to leave and sent out to work at an early age. In today's culture, however, there is an increasing emphasis on the importance of a child's ability to sit still, pay attention and finish things at a very early age. Children compromised in their ability to do so, even if they do not experience any other sort of developmental problem, are effectively unable to integrate into and meet the expectations of our school system.

The issue of definition must also be considered when determining the presence or absence of ADHD in various cultures. A predominant school of thought in Great Britain argues strongly that symptoms of attention deficit are a reflection of conduct disorder (Sandberg, Rutter & Taylor, 1978). For this reason, and because of differences in diagnostic criteria, a higher percentage of conduct disorder is diagnosed in Great Britain, balanced by a lower diagnosis rate for ADHD. In the United States, on the other hand, we choose to view a majority of these symptoms as reflecting ADHD and thus diagnose a higher percentage of children as having ADHD.

It has also been argued that as the tempo of our society increases, there is a greater incidence of attention deficit (McNamara, 1972). Normative data obtained for the revised edition of the Wechsler Intelligence Scale for Children, however, does not support this hypothesis (Wechsler, 1974; Spring, Yellin & Greenberg, 1976). Rather, increased community, professional and parental awareness seem to be resulting in more children being referred, correctly identified and placed in treatment programs (Lambert, Sandoval & Sassone, 1978).

AN HISTORICAL OVERVIEW

Historically, there are allusions in many of the great early civilizations to these childhood problems. The Greek physician Galen was known to prescribe opium for restless, colicky infants (Goodman & Gilman, 1975). In the 1890s, physicians working with brain-injured individuals noticed a similarity in the pattern of inattentive, restless and overaroused behavior exhibited by these individuals and a similar pattern of behavior exhibited in retarded individuals with no history of trauma. They hypothesized that these behavioral patterns in the retarded individuals resulted from some sort of brain damage or dysfunction.

In 1902, Still described a problem in children that he characterized as a *defect in moral control* (Still, 1902). Still noted that this problem resulted in the child's inability to internalize rules and limits, as well as in a pattern of restless, inattentive and overaroused behavior. Still was extremely insightful, noting that this pattern of behavior could have resulted from injury, heredity, disease or environmental experience. He observed that the disorder occurred more frequently in males than in females, something he felt did not happen by chance. He was also quite pessimistic, believing that these children could not be helped and should be institutionalized at an early age.

In the years 1917 and 1918, following a world outbreak of encephalitis, health professionals observed that there was a group of children physically recovered from the encephalitis but presenting a pattern of restless, inattentive, easily overaroused and hyperactive behavior not exhibited before their illness (Hohman, 1922). It was thought that this pattern of behavior resulted from some degree of brain injury caused by the disease process. This pattern of behavior was described as *post encephalitic disorder* (Bender, 1942).

In 1937, a physician by the name of Charles Bradley, while working with emotionally disturbed children in a child psychiatric inpatient setting, experimented with stimulant drugs (Bradley, 1937). In that same year, Molitch and Eccles (1937) investigated the effect of benzedrine on intelligence scores in children. Bradley observed a remarkable response when these children were given benzedrine. For a period of time they calmed down, were more positive, less oppositional, paid attention better and appeared to learn better.

World War II afforded researchers the opportunity to study a wide variety of war wounds, including trauma to the head by various means (Goldstein, 1942). It was discovered that injury to any part of the brain frequently resulted in a pattern of inattentive, restless and overaroused behavior. This research supported the notion that children with this pattern of problems were victims of some form of brain damage or dysfunction. Also at this time, Strauss and his colleagues (Strauss & Lehtinen, 1947) hypothesized that the core problem for these children was distractibility. Strauss believed that if distractions were kept to a minimum, these children would function much better. This led to the introduction of the minimal stimulation classroom, in which teachers wore drab colors, the room remained undecorated and windows were frosted. A special curriculum was also developed. The research literature, however, has never supported this type of intervention as significantly benefiting distractible, inattentive children (Sarasone, 1949).

The 1950s saw a growing use of psychotropic medications. Classes of medications were developed that allowed approximately four-fifths of psychiatrically institutionalized individuals to function in society. Along with this revolution came a renewed interest in the use of medications for children, specifically the use of stimulants for children with attention problems. The disorder was initially identified as one of hyperactivity with secondary problems of limited attention span and impulsivity (Laufer & Denhoff, 1957). By the 1970s, however, research strongly began suggesting that the core problem was not excessive activity but inattention (Douglas & Peters, 1979). This led to a major shift in the focus of research, diagnosis and treatment.

In the 1950s, when efforts were initiated to identify the incidence of this disorder in childhood, teachers who were asked to name all the children in their class presenting with hyperactivity mentioned more than half the males and almost half the females (Lapouse & Monk, 1958). Later studies cited incidence rates as high as 20% (Yanow, 1973).

Today we have become more sophisticated as practitioners. We now ask a series of questions seeking both a consistency in problems among various settings and consensus by a number of raters—including parents, teachers and community-based professionals—concerning the severity of these problems. The practitioner also seeks to determine a statistical difference between the level of the identified child's behavioral problems and those of a similar sex and age population. When these criteria are met, the incidence rate for attention deficit drops to a more reasonable 1 to 6 percent (Lambert, Sandoval & Sassone, 1978). It also appears that a higher incidence of attention disorder, as well as other adjustment and developmental problems in children, occurs in lower socioeconomic areas. This is not surprising given the findings that a percentage of ADHD children become attention-disordered adults, have families, do not integrate well into society, fall to the lower socioeconomic strata and cluster in certain neighborhoods.

On the average, research studies have suggested that attention deficit is approximately five to nine times more prevalent in males than females (Ross & Ross, 1982). It has recently been proposed, however, that when males and females are compared to same-sex normative groups and controls are present for symptoms of hyperactivity and antisocial behavior, there may be an equal occurrence of ADD in both males and females (McGee, Williams & Silva, 1987). Studies suggest that females with this pattern of behavior may present with more mood, affect and emotion problems and with less difficulty with aggression (Kashani, Chapel & Ellis, 1979; Ackerman, Dykman & Oglesby, 1983). Others suggest that ADD females present with greater cognitive and language function impairments (Berry, Shaywitz & Shaywitz, 1985).

Despite the fact that the DSM-III-R has combined the diagnoses of *Attention disorder with and without hyperactivity* into the singular ADHD diagnosis (APA, 1987), there is a volume of literature suggesting that these are very different disorders in children (Lahey, Schaughency, Hynd, Carlson & Nieves, 1987; Edelbrock, Costello & Kessler, 1984; Porrino, Rapoport, Behar, Sceery, Ismond & Bunney, 1983). Researchers have suggested that children experiencing attention problems without concomitant hyperactivity may present twice as frequently in epidemiological studies as attention-disordered hyperactive children (Lahey, Schaughency, Strauss & Frame, 1984).

A higher percentage of hyperactive, attention-disordered children are referred to mental health clinics because of the cluster of aversive problems they present. In comparison to attention-disordered children without hyperactivity, children with attention and hyperactivity problems present as more aggressive, unpopular and guiltless and have greater difficulty with conduct (King & Young, 1982; Pelham, Atkins, Murphy & White, 1981a). The attention-disordered child without hyperactivity is more frequently described as shy, socially withdrawn, moderately unpopular and poor at sports (Lahey, Schaughency, Frame & Strauss, 1985; Lahey et al., 1984). Intelligence testing yielded significantly lower full-scale I.Q. scores and lower verbal I.Q. scores for attention-disordered children with hyperactivity than for those without hyperactivity (Carlson, Lahey & Neeper, 1986). Studies have consistently found that both groups have a higher incidence of depressive behavior, poorer school performance and poorer self-concept than do their same-age peers (Lahey et al., 1984). A recent study also suggested that children experiencing attention and hyperactivity problems score eight to ten points higher on the Conners Questionnaire hyperkinesis index than those experiencing only attention difficulty (Brown, 1985).

DEFINITION OF ATTENTIONAL SKILLS

The brain possesses limited capacity for simultaneous information processing. It relies on a complex process to narrow the scope and focus of information to be processed and assimilated. Attention is a generic term used to designate a group of hypothetical mechanisms that collectively serve this function for the organism (Mesulam, 1985). Over the last 100 years, beginning with James (1890), researchers have identified attentional processes as essential prerequisites for higher cognitive functions.

Researchers and clinicians have been criticized for characterizing the hyperactive child as experiencing a generic attention deficit (Rosenthal & Allen, 1978). Posner and Snyder (1975) described attention as a complex field of study. Although it has been suggested that the field of psychology lacks an adequate definition for attentional skills (Mostovsky, 1970), others have argued that attentional skills can be operationally and statistically defined (Gordon & McClure, 1983). Although many utilize the term *attention* as a homogeneous skill, there are a number of distinct aspects to the attentional process. Taylor (1980) suggested that the statistically weak correlations between various tests of attention suggest that there are distinct and different aspects of attentional skills. It is important for the practitioner to operationally understand these aspects and consider each during the process of evaluation.

A child presenting with difficulty completing two simultaneous tasks, such as listening to the teacher and taking notes, would appear to have a problem with *divided attention*. A child frequently described as daydreaming and often preoccupied with other activities instead of the task assigned by the teacher or parent would be considered to have a problem with *focused attention*. A child easily distracted by extraneous events, such as minor noises in the classroom, would be considered to have a problem with *selective attention*. Surprising as it may seem, this child also appears unable to prioritize and select what is the most important thing to pay attention to in the immediate environment. For example, although the teacher may be standing in front of the room and speaking, the child may be unable to identify this as the most important stimulus in the immediate environment and instead may pay attention to the child sitting next to him. A child unable to remain on a task for a sufficient amount of time to satisfactorily complete the task would be considered to have a problem with *sustained attention*, or *persistence*. Finally, a child unable to perform such tasks as listening for the next spelling word presented by the teacher during a test would be considered to have a problem with *vigilance*, or *readiness* to respond.

There may be different anatomical bases for different aspects of attention (Posner, 1987). In studies measuring the ability of head-injured individuals to pay attention, it has been demonstrated that these attentional skills may not be equally impaired as the result of head trauma (Van Zomeren & Brouwer, 1987). In children experiencing attentional problems, a similar level of variability in attentional skills is observed.

A number of skills closely related to attention must also be defined. *Impulsivity* is best defined operationally as an inability to stop and think before acting, while *reflection* is its exact opposite. For the purposes of this text, *hyperactivity* refers to excessive bodily movement ranging from restless, incessant fidgeting while seated to frantic, seemingly purposeless racing around in the playground. *Overarousal* in this text is used to describe a responsive pattern of emotional behavior, either positive or negative, that is inappropriate in the speed at which it occurs and excessive in the frequency of its occurrence.

DEFINITIONS OF ADHD

It is important for the practitioner to understand and utilize a number of different definitions for this disorder.

The Common Sense Definition

This definition assists the practitioner in understanding the nature of ADHD children's functioning, the complexity of their behavioral problems and the reasons for their inability to respond to more traditional treatment interventions. This definition is based on the hypotheses of Douglas and Peters (1979) and Douglas (1985), which suggest that attention-disordered children experience a constitutional predisposition to experience problems with attention, effort and inhibitory control; poorly modulated arousal; and a need to seek stimulation. This is the definition the practitioner may use to assist parents in understanding the cause of their child's problems. Helping parents understand this disorder is the first and most crucial step in making change.

The *common-sense* definition has four components:

1. *Inattention and Distractibility*. ADHD children have difficulty remaining on task and focusing attention in comparison to non-ADHD children of similar chronological age (APA, 1987). It has been suggested that the average two-year-old can attend in an independent activity without direct supervision—and without a stimulus that is constantly changing, such as television—for approximately 7 minutes; three-year-olds for 9 minutes; four-year-olds for 13 minutes; and five-year-olds for 15 minutes (Call, 1985). From that point on, children's attention span (i.e., their ability to sit and color or play with clay) continues to increase with age. By first grade we expect children to be able to sit and work for an hour at a time. ADHD children additionally have difficulty screening out distracting stimuli in their environment as they attend to a task. At one time it was suspected that distractibility was the core problem (Strauss & Kephart, 1955). We are now aware that distractibility is only a small part of ADHD children's problems. Their inability to remain on a specific task frequently results in their seeking distractions. Thus, attention and distractibility problems combine to negatively affect their ability to remain on task.

2. *Overarousal.* ADHD children tend to be excessively restless, overactive and easily aroused. Their difficulty in controlling bodily movements is especially noted in situations in which they are required to stay put or sit still for long periods of time. They are quicker to become aroused. Whether happy or sad, the speed and intensity with which they go to the extreme of their emotion is much greater than that of their same-age peers. This pattern of behavior frequently frustrates parents because 15 minutes after becoming extremely upset the child has forgotten the upsetting event and moves on to something else. The parent, however, continues to be agitated by the event, cannot understand why the child no longer seems bothered and accuses the child of lacking guilt. As one parent has aptly put it, ADHD children wear their emotions on their sleeves.

3. *Impulsivity.* ADHD children have difficulty thinking before they act. They have difficulty weighing the consequences of their actions before acting and do not reasonably consider the consequences of their past behavior. They have difficulty following rule-governed behavior (Barkley, 1981a). Although they may be well aware of a rule and able to explain it to you, in their environment they are unable to control their actions and to think before they act. This results in impetuous, unthinking behavior and children who do not learn from their experiences. They are frequently repeat offenders. They require more parental supervision and frustrate their parents because of their inability to benefit from experience. As one parent explained, 22 times he asked the child not to get into his tools. The child did so a twenty-third time. The child was able to explain what had been requested, but the immediate need for gratification and the inability to stop and think resulted in a repeated offense. Frequently the parental perspective is to label this behavior as purposeful, noncaring and oppositional, which in reality does not describe what is taking place.

4. *Difficulty with Gratification.* ADHD children have great difficulty working towards a long-term goal. They frequently require brief, repeated payoffs rather than a single, long-term reward. They also do not appear to respond to rewards in a manner similar to other children (Haenlein & Caul, 1987). Rewards do not appear effective in changing their behavior on a long-term basis. Frequently, once the reward and the accompanying structure of the behavior-change program are removed, the ADHD child regresses and again exhibits behavior that was the target of change. It may be that as the result of repeated negative reinforcement, which ADHD children experience, they are not as motivated by positive reinforcement. They learn to respond to demands placed upon them by the environment when an aversive stimulus is removed contingent upon performance rather than for the promise of a future reward.

DSM-III-R Definition

The *Diagnostic and Statistical Manual* of the American Psychiatric Association is currently in its revised third edition, DSM-III-R (APA, 1987), which supersedes the third edition (APA, 1980). The evolution of its definition of this cluster of problems is interesting to follow. This disorder was originally referred to in the second edition as *Hyperkinetic reaction of childhood* (APA, 1968). The third edition greatly expanded the definition and retitled the disorder as *Attention-deficit disorder*. It included attention disorders with and without hyperactivity and a residual category for individuals presenting some symptoms of the disorder currently but whose history clearly demonstrated a period when the full disorder was exhibited.

Despite strong research suggesting a distinction behaviorally between attention-disordered children with and without hyperactivity (Lahey et al., 1987), the authors of DSM-III-R, based on their field studies, chose to collapse the diagnostic criteria into a single diagnostic entity, *Attention-deficit hyperactivity disorder* (see Table1.1). Part of the rationale was based upon the DSM-III-R authors' conclusion that a diagnosis of attention deficit without hyperactivity "is hardly ever made" (APA, 1987, p. 411). Epidemiological studies, however, have not supported this conclusion (Cantwell & Baker, 1985). Critics of the DSM-III-R revision have also noted that the manual does not provide details or results of the field studies (Rutter, 1988). The field studies did not meet the standards of "solid scientific study" (Cantwell & Baker, 1988, p. 527) and the new criteria appear "hastily-derived" and "largely untested" (Werry, 1988, p. 139). Cantwell and Baker (1988) also believe that the present diagnostic criteria for ADHD were poorly selected and do not appear to fit with clinical impressions of many practitioners. Shaywitz and Shaywitz (1988) conclude that there was no empirical evidence to suggest that the revised diagnostic criteria were superior to DSM-III.

The present authors agree with Cantwell and Baker's conclusions. Ten of the 14 criteria in part A of the DSM-III-R ADHD diagnosis relate to hyperactivity, impulsivity or behavior problems. Since 8 of the 14 criteria must be met, it is theoretically possible for a child to be considered ADHD and not present with even 1 of the 4 critical criteria relating to attention problems. In response to a groundswell of clinical complaints, there is a strong likelihood that when published a few years from now, DSM-IV will again revise the diagnostic criteria. The practitioner must be aware that these behaviors of childhood and the problems they cause have consistently affected children and adolescents. However, the label chosen to describe these behaviors and problems will vary based upon the whim of a committee process.

Despite complaints, the DSM-III-R criteria for ADHD represent an attempt to improve the operational definition of diagnostic behaviors. As in the third edition, a child diagnosed as *Attention-deficit hyperactivity disorder* must present with an onset of symptoms before age seven, experience the disturbance for at least six months and not meet the criteria for a *Pervasive developmental disorder*. The third edition specified that these problems may not be the result of retardation, schizophrenia, or severe emotional or behavior problems. The revision indicates that a coexisting diagnosis of ADHD can be made for those populations if the relevant symptoms are excessive for a child's mental age or adjustment difficulty. The revision suggests that a diagnosis of ADHD can be warranted even if it is impossible to determine whether a child's attentional problems result from a disorganized or chaotic environment. The revision also notes that it is important

TABLE 1.1.   DSM-III-R Diagnostic Criteria for Attention-Deficit Hyperactivity Disorder

Note: Consider a criterion met only if the behavior is considerably more frequent than that of most people of the same mental age.

A. A disturbance of at least six months during which at least eight of the following are present:
   1. often fidgets with hands or feet or squirms in seat (in adolescents, may be limited to subjective feelings of restlessness)
   2. has difficulty remaining seated when required to do so
   3. is easily distracted by extraneous stimuli
   4. has difficulty awaiting turn in games or group situations
   5. often blurts out answers to questions before they have been completed
   6. has difficulty following through on instructions from others (not due to oppositional behavior or failure of comprehension), e.g., fails to finish chores
   7. has difficulty sustaining attention in tasks or play activities
   8. often shifts from one uncompleted activity to another
   9. has difficulty playing quietly
   10. often talks excessively
   11. often interrupts or intrudes on others, e,g., butts into other children's games
   12. often does not seem to listen to what is being said to him or her
   13. often loses things necessary for tasks or activities at school or at home (e.g., toys, pencils, books, assignments)
   14. often engages in physically dangerous activities without considering possible consequences (not for the purpose of thrill-seeking), e.g., runs into street without looking

Note: The above items are listed in descending order of discriminating power based on data from a national field trial of the DSM-III-R criteria for Disruptive Behavior Disorders.

B. Onset before the age of seven.

C. Does not meet the criteria for a Pervasive Developmental Disorder.

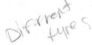

Criteria for severity of Attention-deficit hyperactivity disorder

Mild: Few, if any, symptoms in excess of those required to make the diagnosis **and** only minimal or no impairment in school and social functioning.

Moderate: Symptoms or functional impairment intermediate between "mild" and "severe."

Severe: Many symptoms in excess of those required to make the diagnosis and significant and pervasive impairment in functioning at home and school and with peers.

Diagnostic and Statistical Manual of Mental Disorders: Third Edition, Revised. Copyright 1987 by the American Psychiatric Association. Reprinted with publisher's permission.

to consider a diagnosis of mood disorder before making the diagnosis of ADHD. The DSM-III-R definition also includes general criteria for severity ratings of mild, moderate or severe.

Additionally, the authors of DSM-III-R include a category titled *Undifferentiated attention-deficit disorder*. Although this diagnostic category utilizes a diagnostic number similar to the third edition's diagnosis for *Attention-deficit disorder without hyperactivity*, the *Undifferentiated attention-deficit disorder* is simply described as a diagnosis "for disturbances in which the predominant feature is the persistence of developmentally inappropriate and marked inattention that is not a symptom of another disorder such as retardation or a disorganized, chaotic environment" (APA, 1987, p. 96).

Although the DSM-III-R provides a good description of behavioral problems many children with attention difficulty present, it is inadequate if used in isolation to diagnose the disorder. The American Psychiatric Association also recommends that these diagnostic criteria be used as part of a comprehensive evaluation. As with all psychiatric diagnoses, evaluator ratings are subjective. For this disorder, subjective impressions make diagnosis even more difficult. There is a marked difference in the pattern of these behaviors as exhibited by a 5-year-old as opposed to a 15-year-old. The DSM-III-R criteria, when used in isolation, require extraordinary expertise and understanding of the normal developmental profile of these behaviors at various ages and in response to various stresses. Even when data to meet the DSM-III and DSM-III-R criteria is gathered from a wide variety of sources, including parents, teachers and child interviews, the result appears to be an overinclusion of children with a possible wide variety of problems. Satin, Winsberg, Monetti, Sverd and Ross (1985), in a study screening six- to nine-year-old boys in a general population, found 24% met the DSM-III ADD criteria. Ostrom and Jensen (1988) felt data from this study suggests that over 16% would have met the DSM-III-R ADHD criteria as well. Finally, it appears excessively liberal to allow age seven to be the cutoff for the onset of symptoms. In today's society, the majority of children enter school at age five. It is a well-researched phenomenon that children with unidentified learning problems enter the school system, cannot meet academic demands and in response to the stress placed upon them, may develop a pattern of inattentive, restless behavior (Cunningham & Barkley, 1978a). Jay, a child with a visual processing and a written expression learning disability, presents an excellent example of such a phenomenon.

Jay's infancy, toddler and preschool experiences were fairly benign. His parents were not at all concerned about his ability to function within the school setting prior to his entering kindergarten. Jay is an extremely intelligent child and utilized his exceptionally good verbal skills and visual memory to compensate for other weaknesses, resulting in good integration into the kindergarten setting. By first grade, however, the demands of the classroom changed and the ability to process input visually and produce a written product on an independent basis became increasingly important. Jay's teachers in first and second grade expressed surprise and concern at what they observed to be an increasing pattern of inattention, distractibility, restlessness and off task behavior. Jay's third grade teacher felt certain that Jay was experiencing an attention disorder and suggested the family seek further evaluation. At that point, Jay had begun experiencing a similar pattern of behavior within the home setting as well. An indepth, multi-disciplinary evaluation identified Jay's learning disabilities, his superior intelligence and the fact that on structured assessment Jay had no difficulty with attention, concentration, vigilance or reflection. Appropriate educational intervention and private academic tutorial assisted Jay in understanding the nature of his difficulties, and provided remedial as well as compensatory intervention. Jay's teachers made allowances in the classroom to assist him in using his exceptionally good intellect to compensate for his learning problems. Within a very short period of time, teachers and parents reported a significant decrease in attention and hyperactivity problems.

The majority of children diagnosed as attention disordered present a clear pattern of attention-related problems before entering an organized school program (Barkley, 1981a). It is important for the practitioner to understand this phenomenon and begin the diagnostic process with a careful developmental and social history.

Working Definition

A number of practitioners (Cantwell & Carlson, 1978) and even a pharmaceutical company (CIBA, 1974) have recommended a multicomponent approach to the evaluation and identification of ADD in children. Still others have proposed very limited evaluative components, including just a history from parents and a teacher rating, to confirm the diagnosis of ADD (Sleator, 1982). Rather than prescribing the components of the evaluative process, the present authors have advocated a *working definition* that describes the type of data necessary to make the diagnosis of ADHD (Goldstein & Goldstein, 1985). The working definition will allow the practitioner to make the diagnosis of ADHD with a high degree of confidence. Although many of the items in this definition have been closely researched and identify attention-disordered children with a high degree of reliability, the items as a group have not been tested. As a practitioner you may wish to adapt or modify this working definition, utilizing various questionnaires or assessment procedures that you have found helpful or discriminatory based on clinical experience. The use of the common-sense definition in making the diagnosis of ADHD will be reviewed in depth in Chapter 7. Case examples will be provided to illustrate the complexity of making the diagnosis of ADHD and the need for multiple diagnostic criteria.

In making the diagnosis of ADHD or *Undifferentiated attention-deficit disorder*, it is suggested that the following criteria be considered:

1. *DSM-III-R Diagnostic Criteria.*   Since this is the most utilized and best researched definition we have at this time, it is important for the child to meet these criteria.

2. *Elevated Rating Scales.*   The most commonly used scales specifically designed to measure attention are the Conners Parent's and Teacher's Questionnaires (Conners, 1969). These will be reviewed in Chapters 4 and 5. There are other attention-measuring questionnaires, including the SNAP Checklist (Pelham, Atkins, Murphy & White, 1981b) and the ACTeRS (Ullman, Sleator & Sprague, 1985). Some general adjustment questionnaires such as the Child Behavior Checklist (Achenbach, 1978) and the Personality Inventory for Children (Wirt, Lacher, Klinedinst & Seat, 1977) also contain attention and hyperactivity scales. In the working definition, the child must be at or beyond two standard deviations difference in a negative direction on at least one of these questionnaires in comparison to same chronological age and sex. This criterion must be met by two independent raters, usually the parent and teacher.

3. *Objective Measures.*   Assessment of ADHD has rarely involved direct measures of attention (Ostrom & Jensen, 1988). Chapter 5 will present a wide range of objective, norm-referenced measures ranging from computer-based instruments to simple paper and pencil assessment tasks. The ADHD child should demonstrate difficulty on a selection of such tasks that measure various attentional skills.

4. *Situational Problems.*   Children with attention disorder have been found to have problems of varying severity in at least half of all home and school situations (Barkley, 1981a; Breen, 1986). Gordon, Mammen, DiNiro and Mettelman (1988) found that 72% of a population of children referred for problems with attention and arousal level presented with a consensus between parents and teachers concerning the severity of these problems. These authors suggest that children referred for situational attention problems by only the parent or teacher may have very different reasons for and kinds of problems than those for whom there is a consensus. The inclusion of situational data allows the evaluator to assess the impact of the child's attentional problems upon daily living.

5. *Differential Diagnosis.*   Sufficient historical, behavioral and assessment data is collected to rule out or minimize the contribution of medical or learning problems, language disorders, auditory processing disability, specific intellectual deficits and psychological problems of childhood contributing to attention-disordered symptoms.

DEVELOPMENTAL PROFILE

Although the cluster of problems ADHD children present are homogeneous, each child's presentation is clearly unique. ADHD children at similar developmental stages and ages are also very different from one another. It is therefore important to understand how a similar problem or behavior will present differently at different maturational levels. For example, the thrashing, temperamental infant may develop into the frantic, overactive preschooler, then become the hyperactive school-age child who may not be able to stay seated or remain on task, then become the restless, fidgety adolescent and finally the pacing, overenergetic adult (Ross & Ross, 1982). It is also important to keep in mind that behavior easily overlooked at one particular stage is not well tolerated at another stage. The four-year-old preschooler, unable to pay attention, may be described casually by the teacher as somewhat immature but not significantly different from a number of other children in the classroom. By six years of age, a very similar level of inattentive behavior will be described by the first-grade teacher as a significant problem.

Infants

During their years of research on childhood temperament, Thomas and Chess (1977) and others (Carey, 1970) have described a pattern of temperamental or innate qualities that children bring to the world. These qualities affect their ability to accommodate and meet the environment's expectations. These qualities play a role in determining the manner in which the environment responds to the child as well. Approximately 10% of the population studied were described as having a difficult temperament (Thomas & Chess, 1977). These children tended to withdraw in a negative manner from new stimulation. They had problems with changes in routines. They tended to present with significantly greater negative as opposed to positive mood and had intense reactions to events in their environment. As many as 70% of this difficult infant population developed problems at school age. In a related study, Persson-Blennow and McNeil (1988) found that there was statistically significant individual stability for children evaluated as being of difficult temperament at one or two years of age to six years of age. These authors also concluded, however, that an infant's temperament can change over several years and temperament alone must be used cautiously in an attempt to assess a child's risk for future problems. In a temperament study of slightly older children, three-year-olds were identified using the criteria of negative mood and intense reaction. This population was followed for five years. At that point, all of those children were experiencing school-related problems (Terestman, 1980).

Difficult infants have been referred to as children at risk (Ross & Ross, 1982), primarily because their problems are nonspecific in predicting the type of difficulty they may experience in later childhood. Children in this population may develop learning problems, behavioral excesses, difficulty with socialization or attention disorder. Many may experience a combination of these problems.

Infants at risk typically present with a very high activity level. They are difficult, even for experienced, maternal workers to manage. They may be restless and overactive in their sleep patterns and present a significant challenge during routine care activities, such as dressing and bathing. These are the children that parents describe as rolling off the bed or changing table in a split second.

Research studies additionally suggest that some of these children have a very different pattern of crying. Most children cry at a soundwave frequency somewhere between 400 and 450 cycles per second. Among the at-risk group the cry may be somewhere between a frequency of 650 and 800 cycles per second (Wolff, 1969). Parents describe this child as presenting with a high-pitched, monotonic cry or scream. One parent described the problem as the static or whine of a car radio. Another parent described the problem as analogous to a broken alarm clock. The parent was never quite sure what was distressing the child, when the child would be set off or how to stop the child's crying once it began. During history sessions, parents frequently describe these children as experiencing excessive colic from the day they were brought home. Careful questioning often reveals that the problem is one of excessive irritability and not necessarily colic. Colic does not begin at birth and is frequently routine, occurring at similar times during the day.

Sleep studies suggest that the at-risk population of infants presents with a pattern of sleep similar to premature infants. The pattern is characterized by a three-to-one ratio between rapid-eye-movement sleep (REM) and non–rapid-eye-movement sleep (Ross & Ross, 1982). REM sleep is characterized by irregular patterns of respiration and heartbeat. In older individuals, REM sleep is often described as dream sleep; it is uncertain what the purpose of this pattern of sleep holds for infants. These infants at risk also present with extremely irregular patterns of sleep (Campbell, Szumowski, Ewing, Gluck & Breaux, 1982). It is difficult for them to establish a sleep routine. They may wake repeatedly or suddenly, startle themselves and cry (Nichamin, 1972). This pattern of different sleep may continue throughout childhood for this population of children (Luisada, 1969). At one time, sleep-related problems were considered part of the diagnostic criteria for attention disorder (APA, 1980).

At-risk infants are also frequently described as obstinate, picky and obstructive feeders (Ross & Ross, 1982). They often have difficulty nursing and making the transition from the bottle to regular foods. There is also an unexplained higher incidence of allergy to formula in this group.

Longitudinal studies have suggested that the interaction of a number of variables, including perinatal distress and low socioeconomic status, contributes to a wide range of childhood behavioral abnormalities (Werner & Smith, 1977). In an interesting study of medical problems present in ADD children, Hartsough and Lambert (1985) found that a significant degree of pre- and perinatal medical factors discriminated between a group of ADD and control children. Mothers of ADD children had a significantly higher incidence of poor maternal health during pregnancy, toxemia or eclampsia, postmaturity and longer labor. A significantly higher percentage of the ADD children were the product of their mother's first pregnancy. These mothers also tended to be younger than the mothers of the control children. As infants, in comparison to the control group, the ADD children were significantly different in experiencing four or more serious accidents, delays in achieving bowel control and speech problems. A summary of Hartsough and Lambert's research appears in Table 1.2.

It is easily observed that this pattern of problems, especially if this is the parents' first child, may have a significant negative impact on the relationship those parents will develop with their child. New parents may feel guilty because of their inability to calm and comfort the child. This may result in overly permissive or solicitous behavior. They may feel angry and either consciously or unconsciously reject the child or perceive the child as damaged goods. One parent, after a miserable first week, went so far as to contact the hospital just to make sure she had in fact brought home the right child. D. W. Winnicott (1974) wrote that most mothers are good enough for most children. An infant at risk presents a challenge to even the best and most competent parents. In response to a difficult infant, many parents become frustrated, angry, irritated or anxious. These responses will have a negative impact on the type of relationship that the child and parent are able to develop with each other. An impaired parent-child relationship will certainly have an affect on the child's future development. A disharmony in the early mother-child relationship of children later diagnosed as having behavioral problems consistent with attention deficit has been observed in longitudinal studies (Battle & Lacey, 1972). On top of these problems, we add the potential for negative or inappropriate parenting. Mothers of young, attention-disordered children have also

TABLE 1.2. Medical Problems Present in ADD and Control Children

Variable	ADD	C	X^2
Pre/Perinatal Factors	%	%	
1. Poor maternal health during pregnancy	26.4	16.2	6.45**
2. Young mother (under 20 at birth of child)	16.3	6.7	9.58**
3. At least one previous miscarriage	21.1	24.4	NS
4. First pregnancy for mother	42.7	32.8	4.34*
5. Rh factor incompatibility	14.9	12.4	NS
6. Prematurity (8 months or earlier)	7.9	5.4	NS
7.· Postmaturity (10 months or later)	7.9	1.5	8.44**
8. Long labor (13 hours or more)	24.8	15.7	5.04**
9. Toxemia or eclampsia during pregnancy	7.8	2.5	5.23**
10. Fetal distress during labor or birth	16.9	8.0	7.07**
11. Abnormal delivery	26.6	20.2	NS
12. Low birth weight (under 6 lbs.)	12.2	7.8	NS
13. Presence of congenital problems	22.1	13.2	5.50*
14. Problems in establishing routines during infancy (eating, sleeping, etc.)	54.6	31.7	24.00**
15. Health problems during infancy	50.9	29.2	22.19**
Developmental Milestones			
16. Delay in sitting up	.4	0	NS
17. Delay in crawling	6.5	1.6	5.05*
18. Delay in walking	1.5	.5	NS
19. Delay in talking	9.6	3.7	4.76*
20. Delay in bladder control	7.4	4.5	NS
21. Delay in bowel control	10.1	4.5	4.18*
Childhood Illness and Accidents			
22. Presence of chronic health problems	39.1	24.8	10.47**
23. One or more acute illnesses or diseases in childhood	78.0	79.0	NS
24. Four or more serious accidents	15.6	4.8	9.73**
25. More than one surgery during childhood	27.3	19.5	NS
Childhood Health Status			
26. Poor general health	8.9	2.4	7.79**
27. Poor hearing	11.1	7.6	NS
28. Poor vision	21.6	13.4	4.86*
29. Poor coordination	52.3	34.9	13.92**
30. Speech problems	26.6	14.8	9.27**

*$p < .05$.
**$p < .01$.

Hartsough, C. S. and Lambert, N. M. "Medical Factors in Hyperactive and Normal Children," *American Journal of Orthopsychiatry*, Copyright 1985 by the American Orthopsychiatric Association, Inc. Reprinted by permission of the authors.

been reported subjectively experiencing a higher level of stress in parenting and feelings of lower self-esteem. Mash and Johnston (1983) reported that the greater the level of these two variables, the more inaccurate was the mother's perception of the child's problem. Additionally, the hereditary nature of this disorder frequently results in impulsive, easily overaroused parents bearing offspring with very similar problems. This unfortunate pairing of similar temperament in parents and child places the at-risk infant in even greater jeopardy of beginning a long chain of negative interactions with the environment. These additional factors cannot help but have a cumulative, negative impact on the child's development and personality.

Preschoolers

The overactive, temperamental infant frequently becomes the hyperactive, non-compliant preschooler (Barkley, 1978). The identification of ADHD preschool children is extremely complex. Although the DSM-III-R guidelines provide a ceiling limit of age seven as to when the symptoms must have been observed, they do not provide a lower limit or cutoff under which the diagnosis should be made with caution. Campbell (1985) cautions that the practitioner must draw the line between a three-year-old presenting with age-appropriate behavior that may be typically vigorous and unrestrained and a child presenting a pattern of overactivity, impulsivity and inattention, which is clinically significant. As Campbell notes:

> Preschoolers, who are learning about the world and how to master its complexities, are expected to exhibit boundless energy, to attend readily to the new and novel, and to demonstrate unrestrained enthusiasm and exuberance. When, therefore, does a shift in activity and interest signify curiosity and exploration and when does it reflect a too rapid change in focus and inadequate investment of attention? When does excitable and impatient behavior indicate an age-appropriate need for external support and limit-setting and when does it suggest a failure to internalize standards necessary for the development of self-control?
>
> (Campbell, 1985, p. 407)

The practitioner must be aware that symptoms of ADHD may reflect an exaggeration of age-appropriate behavior in toddlers.

The erratic nature of attention-deficit symptoms and their variability as a function of situation makes the practitioner's job with preschoolers that much more difficult (Whalen & Henker, 1980). ADHD is a disorder in which the severity of the presenting problems results from an interaction of the child with the demands made upon the child by the environment. A multitude of environmental variables can influence the preschool child's behavior. "The child who is an absolute terror in preschool may be relatively restrained when alone with his mother; another hyperactive child may function well in the peer group, but run wild in the supermarket where the temptation to sample everything in sight overwhelms his limited capacity for self-control" (Campbell, 1985, p. 408). The unpredictability of the ADHD child's behavior is extremely frustrating for parents. Perplexed parents are frequently unable to understand the causes of the child's behavior.

Campbell (1985) further points out that "differences in knowledge, attribution, and tolerance levels influence how the child's behavior is construed and whether typical behavior as defined by parents is problematic or problematic behavior is seen as acceptable" (p. 408). Referrals of preschoolers are frequently influenced by the nuisance value of the child's behavior. It is not uncommon to see extremely distressed parents concerned about a child temperamentally not much more difficult than average. The child presents as a challenge to those parents because of their rigid, unrealistic expectations. Conversely, it is also common to see parents perplexed not by the child's abnormal behavior but by the negative response expressed by nonfamilial adults in the child's life. Frequently in those situations the entire family may experience attention disorder. Nothing happens on time or with any organization. The fact that this child presents in a similar manner is not at all distressing to that family.

Additionally, despite the exceedingly large volume of literature in this area, the majority of research has not focused on children under six. Campbell (1985) notes that a similar pattern is reflected in referral for this disorder. Parents concerned about attentional problems in preschoolers are frequently advised that these problems are transient and will be outgrown. Although it is well recognized that some preschool problems do in fact represent transient phases, this has been erroneously interpreted and generalized so that symptoms observed in preschoolers are thought by many practitioners to have little prognostic significance (Robins, 1979). Research data suggests, however, that ignoring these signs, especially in the later preschool years, results in the loss of valuable treatment time (Cohen, Sullivan, Minde, Novak & Helwig, 1981). Studies suggest that 60% to 70% of children later diagnosed as ADD were identifiable by their symptoms during the preschool years (Barkley, 1981b).

A higher percentage of ADD preschoolers present with speech and language problems than of the normal population (Baker & Cantwell, 1987). It has also been repeatedly observed that children experiencing language problems are at a significantly greater risk to develop a wide range of behavioral problems (Cohen, Davine & Meloche-Kelly, 1989; Cantwell, Baker & Mattison, 1981; Cantwell & Baker, 1977). Beitchman (1987) hypothesized that there may be a specific subgroup of language-delayed hyperactive preschoolers. Love and Thompson (1988), in a study of 116 preschool children referred for behavioral problems, found that 56 out of 75 children diagnosed as having a language disorder also met the diagnostic criteria for an *Attention-deficit disorder*. These authors also found that 56 out of 85 children diagnosed initially as experiencing *Attention-deficit disorder* were found to experience a language disorder. Recent preliminary research (Beitchman, Hood, Rochon & Peterson, 1989) found that the risk of psychiatric disorder, especially ADHD, is greatest among children with general linguistic impairment as opposed to those experiencing specific problems with articulation or comprehension.

ADHD children with speech and language problems typically present difficulty in three areas (Ross & Ross, 1982). First, they have difficulty with covert speech. They do not appear to develop the capacity to carry on an internal conversation, to reason and to solve problems. It is unclear if this is a result of their impulsivity or if their lack of internal conversation contributes to the observation of impulsivity. Second, ADHD children with speech and language problems typically have difficulty with overt speech. They do not develop effective communication skills. They tend to impulsively act without thinking and without talking. Finally, these children typically have difficulty changing from a tactile means of dealing with the world to a visual means (Funk & Ruppert, 1984). Infants learning about the world before the acquisition of significant language and the ability to provide verbal labels must touch, feel and taste things as a means of gaining information. Once effective language is established, words can take the place of tactile, sensory input. Typically, ADHD preschoolers continue to need to touch and feel things and people as a means of gaining sensory input from their environment.

ADHD preschoolers are frequently impulsive, noncompliant and fearless. They may present with a combination of boundless energy and poor judgment (Ross & Ross, 1982). They experience more accidental poisonings and trips to the emergency room (Stewart, Thatch & Freidin, 1970). The irregularity of their behavior creates a marked degree of family stress and tension for all family members. Often, neither the threat of punishment nor the promise of reward has an impact on the child's behavior. Parents frequently misinterpret the child's repetitive inability to benefit from intervention as purposeful rather than the result of impulsive, nonthinking behavior.

During the preschool period, most children are developing basic, foundational social skills. ADHD preschoolers frequently do not. Although they frequently have not developed well-set negative patterns of social interaction, they are simply unable to integrate effectively with their peers. Only one out of five comparison children present with similar problems (Campbell & Cluss, 1982). These authors also found that inattentive and hyperactive children demonstrated disproportionate rates of aggressive interactions with their peers.

Middle Childhood

By school age, the ADHD child begins to venture out into the community and no longer has the family to act as a buffer. Behavior once dismissed as immature is no longer tolerated or accepted. Within the home setting, the child is a negative force with the inconsistency in his behavior continuing to act as a family stress. The ADHD child is typically perceived by his siblings as the source of family problems. A pattern of negative reinforcement intensifies. Frequently, ADHD children are described as beginning but never completing tasks. This results in parents acting as negative reinforcers, bringing the child back to task and leaving once the task is begun. The parents' attention to the child's off-task behavior acts as an aversive consequence that is then removed when the child returns to task. This is the operational definition of a negative reinforcement. The child is then a victim of his temperament that makes it difficult for him to persist on task and a victim of his learning history that reinforces him for beginning but not completing tasks. A similar pattern of difficulty develops at school. In the school setting, the teacher's negative reinforcement tends to focus on the misbehavior rather than on the termination of the behavior. This may further disrupt the classroom by having a disinhibitory effect on other children for whom the competing task of schoolwork is only slightly more attractive than watching the ADHD child (Ross & Ross, 1982).

It has been argued that attention-disordered children are intellectually less competent than their same-age peers (Palkes & Stewart, 1972). The experienced practitioner, however, is well aware that the interpretation of normative tests must be based on an understanding of the child's approach to those tests. Typically, attention-disordered children present with a normal range of intellectual skills; weak performances on specific tasks result from the impact of impulsivity and inattention on test taking rather than an innate lack of intellect (Ross & Ross, 1982). Attention-disordered children appear to present with a similar range of intellectual skills as the normal population (Prinz & Loney, 1974; Loney, 1974). The more intelligent ADHD child often manages to survive during the elementary school years and may not be referred for problems. His superior intellect allows him to compensate for his inability to remain on task. This child may not work very long, but the time he spends on task results in a completed, frequently correct product. In junior high school, however, even the intelligent ADHD child cannot consistently keep up with the educational demands. It is frequently during the junior high school years that intelligent ADHD children are recognized as experiencing attention-related problems that may be interfering with their school performance.

Earlier research suggested that ADD children underachieve academically in elementary school relative to their same-age peers (Cantwell & Satterfield, 1978; Minde, Lewin, Weiss, Lavigeuer, Douglas & Sykes, 1971) and experience a higher incidence of learning disabilities (Lambert & Sandoval, 1980; Silver, 1981). Safer and Allen (1976) estimated problems with hyperactivity in 80 percent of a learning disabled population. Holborow and Berry (1986) estimated 41 percent of a learning disabled population exhibited symptoms of ADD. Yet Halperin, Gittelman, Klein and Rudel (1984), found that only nine percent of a sample of 241 ADDH elementary school childern had a reading disability. A more recent study has suggested that during the elementary school years a majority of ADD children achieve as well as the normative population. Shaywitz (1986) followed a population of 445 children from kindergarten through third grade. Eleven percent of the ADD children were classified as learning diabled in either reading or arithmetic. Conversely, 33 percent of learning disabled children in this sample satisfied the diagnostic criteria for ADD. Shaywitz concluded that these findings suggest that although the majority of ADD children do not experience specific learning disability, the small percentage of ADD children that are learning disabled constitute a significant group of the learning disabled population. Shaywitz and Shaywitz (1986) conclude that although the overlap between learning disability and attention deficit is real, "it is not reasonable to believe that all, or even a majority of ADD children have LD" (p. 457). They further conclude that although many investigations indicate a relationship between learning disabilities and attention deficit, the nature of the relationship has not been well defined, and these are two separate disorders in that one does not necessarily predict the other. For the purposes of this text children with a learning disability are considered to experience one or more specific cognitive deficits that impair the ability to learn. Non–learning-disabled ADHD children described as underachieving have the capacity and potential to learn but may not do so because of the cumulative impact of impulsivity and inattention. Day in and day out the classroom performance of ADHD children may not reflect their capabilities or actual skill attainments. It is therefore reasonable for the practitioner to assume that although there is a higher incidence of learning disabilities among children with ADHD than in the normal population, not all inattentive children present with learning problems (Cantwell & Satterfield, 1978). Conversely, the majority of learning-disabled children do not experience ADHD. By the later school years, however, the cumulative impact of the child's temperamental quality and an inability to complete tasks has a negative effect on academic achievement. This pattern may begin in the first few years of school. Meichenbaum and Goodman (1969) found that impulsive kindergarteners performed more poorly than reflective kindergarteners on a range of basic cognitive skills. Achenbach (1975) defined associative responders as children who tend to impulsively free associate on intellectual and achievement tasks. These children performed more poorly at school and because of their inability to develop effective reasoning skills began demonstrating a slow but cumulative decrease in intellectual development and achievement. Eventually, the lack of these skills, as well as a lack of practice in effectively utilizing whatever skills have been acquired, further impairs intellectual and academic achievement.

In the classroom setting, ADHD children are typically described as daydreaming. Careful observation suggests that these children are not daydreaming but simply interested in tasks other than what the teacher may be focusing upon (Douglas, 1972). They typically engage in significantly more nonproductive activity during work and free time than their same-age peers. Their uneven, unpredictable pattern of behavior and work completion is equally distressing to the classroom teacher. A child may complete a task one day but be unable to complete a similar task the next day. The resulting interpretation is that the child can do it but simply needs to try harder. For ADHD children this is a misinterpretation that frequently results in increased pressure by the teacher on the child. The result is a marked degree of frustration for both the teacher and child when the task is not completed.

Inattentive children are well aware of their classroom inabilities (Glow & Glow, 1980). Sociometric studies frequently point to the ADHD child not being chosen by peers as best friends, as partners in activities or as seatmates. Studies in which children with no previous knowledge of each other were placed together for play periods resulted in the majority of those children, after the play period, nominating the ADD child as the child they did not want to play with again (Pelham & Milich, 1984). The ADHD child also has a coercive effect on teacher behavior. Campbell, Endman and Bernfeld (1977) found that the overall rates of negative teacher-child interactions involving normal students were higher in classrooms that contained children experiencing significant attention problems. Teachers have also been found to be more intense and controlling in interactions with attention-disordered boys than with other male students (Whalen, Henker & Dotemoto, 1981).

Socially, ADHD children may be immature and incompetent. Even their best efforts frequently fail. They lack basic social skills. Their social-skill deficit results in a pattern of high-incidence, low-impact behaviors. They may be incompetent in their ability to join an ongoing conversation or take turns. These are not terribly aversive behaviors but result in the ADHD child being less popular and not well accepted. Some ADHD children also present with a pattern of low-incidence, high-impact behaviors. These are frequently aggressive behaviors that may not occur with great frequency, but result in the ADD child being more rejected and disliked by others (Pelham & Milich, 1984). An in-depth review of the socialization process and the problems ADHD children experience will be presented in Chapter 12.

Adolescence

Research studies suggest that many of the primary symptoms of attention deficit may diminish in intensity in adolescence (Weiss & Hechtman, 1979). A review of related research, however, indicates that inattentive adolescents continue to experience significant problems (Milich & Loney, 1979). In some studies, 20 percent (Sassone, Lambert & Sandoval, 1982) to 60 percent (Satterfield, Hoppe & Schell, 1982) were involved in antisocial behavior, while the normal occurrence is 3 to 4 percent Loney (1986) points out that the high prevalence of anti-social problems may reflect the intital co-morbidity of ADD with conduct disorders. In other studies, 35 percent were suspended from school at least once, while the normal occurrence is 8 to 10 percent (Ackerman, Dykman & Peters, 1977). Finally, at this point four-fifths are behind one or more years in at least one basic academic subject (Loney, Kramer & Milich, 1981; Cantwell & Satterfield, 1978). These studies consistently suggest that the secondary problems of ADHD may persist, intensify and become increasingly complex in adolescence (See Figure 1.1.)

We now recognize that normal adolescence may not be as terrible a period of turmoil as once thought (Nicholi, 1978). Successful passage through these years is typically based on achievement either academically, socially or in extra-curricular activities such as athletics. ADHD children have histories of not succeeding in any of those areas. Even the athletic ADHD adolescent may have difficulty remaining on a team, not for lack of competence but because of an inability to show up on time for practices and follow the coach's instructions closely.

Research has suggested that a significant proportion of inattentive adolescents may present with symptoms of depression (Cantwell, 1979) and problems maintaining social contact (Waddell, 1984). Inattentive adolescents may lack confidence, experience feelings of helplessness (Battle & Lacey, 1972), and experience problems maintaining social contact (Waddell, 1984). Given their long history of not succeeding and not meeting the expectations of the environment, this is not a surprising pattern. Zagar, Arbit, Hughes, Busell and Busch (1989), in a sample of almost 2,000 adjudicated delinquents with an average age of 14 years, found that 9 percent of the sample met the diagnostic criteria for ADD-H while 46 percent met the diagnostic criteria for ADD without hyperactivity. The ADD-H adolescents also showed greater scholastic delays than the ADD group.

ADHD adolescents present a significant challenge for the practitioner. Their patterns of interaction with the environment are frequently well entrenched. They are often unwilling to accept responsibility for their problems and resistant to

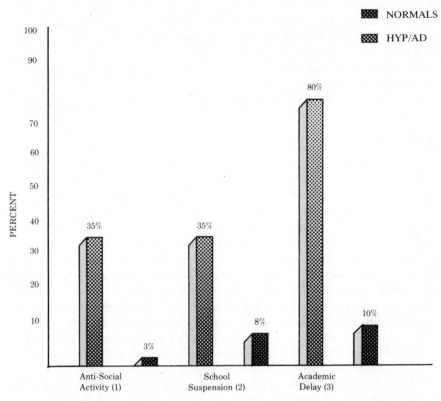

Figure 1.1 Antisocial activity, school suspension and academic delay of ADHD adolescents: (1) Sassone et al. (1982) and Satterfield et al. (1982); (2) Ackerman et al. (1977); (3) Loney et al. (1981).

treatment. In treatment, the initial hurdle with ADHD adolescents is convincing them to be active, as opposed to passive, participants.

Adulthood

The majority of early adulthood studies of attention problems were retrospective (Shelley & Riester, 1972; Bellak, 1979). Frequently, these studies observed groups of adults experiencing problems and attempted to develop a causal relationship between attention problems in childhood and adult difficulty. There are now a number of studies that have followed attention-disordered children through adolescence and into adulthood. There is a consensus that a majority of inattentive children, one-half to two-thirds, outgrow the core symptoms of attention disorder by adulthood (Gittelman et al., 1985). As a group they tend to blend into society. Approximately one-third continue to present a very clear pattern of attention-disordered behavior as adults. This group presents with a significantly higher incidence of achievement, vocational, antisocial, psychiatric and marital problems than the normal population. As many as half of this group may be alcoholics (Gittelman et al., 1985). Some adult-outcome studies have suggested that as many as 25% may exhibit antisocial personality problems (Weiss & Hechtman, 1986; Borland & Hechtman, 1976). It is encouraging to note that Kramer and Loney (1982), in an in-depth review of the literature concerning attention deficit and substance abuse, concluded that it had not been demonstrated that individuals with history of attention deficit were more involved with illicit drug use and alcohol consumption than other individuals and that when differences were reported they usually involved alcohol. The authors observed, however, that failure to find major differences might also reflect limitations in the current state of research design.

PREDICTING OUTCOME

The toughest question a practitioner must answer is not "What's wrong with my child?" but "How will these problems affect my child when she grows up?" and "What kind of an adult will he be?" Studies following inattentive children over multiple-year periods suggest that those children receiving a multi-disciplinary program of intervention demonstrate better adjustment than children receiving no intervention or singular intervention (Satterfield, Satterfield & Cantwell, 1981). A multidisciplinary program of intervention provides assistance to the child or family for home, school, social or psychological problems. Chapter 8 will provide an overview of and a rationale for the successes and failures in the research dealing with multidisciplinary treatment for ADHD children.

Although the adult literature suggests that at least two-thirds of ADHD children generally outgrow the core symptoms, this does not mean that their personalities have not been affected. This also does not mean that they will achieve as much as they might be expected to based on estimates of their intellect or family history. The years of ADHD problems certainly take their toll on adult outcome. There are, however, a number of general variables that are used with children to predict outcome in adulthood. These predictors are generally independent of a specific type of childhood problem.

1. *Intelligence.* It is accepted that more intelligent individuals make a bet- ter adjustment to adult life, attain higher vocational status and as a group are better adjusted emotionally. ADHD children with higher intellect appear to fare better than their counterparts with average or below average intelligence.

2. *Socioeconomic Status.* Lower SES families have a higher incidence of poor medical and nutritional care for their offspring, tend to be less educated concerning appropriate child rearing and are more likely to experience psychiatric problems. Higher SES parents are more likely to seek and follow through with treatment. Additionally, children from higher SES families tend to grow up and obtain a level of status similar to or better than their families. Since a percentage of ADHD children have parents with very similar problems, many of those families tend to fall to the lower socioeconomic strata, thereby providing further negative impact on adult outcome for their children. Trites (1979) found that as many as

one out of every four children in lower socioeconomic areas of Ottawa, Canada presented significant symptoms of attention deficit. It has also been suggested that low SES parents are more inconsistent in their parenting than are higher SES parents (Paternite, Loney & Langhorne, 1976). Lower SES parents are more likely to have difficulty in setting appropriate consequences for behavior and may use excessively aggressive punishments. Lower socioeconomic status has also been found to correlate with childhood aggression (Paternite & Loney, 1980).

3. *Socialization.*   In all likelihood, the best single predictor of adequate emotional adjustment in adulthood is the ability to develop and maintain positive social contacts and friendships in childhood (Milich & Landau, 1981). ADHD children with a history of generally positive social interaction frequently adapt better to their attentional problems and to the daily frustrations of home and school.

4. *Activity Level.*   Studies have suggested that there is an inverse relationship between the degree of hyperactive behavior in elementary school and academic achievement in high school. The more hyperactive the elementary school child, the more likely high school achievement will be negatively affected (Loney et al., 1981). It may be that the hyperactive symptom is a general marker of the severity of the ADHD child's problems. More severe ADHD children would be expected to have greater achievement problems in later school years.

5. *Ability to Delay Rewards.*   Mischel, Shoda and Rodriguez (1989), based on a comprehensive review of the literature, have suggested that children who are more competent at delaying rewards tend to develop into adolescents who perform better on tests of intelligence, have greater success resisting temptation that may result in problems, demonstrate more appropriate social skills and have higher achievement strivings. Those children who are more competent at spontaneously developing effective strategies to delay gratification and increase self-control have also been reported as less aggressive than children matched for similar problems who are unable to generate or master these strategies (Rodriguez, Shoda, Mischel & Wright, 1989).

6. *Aggression.*   Aggression is considered a secondary symptom of attention deficit that is closely related to parenting style and socioeconomic status (Conners & Wells, 1986). One of the best single predictors of antisocial behavior and poorly adjusted emotional status in adolescence is a history of aggressive behavior in younger childhood (Loney, 1980a). It appears that once a child develops a pattern of aggressive behavior it is extremely difficult to extinguish. As a society, we tend to deal with aggressive behavior aggressively. It is therefore not surprising that in our attempts to extinguish aggressive behavior in children, we may in fact be reinforcing this very same pattern of behavior.

In the past it was thought that aggression was a primary component of attention disorder. It has been well established that aggression is an independent variable that may or may not occur with attention deficit and tends to occur more frequently if hyperactivity symptoms are present (Loney & Milich, 1981). Shapiro and Garfinkel (1986) found in a nonreferred elementary school population a prevalence rate of 2.3 percent for inattentive, overactive symptoms, 3.6 percent for aggressive and oppositional symptoms, and 3 percent for both sets of symptoms. Concentration problems, impulsivity and excessive motoric behavior were associated with both groups of children. The Conners Teacher's Rating Scale was the only questionnaire that could differentiate the three groups. Other measures alone, including a child interview, attentional test battery or school performance, could not validate the diagnostic distinction.

The elementary school attention-disordered child with a pattern of aggressive behavior presents a poor prognosis for appropriate adjustment in adolescence (Loney et al., 1981; August, Stewart & Holmes, 1983). Garfinkel (1989) reported that approximately two-thirds of children with ADHD present co-morbid external-izing problems. Of this group, approximately half appear to have marked problems with aggression. This aggressive sub-group appears at greater risk for alcoholism and antisocial behavior into adulthood. The practitioner must be alert to this prob-lem and intensively work to extinguish aggressive behavior before the child enters junior high school. Studies also suggest that interventions for ADD are typically not effective long-term in reducing aggressive behavior. Aggression must be dealt with as an independent problem of childhood (Stewart, 1980).

7. *Family Mental Health.*   Families with multiple generations of ADHD, as well as more serious psychiatric problems, tend to be extremely difficult to deal with in treatment. Although these parents may be unhappy with their ADHD child, they frequently lack skills, persistence, and the ability to stick with a practitioner and a treatment program. A history of psychiatric problems in a family increases the likelihood that the inattentive child will grow up and present with a similar or related set of problems (Weiss, Minde, Werry, Douglas & Nemeth, 1971). Robins (1979) suggested that overall social adjustment of parents is also a contributing factor to the severity of childhood problems. When social class was controlled, parents of delinquents appeared less educated, made less use of available health services and demonstrated less ability to obtain and hold a job than parents of nondelinquents. These factors may suggest that overall this group of parents of delinquents may not be as well adjusted or cope as well in effectively parenting their children. It would be likely that an ADHD child or adolescent would not fare as well with such parents.

It is important to acquaint parents with these predictor variables. It is rare that a child does not have some of these variables predicting a positive outcome into adulthood. The data can assist parents in a motivational way. The data can also assist parents, especially with problems of aggression, by educating them as to the seriousness of this pattern of behavior and the need for intensive intervention.

SUMMARY

This chapter reviewed the history and definition of attention disorders and the development of children experiencing attention-related problems. The volume of research in this area sensitizes the practitioner to the complex and multiple effects attention-related problems have on all areas of a child's functioning and interaction with the environment. With this background in place, hypotheses of causality will be reviewed in Chapter 2.

CHAPTER 2

Etiology

In this chapter, etiology of *Attention-deficit hyperactivity disorder* will be considered from two perspectives. It has been suggested that ADHD may result from heredity or from a variety of prenatal or postnatal environmental factors. Commonly suspected causes have included toxins, developmental impairments, diet, injury and ineffective parenting. It has been suggested that these potential causes affect brain functioning, and ADHD can also be considered as a disorder of brain function. This chapter will review brain function and suspected causes of ADHD in order to provide an academic and medical framework for understanding this disorder.

BRAIN INJURY

In the early twentieth century, the cluster of symptoms now called ADHD was hypothesized to relate to brain trauma (Still, 1902). This theory gained wide acceptance, and a wide range of behavioral and cognitive problems were diagnosed in children and adults who had suffered encephalitis. Most children with these symptoms, however, did not have definite brain injury (Bond & Partridge, 1926; Ebaugh, 1923; Hohman, 1922). The concept of minimal brain dysfunction (MBD) emerged and was applied to a large group of children who had MBD symptoms but did not have obvious neurological signs of injury. This concept was based on the theory that a lesser degree of injury could cause observed behavioral changes without other signs of brain injury (Knobolc & Pasamanick, 1959). The overwhelming majority of children with ADHD symptoms could then be considered as being the victims of a minimal degree of brain injury and their ADHD symptoms the result of mishaps in pregnancy, labor or delivery or of later illness or injury. Most families with children manifesting attention-deficit symptoms could point to one difficulty or another, during or after the pregnancy, as the cause of the child's problem. As a result, the theory that mishaps of pregnancy, labor or delivery or other brain injury was the major cause of attention-deficit symptoms was widely held through the 1950s.

Scientific evidence was required to disprove this theory, which seemed to result from everyday logic. Routh (1978) reported that there was little evidence to support the view that brain damage was a major cause of attention deficit. Other studies found that a very small percentage of children with histories of attention deficit also had histories suggesting brain injury (Stewart & Olds, 1973). Major studies did not find a significant relationship between severe perinatal stress and later adjustment (Werner, Bierman, French, Simonian, Connor, Smith & Campbell, 1968).

One of the largest of these pregnancy studies, the Collaborative Perinatal Project of the National Institute of Neurological and Communicative Disorders and Strokes, was a multicenter, cooperative effort studying the outcome of 55,000 pregnancies. Detailed records of all aspects of pregnancy, labor and delivery were recorded, and psychological, neurological and medical follow-up examinations were carried on during the development of the child. At birth, every child was evaluated for movement, tone, color, respiratory effort and heart rate. The results of this evaluation when totaled was the Apgar score, which is a measure of the health of the baby at birth. Nelson and Ellenberg (1979) reported a study correlating the Apgar scores and long-term neurological follow-up for this large group of children. They found that there was no correlation between symptoms of attention deficit and Apgar scores. Large numbers of children with severe difficulty at the time of birth developed no attention-deficit symptoms, and some children without difficult delivery developed severe symptoms of attention deficit. The observation of large numbers of children in the Collaborative Perinatal Project Study demonstrated that in an individual instance, a history of difficulty with delivery alone would not be sufficient to establish birth injury as the cause of ADHD.

The theory that some children develop ADHD and other mild developmental problems as the result of brain injury has regained some scientific support. Delaney-Black et al. (1989) followed 49 children born with a high red blood cell count and hyperviscosity (poor blood flow as the result of excessive red blood cells, possibly causing damaged blood vessels in the brain). At seven years of age, this group of children was found to have lower spelling and arithmetic achievement as measured on the Wide Range Achievement Test than similar children who had not had a high red blood cell count and hyperviscosity at birth. The authors concluded the lower achievement scores were the result of the hyperviscosity. Hartsough and Lambert (1985) analyzed prenatal, perinatal and developmental factors for groups of ADD and normal children. A significantly higher incidence of fetal postmaturity, toxemia or eclampsia during the pregnancy and long labor occurred in the ADD group. The authors concluded, however, that these "medical variables have minor etiological significance as compared to other factors in the generation of hyperactivity" (p. 200).

The possibility that some children suffer ADHD as the result of perinatal injury has been supported in an emission-computed tomography (SPECT) blood-flow study (Lou, Henriksen & Bruhn, 1984). When radioactive xenon gas is inhaled, radioactivity is emitted from the brain proportional to the blood flowing through the region. Thirteen children were studied with this technique. Eleven of the children had been diagnosed as ADD. The authors found a consistent pattern of decreased blood flow in the basal ganglia and in the border zone or space between major arterial distributions within the brain. Treatment with methylphenidate increased the perfusion to these areas, as well as improving ADD symptoms as judged by clinical observation. The authors suggested that the data presented supported the hypothesis that early hypoxic ischemic brain injury may be involved in a substantial percentage of patients with attention deficit.

This study of brain blood flow shows a physiological difference between children with attention deficit and normal children. In addition, it demonstrates a change in blood flow related to clinical improvement with medication. The small number of children and the fact that no standard diagnostic criteria were used, however, make any conclusions drawn from this study preliminary and tentative. In addition, there is no evidence presented to show that the variation in blood flow has a direct relationship to early hypoxic ischemic brain injury. Nevertheless, this blood-flow study adds to the large body of information demonstrating that children with attention-deficit symptoms are physiologically different from other children.

REFINED SUGAR

Refined sugar has been suggested as a cause of attention deficit, often as a result of uncontrolled or anecdotal reports. These accounts are difficult to interpret. For example, a parent who experienced considerable difficulty with her eight-year-old son after an extended birthday party reported long hours of stimulation by a large group of friends and then a sleepless night. She concluded, however, that her son must be sensitive to sugar because he had a piece of chocolate cake during the party. Other variables such as the sleeplessness and excitement of the party may have been more important to the subsequent difficulty with behavior than the chocolate cake, but without a carefully controlled environment it is difficult to be certain. Studies that control these factors were needed to determine whether diet is a cause of ADHD symptoms.

A group of carefully controlled studies have been completed. Twenty-one boys, selected because they were reported by their parents to respond adversely to sugar, were studied by Behar, Rapoport, Adams, Berg and Cornblath (1984). A placebo blind challenge with sugar drinks revealed the possibly surprising result of a slight but significant decrease in observed motor activity three hours after the sugar challenge. Two additional studies of sucrose ingestion and behavior in hyperactive boys were presented by Wolraich, Milich, Stumbo and Schultz (1985) and a third by Milich and Pelham (1986). Careful dietary control with 1.75 gram/kg of sucrose or placebo (aspartame in equivalent sweetness) was presented. The results of all three studies revealed no difference in the boys' performance on the challenge days.

Would a greater effect from the sugar have been seen if the boys had been allowed to use any amount of sugar they wanted? Kaplan, Wamboldt and Barnhardt (1986) allowed children to select any amount of sweetened breakfast that they desired. On some days they were given aspartame sweetener and on others, sucrose. Conners rating questionnaires were used to evaluate behavior. In addition, some children received methylphenidate and others did not. The study was able to distinguish between methylphenidate and non-methylphenidate treatment but was not able to distinguish the aspartame condition from the sucrose condition.

The authors believed the study had additional significance because the children could use any amount of sugar they desired. Under these conditions, differences of behavior produced by methylphenidate were apparent, but no differences in behavior caused by aspartame versus sucrose were seen.

These studies provide evidence that dietary sugar does not cause ADHD symptoms to worsen in groups of children. While it is impossible to prove sugar *never* worsens behavior in *any* child, carefully controlled studies fail to demonstrate that sugar ingestion by children is a significant contributor to the problem of attention deficit.

FEINGOLD DIET

In relation to ADHD, other foods or food additives have received possibly even wider interest than sugar. Feingold (1974) hypothesized from anecdotal observations that ingestion of certain commonly occurring foods and additives contributed to behavioral deterioration. He was concerned about artificial colors and a group of certain food constituents called "natural salicylates." The latter are compounds that are chemically related to salicylic acid. They are found in many fruits and other common foods. Feingold postulated that the elimination of these from the diet would produce substantial improvements in behavior. Again, to support this he cited anecdotal evidence. In order to eliminate these substances, a complex dietary restriction was required. Many foods commonly eaten by and readily available to children would be prohibited by such a diet.

Studies of artificial colors and other additives were conducted by Conners (1980). He first placed children on a controlled diet free of certain additives. During this time, he evaluated their behavior with the Conners Parent's Questionnaire to determine the severity of symptoms. He next reintroduced the possibly offending substances in a double-blind manner. Every day the children received a cookie. Some days it contained a full day's supply of food additives, and some days it contained none of these substances. In this way, both the subjects and the examiners did not know whether the children had received the additives. Conners' first observations suggested that there was a substantial improvement in symptoms when the diet was undertaken. This information could be used by advocates of the diet program. However, when the offending substances were reintroduced, there was no clear deterioration of behavior. This would suggest that the improvement seen on the diet was unrelated to the specific dietary exclusion. As a result of this group of studies, it was concluded that there is no clear evidence implicating artificial salicylates and food additives as a substantial cause for attention deficit.

Some studies, however, suggest that food additives may play a role in attention deficit. Swanson and Kinsbourne (1980) found that 85 percent of a group of 20 medication-responder hyperactive children experienced adverse effects after ingestion of food dye in a double-blind crossover study. Egger, Carter, Graham, Gumley and Soothill (1985) found that after ingestion of a combination of dyes and preservatives 79 percent of 28 children referred for suspected food-based behavior problems suffered behavioral deterioration. Lester and Fishbein (1988) suggest several reasons the earliest studies may have produced false negative results. First, the dosage of dyes may have been too low in studies conducted before 1980. Second, the combination of preservatives found in normal diets but not in test situations may be needed to produce behavioral symptoms, and third, artificial flavors, which outnumber dyes, may also be important precipitants of behavior change.

A study of preschool-aged boys by Kaplan, McNicol, Conte, and Moghadam (1989) further supports the hypothesis that diets eliminating multiple offending agents are effective at improving behavior. Twenty-four hyperactive preschool boys were studied. All foods were provided by the investigators. They eliminated not only artificial colors and flavors but also chocolate, monosodium glutamate, preservatives, caffeine and any substances that families reported might affect their specific child. The diet was also low in simple sugars and was even milk-free if the family reported a history of possible problems with cow's milk. More than half of the children, based upon Conners Parent Questionnaires, were reported to improve on the diet but not on the placebo. In addition, halitosis, night awakenings and sleep latency, or time to sleep onset, were improved. The authors believed their diet had a stronger effect than previous challenge studies because they eliminated many offending agents.

In 1986, when Wender wrote her review of food additives, the conclusions were clear. Only one study suggested a significant effect of food additives. Subsequently, however, at least two additional studies have reexamined the question. The new approach looks at the combination of many substances and studies children on such restricted diets that all their food must be supplied by the examiner. Only further research will determine if this approach has any relevance to the daily lives of most ADHD children.

LEAD

Lead is a trace element that has no known use in the human body. Ingested flakes of lead paint can poison the energy production within brain cells. As the brain becomes more and more swollen, general brain function decreases and thinking becomes confused. Convulsions can occur, and swelling can progress to brain injury and death (Byers, 1959).

Can lead intoxication too mild to produce brain swelling and convulsions cause attention-deficit symptoms? de la Burde and Choate (1975) presented a collabora-tive study of 67 seven-year-old children. These children had a history of eating plaster and paint when they were between one and three years of age. At that time their qualitative urinary coproporphyrin tests were positive (suggesting lead poisoning), and they had elevated blood lead levels (.04 mgs/dl and above) and/or radiological findings suggesting lead poisoning but no clinical symptoms. At age seven their performance on a series of psychological tests was compared with those of 70 children of the same age and socioeconomic background who did not have significant exposure to lead. Lead-exposed children had deficits in global I.Q. and associative abilities, in visual and fine motor coordination and in behavior. School failure resulting from learning and behavior problems was more frequent in the lead-exposed than in the control group. The question remained, however, whether the children had problems as a result of lead or had ingested lead as a result of abnormal behavior.

The relationship between lead level and I.Q. in a group of children exposed to lead in the environment was studied by Landrigan,Whitworth, Baloh, Staehling, Barthel and Rosenbloom (1975). Forty-six symptom-free children, aged 3 to 15, with blood lead concentrations of 40 to 68 (mean 48 micrograms per 100 ml.) and 78 ethnically and socioeconomically similar controls with levels less than 40 (mean 27) were compared. All the children lived within 6.6 kilometers of a large lead-emitting smelter. "Testing with Wechsler Intelligence Scales for school children and preschool children showed age-adjusted performance I.Q. to be significantly decreased in the group with higher lead levels (mean scores WISC or WPPSI: 95 versus 103). Children in the lead group also had significant slowing in a finger-wrist tapping test" (p. 708). Full-scale I.Q., Verbal I.Q. and hyperactivity ratings were unchanged by lead exposure. This study suggests that for this group of children living in a high-lead environment, higher blood lead levels are associated with lower performance I.Q.

Possibly the most ambitious study of lead was reported by Needleman, Gunnoe, Leviton, Reed, Peresie, Maher and Barrett (1979). The authors studied 3329 children attending first and second grades in two Massachusetts towns, Chelsea and Summerville. Voluntary collection of shed teeth was obtained in 70 percent of the children. The 10 percent of the children with the highest concentration of dentine lead and the 10 percent with the lowest were chosen for analysis. Four or five years earlier, blood readings had been taken in 23 children with high lead levels and 58 with low lead levels. When lead levels in shed teeth were compared with earlier determinations, there was a significant correlation between previous blood lead levels of the high-tooth-lead and low-tooth-lead groups. The blood lead level of both groups was well within normal limits. When I.Q. was evaluated, a strong correlation was seen between Full-Scale WISC-R I.Q. and lead level. The low-lead group had an I.Q. score over four points higher than the high-lead group. Significant correlation was also seen with three measures of auditory and verbal processing on attentional performance and with most items of a teacher's behavioral rating.

These findings suggest that there may be a group of children with attention-deficit, behavior or developmental symptoms that are at least in part the result of lead exposure. How much of the behavior and learning problems is caused by other differences in the two groups (such as genetic influences evidenced by poor parental education in the high-lead group) or by sample bias (higher percentage of males than females in the high-lead group) is yet to be determined. The significant correlation between blood and dentine lead levels on the one hand and Full-Scale I.Q., verbal and auditory processing reaction time or behavioral ratings on the other, suggests that lead may be a significant contributor to ADHD symptoms.

It is difficult to know what should be done as a result of these studies. Long-term longitudinal studies continue to investigate the relationship between lead level, cognitive development and behavior (Wyngaarden, 1988). There is no evidence that treatment for lead poisoning would improve the performance of the children with the higher dentine lead levels. In addition, there was substantial performance overlap between the two groups. Finding slightly above average lead level in either blood or teeth could not be used to help diagnose ADHD. Without understanding how these children came to acquire higher lead levels, one cannot judge which public health measures would be effective in preventing the problem. Nevertheless, there is a disturbing suggestion of a relationship between lead ingestion and learning and attentional problems. There may be some children in whom lead is a contributing factor to attention deficit.

ADHD SECONDARY TO MEDICAL PROBLEMS

Some children exhibit ADHD symptoms as a result of unrelated medical illness (Wender, 1987). Possibly the term ADHD does not apply to the inattentive, distractible, variable and impulsive behavior seen in children with certain medical illnesses. The role of the physician in the differential diagnosis of ADHD can be seen from many different points of view. Cantwell and Baker (1987) reviewed the "diagnostic processes in making the differential diagnosis of hyperactivity" (p. 159). They presented the view that the primary care physician will be able to conduct an initial evaluation and make an active differential diagnosis. They separated clinical psychiatric disorders, developmental disorders, physical and neurological disorders and psychosocial and environmental factors from birthweight, various forms of pre-, peri- and postnatal difficulties (such as very difficult deliveries, asphyxia and maternal infection during pregnancy), movement disorders (e.g., Sydenham's chorea), hyperthyroidism, infection with pinworms and sleep apnea. Cantwell and Baker argue that the diagnosis of ADHD is not appropriate to characterize the impulsive, inattentive and distractible behavior seen in children with these medical conditions.

Otitis Media

An association between otitis media (ear infection) and ADHD has been reported by Hagerman and Falkenstein (1987). In an intriguing retrospective study, the incidence of previous otitis media infection in children who had been diagnosed as being hyperactive by Conners Parent's or Teacher's Questionnaires or DSM-III criteria was compared with the incidence of otitis media reported in children who presented with the problem of school failure but were not hyperactive. The two groups seemed comparable in other respects. Of the group of children with hyperactivity, 94% had a history of three or more ear infections, whereas only 50% of the nonhyperactive school-failure children had three or more infections. Of the hyperactive group 69% had a previous history of more than ten infections, whereas only 20% of the nonhyperactive group had more than ten infections. The data presented showed only an association, not a causal relationship. It is possible that hyperactive children in the study tended to be more irritable as infants. If that was the case, one might wonder if a screaming child is more likely to develop otitis or is possibly more likely to have it diagnosed.

Anemia

Correlations of medical abnormality with attention-deficit symptoms have included iron-deficiency anemia. Webb and Oski (1973; 1974) studied teenage males and found a correlation between anemia and personality disturbance, conduct problems, feelings of inadequacy and immaturity. While iron deficiency has not subsequently been shown to be a common cause of attention-deficit symptoms, one must keep in mind the possibility of medical problems as a cause of ADHD.

Seizure Disorders (Epilepsy) and Medication for Its Treatment

Whether epilepsy itself causes ADHD, or an underlying brain injury causes both epileptic seizures and ADHD remains an unanswered question. Goulden and Shinnar (1988) reported that the behavior disorders seen in mentally retarded children or children with cerebral palsy are unrelated to the presence or severity of seizures. They studied a group of 51 children with epilepsy and evaluated behavior disorders in comparison with severity of cerebral palsy and mental retardation. The authors concluded that "this study found no association between the presence of epilepsy and behavior disorder in children with mental retardation and cerebral palsy. The high incidence of behavior disorder in this population would appear to be a reflection of the underlying brain injury" (p. 57).

Some authors argue, however, that there is a correlation between epilepsy and behavior problems. A group of 110 children with epilepsy showed significant differences in motor speed, impulsivity and inattention when compared with 152 normal children (Mitchell, Chavez, Zhou & Guzman, 1988). However, no difference was seen on tests, including the Conners questionnaires, between children taking antiepileptic drugs and those who were drug-free. In addition, performance on a microcomputer-based video game showed no change with varying levels of medication, including phenobarbital and carbamazepine (Tegretol®). The authors were able to conclude that "children with epilepsy have significant deficits in reaction time, attention and impulsivity compared to normal peers, even eliminating children with low I.Q" (p. 45). Generalized absence epilepsy produces spells of staring and inattention during a seizure. This condition must be diagnosed and treated differently from ADHD. Additional information concerning this disorder is presented in Chapter 3.

Medications used to treat epilepsy may cause some ADHD symptoms in some children. Phenobarbital and diphenylhydantoin (Dilantin®) are common medications used in the treatment of epilepsy. According to a study by Pellock, Culbert, Garnett, Crumrine, Kaplan, O'Hara, Driscoll, Frost, Alvin, Hamer, Handen, Horowitz and Nichols (1988), 30 children changed from phenobarbital or diphenylhydantoin to carbamazepine showed significant improvement in color naming, finger oscillation, continuous performance time, reaction time, digit vigilance and

Conners Parent's Questionnaire total score. The authors concluded that "significant cognitive and behavioral effects may be produced by antiepileptic drugs in some patients" (p. 79).

Fragile-X Syndrome

A genetic deficit known as fragile-x syndrome has been associated with ADHD. A fragile site on Q27 of the x chromosome gives this syndrome its name. Clinical symptoms include large ears and testes in males. Most children with fragile-x are mentally retarded. Hagerman, Kemper and Hudson (1985) report four boys who were not retarded but had learning disabilities and attentional problems associated with fragile-x syndrome. Their report points to a group of children whose learning disabilities and attentional problems apparently result from a definable genetic defect. The abnormal chromosome is the presumed cause of the learning and attention problems seen in these four children. Because chromosome studies are ordinarily not performed on most children with attention deficit, it is difficult to be certain how common this syndrome is. The lack of additional reports, however, would suggest that this chromosome defect is an uncommon cause of ADHD symptoms. Further studies will be needed to determine if this is an isolated finding. Presence of unusual features might warrant evaluation with chromosome studies to determine whether fragile-x is present. While some improvement in genetic counseling might be possible if the fragile-x was discovered, at this point not enough is known about the children with ADHD and fragile-x to comment on changes in treatment or expectation of outcome for this group.

ADHD SECONDARY TO NONMEDICAL PROBLEMS

It has been suggested that attention-deficit symptoms are the result of difficulty with learning (McGee & Share, 1988; Cunningham & Barkley, 1978a). In support of this theory have been the findings of Whalen, Collins, Henker, Alkus, Adams and Stapp (1978), which suggest that attention-deficient children function better if their academic tests are not challenging but demonstrate increasing difficulty as task-complexity increases; Henker and Whalen's (1980) suggestion that inattentive children perform better on self-paced tasks than when they are required to work at a pace set by others; and suggestions by Battle and Lacy (1972) that the inattentive child functions best when frustration is kept to a minimum. It follows that the successful treatment of learning difficulties may result in resolution of the ADHD symptoms. For example, McGee and Share (1988) point out that reinforcement contingent on academic productivity has been shown to increase the quality and quantity of academic output in disruptive children. This body of research provides evidence that there may be a subgroup of learning-disabled children who develop ADHD symptoms as the result of school frustration.

Other behavioral problems of childhood, such as depressive and oppositional disorders, as well as other cognitive problems involving memory, achievement, language, auditory processing and general intelligence, can produce symptoms similar to ADHD. These problems are discussed further in Chapter 7.

HEREDITY

The majority of children with learning and attention problems are found to have none of the specific etiologies mentioned above. A positive family history of ADHD symptoms, however, is a common finding. In many children, one of the close family members, such as the father, has had symptoms of attention deficit in childhood. Hyperactivity was noted in the parents of hyperactive children four times as commonly as in those of controls in studies by Morrison and Stewart (1971) and Cantwell (1972).

Twin studies often help differentiate genetic and environmental factors. Monozygotic (identical) twins have identical genetics since they both originate from the same fertilized egg. However, dizygotic (fraternal or nonidentical) twins differ from each other genetically since they arise from separate eggs fertilized by different sperm. Monozygotic twins raised in different environments (adopted by different sets of parents) will develop similar genetically determined characteristics. Willerman (1973) studied 93 sets of twin girls. If one identical twin was hyperactive, the other was more likely to be hyperactive. Very few of the genetically different, dizygotic twins were both hyperactive. This finding suggests a strong element of heredity, at least in this group of twin girls.

Lahey, Pelham, Schaughency, Atkins, Murphy, Hynd, Russo, Hartdagen and Lorys-Vernon (1988) studied parental psychopathology in children with conduct disorder and hyperactivity. They concluded that when conduct disorder and ADHD occur together, markedly more aggression and illegal activity in both fathers and children is seen. They also concluded that there is probably a familial pattern of transmission of ADHD. Several studies have shown that attention deficit may be more common in the fathers and uncles of attention-disordered children than in the relatives of children without attention disorder (Cantwell, 1972; 1975; Morrison & Stewart, 1971). The tendency for attention deficit to run in a family was further suggested by Stewart, DeBlois and Cummings (1980). When attention-disordered children are adopted and raised by biologically unrelated families, inattentive symptoms are not more common in the nonbiological relatives (Morrison & Stewart, 1973; Cantwell, 1975). Heredity appears to represent the most common identifiable cause of ADHD.

BRAIN DYSFUNCTION AS THE CAUSE OF ADHD

Abnormality of behavior can be considered from the point of view of abnormality of brain function. An animal model of ADHD has been created by injuring the chemical brain system of animals. Figure 2.1 represents the chemical structures

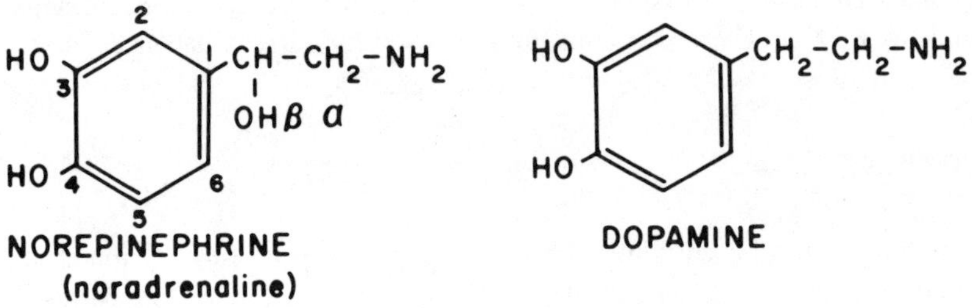

Figure 2.1 Chemical structure of dopamine and norepinephrine. From Snyder, S.H. and Meyerhoff, J.L. How Amphetamine Acts in Minimal Brain Dysfunction. Copyright 1973. *Annals of New York Academy of Sciences*. Reprinted with permission of the publisher and authors.

of dopamine and norepinephrine. Other studies of brain chemicals released into spinal fluid and blood suggested brain chemical changes in ADHD children. A brain model for ADHD helps to understand ADHD in terms of brain function.

Animal Model

Animal studies give important clues to the cause of illness observed in humans. If an animal equivalent or animal model of illness is discovered or created, the cause of the animal illness may be similar to that of humans. The more features seen in the animal illness that correspond to the human disorder, the better are the insights of cause and treatment learned from the animal model.

An animal model of attention deficit based on dopamine has been developed by Shaywitz, Hunt, Jatlow, Cohen, Young, Pierce, Anderson and Shaywitz (1982). An infant rat is administered a chemical that seeks out and selectively destroys dopamine nerve endings. The chemical (6-hydroxydopamine) is administered into the spinal fluid at the base of the skull. Rapid and permanent reduction of brain dopamine to concentrations of 10% to 25% of that in controls is produced. Some other brain chemicals, notably norepinephrine and serotonin, remain unaffected.

As the rats develop, they go through a period of time while they are immature during which they demonstrate increased activity and increased difficulty learning. As they mature, the hyperactivity resolves, but they continue to have difficulty with certain types of learning tasks. The hyperactivity and learning problems seen in the dopamine-depleted rat pups improved with amphetamine (Shaywitz, Yager & Klopper, 1976) and methylphenidate (Shaywitz, Klopper & Gordon, 1978), and exacerbation of the hyperactivity was produced by administration of phenobarbital (Shaywitz & Pearson, 1978). The rat pups also had difficulty with a novel environment (Shaywitz, Gordon, Klopper, & Zelterman, 1977). Environmental manipulation (being raised with normal litter mates) was shown to improve motor activity in the avoidance performance of these rats as well (Pearson, Teicher, Shaywitz, Cohen, Young & Anderson, 1980).

In the animal model, increased activity and difficulty with certain kinds of learning are produced not by damage to a specific location of the brain but by damage to the nerve-cell endings that deliver dopamine in their locations throughout the entire brain. This lends substantial support to the concept that a dysfunction of dopamine-containing neurons is the underlying structural defect that results in the clinical syndrome of attention deficit.

Metabolic Studies on Human Subjects

Chemicals such as dopamine flow from the brain to the cerebrospinal fluid (CSF) that surrounds the brain. CSF can be obtained in living subjects and reflects chemical change within the brain. Shaywitz, Cohen and Bowers (1977) demonstrated that changes in dopamine metabolism, as measured in spinal fluid, could be found in children with MBD. The presence of changes in dopamine rather than serotonin metabolites raised the suspicion that dopamine was the principal system involved with the chemical changes of attention deficit.

Homovanillic acid (HVA) is a dopamine metabolite; 5-hydroxyindolacetic acid (HIAA) is a metabolite of serotonin. Shetty and Chase (1976) studied HVA and HIAA levels in spinal fluid of 23 children, aged 2 to 13 years. They found that the base levels of the dopamine and serotonin metabolites (HVA & HIAA) were identical but that the level of the dopamine metabolite (HVA) was substantially reduced by dextroamphetamine treatment and the "amount of HVA correlated closely with the degree of clinical improvement. These results support the view that an alteration in central dopamine mediated synaptic function may occur in children manifesting the hyperactive syndrome" (p. 1001).

Chemical metabolites or breakdown products of brain chemicals are found excreted in urine. Changes in chemical composition of this readily available substance may reflect changes in brain chemical composition. Shekim, Sinclair, Glaser, Horwitz, Javaid and Bylund (1987) studied norepinephrine and dopamine metabolites excreted in urine of hyperactive and normal children. They found subtle correlations between dopamine metabolites and various behavioral and academic qualities.

Not all authors find dopamine the major chemical involved in attention deficit. Shekim, Dekirmenjian and Chapel (1977) studied excretion of dopamine metabolites as well as norepinephrine metabolites with the administration of amphetamine. Boys 7- to 12-years-old, diagnosed as displaying hyperkinetic reaction of childhood by DSM-II criteria were studied. Changes in urinary metabolite excretion suggested noradrenalin rather than dopamine was being changed. The authors reviewed 11 studies that suggested the importance of the noradrenalin system and the interconnection of the noradrenalin and dopamine system in controlling behavior. Raskin, Shaywitz, Shaywitz, Anderson and Cohen (1984) attempted to explain some of the conflicting reports by proposing a mechanism of feedback inhibition of norepinephrine- and dopamine-containing neurons. Starke and Montel (1973) report that clonidine, which has been effective in treating attention-deficit symptoms in some children, also acts to decrease the release of norepinephrine. The authors cite two studies (Bunney & Aghajanian, 1976; Huang & Maas, 1981) showing that at low doses clonidine actually inhibits firing of norepinephrine- and dopamine-containing neurons (p. 394).

Attempts to show that ADHD is the result of a change in dopamine or noradrenalin may suffer from oversimplification. The interconnection of dopamine, noradrenalin and serotonin systems raises the possibility that a change in the function of the dopamine system may be reflected as decreased or increased performance of a different chemical system, such as the noradrenalin or serotonin system. To understand this, consider the hypothetical change in dopamine in hyperactive children. Say that hyperactive children are found to have a lower level of dopamine in the brain. At first this might seem to imply that dopamine is responsible for hyperactivity. However, a possible alternative explanation is that dopamine changes were a reaction to the hyperactivity. In other words, another system, such as the noradrenalin system, would be responsible for the hyperactivity and in response to the noradrenalin change, dopamine metabolism would change. In this hypothetical example, the change in dopamine metabolism would represent a secondary response of the brain in an attempt to compensate for the primary change.

Data presented on the interaction of dopamine and norepinephrine remind us that these systems are complex and that simple measurements of increased and decreased levels do not suffice to explain the workings of the catecholamine systems. Nevertheless, the finding that metabolism of these chemicals is changed in children with attention-deficit symptoms and that these chemical systems are changed by medications that improve the symptoms of attention-deficit lead to the important conclusion that the chemical systems that have their nerve-cell bodies in brain-stem nuclei are important factors in ADHD.

Other models of ADHD have been proposed. Injury to the right cerebral hemisphere in adults produces a syndrome of neglect of the left side, spatial discrimination difficulties and other characteristics. Sunder, DeMarco, Fruitiger and Levey (1988) felt that a group of children who were poorly responsive to medication showed a group of testing characteristics defined as a "developmental right-hemisphere-deficit syndrome" (p. 68). In a preliminary report, they presented 20 children characterized by ten-point disparity between WISC-R verbal and performance I.Q., weakness on picture completion and object assembly subtests, impaired design copying, low math computation, and reading comprehension one grade below oral word recognition. Of these 20 children, 75% were also described as apraxic (poor fine motor skills) and 75% had attention deficits that did not respond well to a trial of medication. Of these children 75% also had significant social and emotional difficulties beyond hyperactivity. Further evaluation of this collection of symptoms may prove useful in defining a group that can be expected to be unresponsive to medication.

DeMarco, Sunder, Batts, Fruitiger and Levey (1988) suggested that the Boder test of reading-spelling patterns can by itself identify children of whom 80 percent will fall into the right-hemisphere deficit syndrome. Voeller and Heilman (1988) presented additional information concerning the relationship of attention-deficit disorder and right-hemisphere function. They initially showed that cancellation tasks suggested right-hemisphere dysfunction in ADHD children. These authors studied motor impersistence in children with ADHD in such tasks as sustaining a movement (tongue protrusion, right lateral gaze, central fixation). They found that ADHD children had significantly more difficulty with these tasks. They suggested that "if the mechanisms producing motor impersistence in children are similar to those in adults, this study provides further support for the postulate that ADHD may be related to right-hemisphere dysfunction" (p. 71). These preliminary results suggest the possibility of defining a subgroup of ADHD children who may not respond as well to stimulant medications and may require a different therapeutic approach. However, it is too early to be certain from these preliminary studies.

Concepts such as underarousal and overarousal have been reviewed by Ross and Ross (1982). Attempts to find the physiological basis for overarousal and underarousal theories have met with limited success. Understanding the cause of attention deficit from the point of view of the brain as a neurological organ has interested many researchers. The frontal-lobe dysfunction model was summarized by Conners and Wells (1986). Levine (1987) proposed an understanding of attention deficit as a dysfunction of multiple control systems. These nine systems include vocal, sensory, associative, appetite, social, motor, behavioral, communicative and affective control. Levine reviewed different etiologies affecting a variety of the control systems and viewed understanding the symptoms as well as the treatment related to these control symptoms as essential. Zametkin and Rapoport (1987), in a comprehensive review concerning the neurobiology of *Attention deficit disorder*, observed that the "large number of efficacious drugs do not support any single neurotransmitter defect hypothesis, and no current model can account for the abundance of positive findings" (p. 676). Table 2.1 presents a summary of neuroanatomical hypotheses of ADHD symptoms.

A BRAIN MODEL OF ADHD

The model that will be presented may help to explain both some of the conflicting information concerning experimental work on attention deficit and the mechanism of drug action. The brain is often divided anatomically into three parts—the cerebral hemispheres, brain stem and cerebellum. The cerebellum, which is involved with balance and coordination, is not considered to have a major role in thinking or behavior and will not be considered further.

Within the cerebral hemisphere, information from primary sensory organs, such as the eyes, the nose, the skin and the ears are converted into electrical impulses that are sent to specific areas of the cerebral cortex. Figure 2.2 represents several locations for cognitive function within the brain. Note that, as this is a midsagittal section, the temporal lobes are not seen. There is a primary area for sensory information for each of the senses: the occipital region for visual information; the temporal region for hearing and sound; the parietal, postcentral region for touch; and the portion of the frontal lobes just above the eyes for the sense of smell. Injury to these areas produces a specific set of symptoms involving inability to utilize these primary sensory modalities.

Other areas of the cerebral hemispheres involve translating primary sensory input into symbolic function or preparing a response. These areas, called association

TABLE 2.1. Neuroanatomical Hypotheses of Dysfunction in Attention Deficit Disorder with Hyperactivity

Investigator	Hypothesis	Test
Laufer and Denhoff, 1957	Diencephalic dysfunction (thalamus, hypothalamus)	HA have lower photometrazol seizure
Knobel et al., 1959	Cortical "overfunctioning"	
Satterfield and Dawson, 1971	Decreased levels of reticular activating system excitation	See text
Wender, 1971, 1972	Decreased sensitivity in limbic areas of positive reinforcement (medial forebrain bundle; hypothalamus; NE)	Multiple medication trials
Conners et al., 1964	Lack of "cortical inhibitory capacity"	
Dykman et al., 1971	Defect in forebrain inhibitory system over ventral formation + diencephalon	
Hunt et al., 1985	Locus coerulens dysfunction (hypersensitive alphapostsynaptic receptor)	Clonidine growth hormone response
Lou et al., 1984	Central frontal lobes, anterolateral, posterolateral Caudate region	Cerebral blood flow
Gorenstein and Newman, 1980	Dysfunction of medial septum, hippocampus orbito-frontal cortex	Animal lesion studies
Porrino et al., 1984	Nucleus acumbens	Animal studies 2-D-G studies with low-dose stimulants
Mattes, 1980	Frontal lobe	Speculation
Gualtieri and Hicks, 1985	Frontal lobe	Speculation
Arnold et al., 1977	Nigrostriatal tract	Amphetamine Rx
Chelune et al., 1986	Frontal lobe	Neuropsychiatric testing

Zametkin, A. J. and Rapoport, J. L. "Neurobiology of Attention Deficit Disorder with Hyperactivity: Where Have We Come in 50 Years?" Copyright 1987 by the *American Academy of Child and Adolescent Psychiatry.* Used by permission of the publisher and authors.

areas, are usually adjacent to the primary sensory or motor areas and lie in the parietal-occipital, frontal and temporal parietal region. Some of these association areas, when injured, prevent the codification and understanding of primary sensory information. For example, an injury to the parietal lobe adjacent to the occipital lobe would result in disturbance of the association and understanding of visual information. The inability to understand words written on the page would be the result of a lesion in the association area in the parietal-occipital region. A learning disability can, insofar as it represents an inability to move information, be viewed as a failure of these areas of the cerebral hemispheres.

The brain stem is an elongated part of the brain that extends from the spinal cord into the base of the cerebral hemispheres, including the hypothalamus. This part of the brain contains, among other things, groups of nerve cells that have regulatory function. For example, small groups of nerve cells are important for regulating blood pressure, breathing rate, appetite and other automatic functions. Disruption

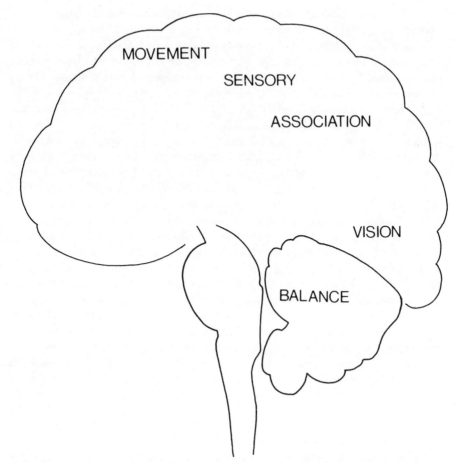

Figure 2.2 Mid-sagittal section representing several locations for cognitive functions within the brain.

of other groups of cells in the brain stem will result in total body paralysis and inability to awaken from a deep sleep or coma. Many of the nuclei in the brain stem work to regulate and modulate functions of other parts of the brain and body. For example, the hunger and satiety centers do not affect the ability to chew or swallow but do regulate interest in acquiring and ingesting food. Other brain stem and hypothalamic centers regulate tiredness and wakefulness, temperature, heart rate, blood pressure, sensitivity to pain and many other functions.

Other groups of cells make certain chemicals, including dopamine, noradrenalin and serotonin. They then distribute these chemicals through connections called axons to all other areas of the brain. Dopamine is transferred from the substantia nigra of the midbrain to many other areas of the brain. In addition, noradrenalin made in the locus ceruleus of the pons in the brain stem and serotonin made in neurons located in the raphe nuclei in the medulla, another part of the brain stem, are also transferred to all areas of the brain. For example, dopamine made within the nerve cells of the substantia nigra in the brain stem travels to the basal ganglia. Disruptions in dopamine pathways results in the clinical symptoms of Parkinson's disease, including stiffness and decreased movement. It is possible to improve the functioning of this dopamine system with a medication, L-dopa, which is converted into dopamine by nerve cells. As a result, improvement in the dopamine system and the symptoms of Parkinson's disease can be achieved.

Attention and concentration is not an all-or-nothing phenomenon. There are situations when one would appropriately be inattentive. For example, a person walking on a lonely and deserted inner-city street would react to the rustling of paper a few feet away by looking in the direction of the rustling paper. In different circumstances, for example when sitting in a classroom, a person would try to concentrate on the teacher, and the same rustling of paper would, under normal circumstances, not cause a break in concentration. Most students are able to adjust their attention and concentration ability so that they can be distracted in certain situations and yet have a focused attention in other situations.

The attention system that allows this change of concentration and distractibility does not represent a single group of neurons or a single microscopic, anatomical location. It projects to all areas of the brain and modulates a change in state from intense concentration to easy distractibility in normal subjects. When it is functioning well, a child will be able to pay attention to the teacher at one time and at a different time be sensitive to distractions. When this system works well, it enables the child in the classroom to concentrate on listening to the teacher and to exclude rustling papers and noises. A few minutes later this same child might be pitching in a baseball game where it is necessary to concentrate both on the batter and catcher, as well as to listen for distractions such as a player stealing second base. The attention system allows the normal subject to change concentration and attention as necessary across a wide spectrum from intense concentration to a high degree of sensitivity to outside distractions.

The attention system may coordinate several groups of nerve cells, possibly dopamine, noradrenalin and serotonin cells. Additional limbic, right-hemisphere and frontal cells are most likely part of this system. It need not have a single microscopic physical location in order to be a functional coordinating system. It most likely utilizes the dopamine neurons whose cell bodies lie in the brain stem but may also utilize other brain stem neurons, including noradrenalin neurons whose cell bodies lie in the locus ceruleus and the serotonin neurons whose cell bodies lie in the midline raphe nuclei of the medulla. The projections of these neurons to all areas of the brain would be important for a regulatory system, the purpose of which is to modulate whole brain activity.

This model may help in understanding some of the complex and conflicting information concerning attention and concentration and the symptoms of *Attention-deficit hyperactivity disorder*. Figure 2.3 represents a diagram of the brain, indicating a brainstem center and its communication with other areas of the brain. Attention and concentration is variable in normal subjects. A wide range of possible levels of concentration and activity is needed. A normal subject must be able to act quickly without deliberation in emergency situations and yet restrain

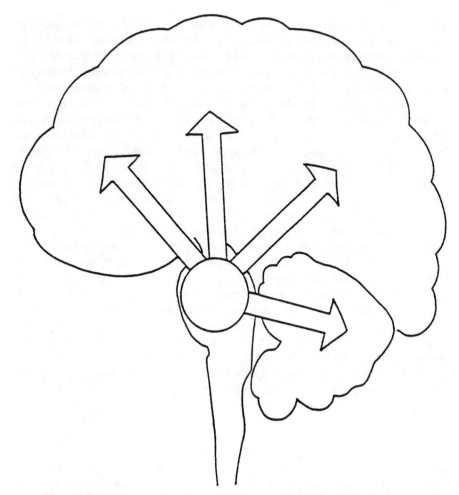

Figure 2.3 Brain stem center and its communication with other areas of the brain.

the impulse to act in other situations. An attention system projecting to all areas of the brain could inhibit impulsive activity in some situations and facilitate it in others. A normal child must be able to sit quietly in a classroom at one time and run explosively at another on a playing field. The brain stem center projections to motor areas, both basal ganglia and cortex, would allow this kind of change by inhibiting motor activity and restlessness at one time, but releasing it at another. This model of brain function would suggest that changes in normal attention, concentration, motor activity, restlessness and impulsive behavior can be viewed as resulting from different "settings" of the attention center.

The attention system must communicate with all areas of the brain as changes in motor activity, restlessness and concentration involve all areas of the brain. The presence of dopamine, noradrenalin and serotonin nerve cell bodies grouped in brain-stem nuclei projecting to all areas of the brain would be compatible with this function. The large body of biochemical information suggesting that injury to dopamine neurons produces attention deficit is consistent with the attention center utilizing the dopamine system to effect changes in state of the entire brain. The attention center may utilize noradrenalin and serotonin as well as dopamine.

Connections between the brain stem, frontal and limbic systems, and right hemisphere neurons also give and receive input. In this way, data suggesting that other chemical systems, such as noradrenalin, and serotonin and other anatomic locations, such as the frontal lobes or right hemisphere, are involved is consistent with the attention-center concept.

The clinical disorder of ADHD can be seen as a dysfunction of the attention system. A disorder in the mechanism for setting the level of the system would produce situations where the subject was always set on a high or low degree of concentration; a high or low degree of restlessness and impulsivity; a high or low degree of motor activity. The system that was working ineffectively might produce responses that were variable and unpredictable. A poorly functioning center might sometimes produce an appropriate and sometimes an inappropriate level of concentration, restlessness, motor activity or impulsivity.

In addition to the regulatory neurons, the functioning of the attention system requires an intact delivery system to transfer the message to other parts of the brain and receptors to receive these messages. The messages might be sent out appropriately from the brain stem through dopamine or noradrenalin neurons, but if the dopamine nerve endings located throughout the brain were not functioning, the system would be ineffective. There might be difficulty with synthesis of the proper amounts of the neurotransmitter, or there might be difficulty with the receptors in various parts of the brain. Dysfunctions anywhere along the pathway from the regulatory center to the receptors scattered throughout the brain would produce lack of effectiveness of the system. The attention system consists of multiple parts, including a central core of nerve cell bodies, axons projecting to all areas of the brain and nerve endings that act through chemical neurotransmitters and receptors throughout the brain to respond to the messages delivered by the neurotransmitters. A breakdown in any of these parts would produce symptoms of poor functioning of the system.

This model can be used to understand various kinds of data concerning attention-deficit symptoms. Treatments that improve the functioning of the nerve-cell bodies, axons, nerve endings, neurotransmitters or receptors would result in improvement of the system. Injury to dopamine nerve endings by 6-hydroxydopamine in rat pups produces symptoms of distractibility and hyperkinetic behavior. From the point of view of the attention system, the destruction of the dopamine nerve endings would mean that messages sent by the nerve cell bodies in the brain stem would have no effect because the neurotransmitter would never be released. Methylphenidate, amphetamine and other chemical agents that improve ADHD symptoms could act to improve the functioning of the nerve-cell bodies in the brain stem or the release of neurotransmitter in the nerve endings to improve sensitivity of the postsynaptic receptors. The high degree of variability of ADHD symptoms could be seen as a variability in effectiveness of the attention system. The complex system of nerve-cell bodies, axons, nerve endings and postsynaptic receptors can be seen as working well at some times and working poorly at others, either for day-to-day or situation-to-situation variability.

The attention-system model allows us to understand why treatment of attention disorders usually does not help learning disabilities. Learning disabilities can be seen as dysfunctions of cerebral cortical function as opposed to poor function of the brain-stem regulatory centers. Chemical agents such as methylphenidate or amphetamine, which improve the attention system, would not improve the function of cortical neurons.

The attention system regulates a child's ability to concentrate on read-ing, whereas the cerebral cortical centers would determine the child's reading comprehension. Improving the attention center might improve a child's interest in reading or his receptivity to reading, which may secondarily improve his reading skill. The attention-system concept explains why ADHD is a separate problem from a learning disability and why medications that improve attentional skills may have little direct affect on learning.

SUMMARY

This chapter presented two ways to view the cause of ADHD. Causes of ADHD can be seen as the result of environmental factors, including heredity. Commonly suspected factors have been disproven by scientific research. Despite intense efforts to demonstrate the effect of sugar on behavior, well-controlled studies have con-sistently failed to show that dietary sugar is a significant cause of ADHD behavior. The Feingold hypothesis that food additives and natural salicylates cause ADHD symptoms has also been subjected to scientific study. These substances, called environmental toxins by some, have usually not been shown to have a significant effect upon the behavior of groups of ADHD children. Birth injury, as reflected in Apgar scores, does not correlate with subsequent development of ADHD.

Some medical factors can cause ADHD. Iron-deficiency anemia as well as other medical illnesses can cause a secondary decrease in brain function and an increase in ADHD symptoms. Some evidence suggests ADHD children are more likely to have suffered frequent ear infections in infancy. Medications such as phenobarbital and Dilantin have been implicated.

A group of provocative studies on the relationship between lead ingestion and ADHD are troublesome. While they seem to show that there is some correlation between lead and behavior, the frequency and severity of this problem and the means of correcting it still need to be studied.

Some data suggesting a correlation between learning and behavior problems and early medical problems such as hyperviscosity, fetal post-maturity, toxemia and eclampsia during pregnancy and low blood flow has been presented. ADHD has been the major problem suffered by a few children with fragile-x chromosomal defect, although nearly all fragile-x children are mentally retarded. Children with encephalitis may develop ADHD symptoms. This group was possibly the first to stimulate scientific thinking concerning brain injury as the cause of ADHD symptoms. Taken as a group, however, all these causes account for only a small number of the children who suffer from ADHD.

Studies of heredity suggest that at least one component of the cause of ADHD is inheritance. Studies show a fourfold increase in ADHD in the fathers of ADHD boys. If one identical twin develops ADHD, the other carries a significantly increased risk of developing ADHD.

Considering the brain as a bodily organ, the cause of ADHD can be viewed in terms of organ dysfunction. Studies from human and animal subjects suggest that chemical pathways utilizing dopamine neurons that originate within brain stem nuclei help to modulate attention. Other studies suggest right hemisphere, frontal-lobe or other chemical system components. The attention system can be considered to consist of a brain-stem center composed of dopamine, noradrenalin and serotonin neurons that, with the help of frontal and/or right hemisphere input, project to all areas of the brain. This system adjusts the sensitivity of the brain to stimuli and regulates the degree of activity, attention and concentration as well as the degree of impulsivity. ADHD children are unable to appropriately modify their degree of attention, concentration and impulsive actions. From this point of view, the cause of ADHD is the dysfunction of this attention system.

PART 2

Multidisciplinary Assessment of Attention Disorders

The chapters in this section provide a framework for the comprehensive and multidisciplinary evaluation of attention and arousal-level problems in children. This type of assessment is essential because the symptoms characteristic of *Attention-deficit hyperactivity disorder* may also be caused by a variety of other medical, developmental and psychological problems.

Chapter 3 presents an overview of the physician's role in the evaluation. Evaluative markers that some physicians utilize in assessment, such as minor congenital anomalies and neurologic soft signs, will be presented and explained. Alternative medical conditions, such as epilepsy and thyroid dysfunction, that could cause symptoms of attention difficulty will be reviewed in an effort to assist in the process of differential diagnosis. Medical tests such as electroencephalography, computerized tomography and magnetic resonance imaging and their relationship to the diagnosis of attention and arousal-level problems will be explained. Guidelines will be provided to assist the practitioner in determining if a child poses a higher than normal risk for medication treatment. The chapter will also include guidelines for the medical evaluation of the child with suspected ADHD.

Chapters 4 and 5 present and review a model for collecting a social and developmental history, qualitative data and quantitative, norm-referenced data concerning the child's functioning within the home and school setting. Chapter 6 provides a model for effective assessment of attentional skills and specific individualized problems children may experience. Guidelines to assist psychologists and evaluators with behavioral observation, academic testing and intellectual assessment are presented. Objective assessment instruments that may assist in the evaluation of impulsivity and attentional skills are reviewed.

Chapter 7 provides a framework for the practitioner to integrate all of the data in an attempt to accurately make the diagnosis of ADHD. Numerous case studies and clinical observations are provided at the close of the chapter to assist the practitioner in developing sensitivity to the issue of differential diagnosis and the complex interaction between ADHD and other disorders of childhood.

CHAPTER 3

Medical Evaluation

It often appears that no two observers agree on the role of the physician in the care of children with *Attention-deficit hyperactivity disorder*. What is the role of the physician, medical testing and medical examination in the diagnosis of children with ADHD? This chapter will help the practitioner, both physician and nonphysician, develop an understanding of the basis for the medical diagnostic evaluation.

THE PHYSICIAN'S DILEMMA

The medical evaluation for a child with ADHD symptoms differs from that of a child with most other common illnesses. For example, when a child is brought to see the physician because of fever and ear pain, a few minutes of questioning concerning the history and a few minutes of examination may determine the cause of the symptoms to be a middle-ear infection. If that same child were to see the same physician for evaluation of school difficulty, the diagnostic process would be more complex. When the patient or physician expects a few simple questions to suffice for an adequate history, a brief examination or a few laboratory tests to suffice for adequate testing and a simple prescription to be an adequate treatment, both the physician and family may find understanding and treating children with ADHD more difficult than expected. The complexity of information required to make the diagnosis and develop medication and nonmedication treatment options is greater for ADHD than for most medical illnesses.

When a child comes to the physician with a fever and a question of an ear infection, the physician performs tests, including an ear examination, possibly a white blood count and temperature examination, as well as inquiring about a history of ear pain and other symptoms. The physician then makes the determination as to whether an ear infection exists. The prescribed treatment, possibly involving decongestants and antibiotics, can be written out on one or two sheets of a prescription pad. Parents are instructed on fulfilling the prescribed treatment, which may involve administering a set number of medication tablets for a specified period of time and observing for improvement in symptoms. A follow-up exam to recheck for the ear infection is usually sufficient to see the resolution of the problem. The physician is able, in a brief period of time, to take an appropriate history, perform needed diagnostic studies with his own hands, prescribe the simple and effective treatment and explain both the disease process and the treatment to the family.

This process may be appropriately completed in its entirety from start to finish in 15 minutes. The patient, the family and the physician all may feel comfortable that a proper evaluation and treatment of the problem has been accomplished.

Attention deficit does not fit into this mode of medical evaluation and treatment. The information required to make a proper diagnosis cannot be obtained simply as a result of a brief conversation between the physician and a parent or the physician and the child. Important information is often obtained from parents, teachers, siblings and others. Diagnostic tests are often not simple to order, perform or interpret. The diagnostic testing must be based upon history and other ancillary information, and interpretation of these studies requires discussion with the family and often teachers and other personnel as well.

A demonstration of these principles is reflected in a study by Brunquell, Russman and Lerer (1988) that examined mental-status testing by child neurologists in children with learning disorders. In a survey of 128 child neurologists, mental-status testing was divided into six categories, including fundamental processes, language, memory, constructional ability, higher cortical functions and related cortical functions. The authors found a progressive decline in testing frequency with increasing complexity of mental-status category. They concluded that higher and related cortical functions are tested significantly less often than other categories of mental-status function in children with learning problems and that the diagnosis ascribed to a child with learning problems is based on findings other than those provided by the mental-status exam.

In children with suspected ADHD the physician's direct observations may be misleading. Two anecdotes may be helpful in illustrating this point. A child who was functioning well in school and at home without symptoms of ADHD became quite restless when the doctor was delayed by an emergency. After sitting in the waiting room for two hours anticipating the possibility of getting a shot, the eight-year-old became anxious, hyperkinetic and impulsive. Even though the child was there for a routine examination and immunization visit, the physician watching his orderly examining room rapidly deteriorate commented to the mother, "Don't you know your child is hyperactive?"

Other situations may also lead to an incorrect conclusion. A child with a severe ADHD problem became acutely anxious when the white-coated physician entered the room. The child's eyes widened and his heart raced as he sat on the exam table in fear of the physician. After ten minutes of listening to the mother's description of the severe ADHD symptoms and observing the child frozen to the table, the physician remarked, "He seems all right to me; you must have the problem, not him."

After experiences such as the ones mentioned above, the physician may adopt one of two extreme positions. He may decide to prescribe medication such as Ritalin® on a "trial" basis for all children with the complaint of learning or behavior problems, saying to the parent, "Your child is having difficulty in school? Try this medication." Another response to the frustration of dealing with ADHD could be a physician who refuses to participate in diagnosis or treatment of ADHD, telling the family something such as, "Your child is having difficulty in school? . . .There is nothing I can do. I am a physician." Neither approach is likely to prove satisfactory. The first approach exposes children to possibly unnecessary medication and overlooks the importance of nonmedication interventions. The second overlooks an enormously effective treatment modality, medication intervention.

The nonmedical practitioner, such as the teacher, psychologist or other therapist, also needs to understand the role of medical evaluation in the diagnosis and treatment of children with ADHD. Understanding which questions medical evaluation can answer will lead to improved and more effective treatment of the ADHD child by decreasing the frustration often experienced by nonmedical practitioners who are also working with the child. Physicians with appropriate training and expertise may choose to expand their role beyond what is described here as the medical evaluation. A physician may choose to undertake every aspect of the diagnosis and treatment of ADHD children. As many of the techniques of evaluation and treatment outside the medical evaluation are more commonly not within the physician's training and expertise, he or she may choose to work with one or more nonmedical practitioners, such as a psychologist or educational specialist, to accomplish the other aspects of the evaluation. The physician, along with the patient, parents, siblings and such others as teachers, psychologists, social workers, speech therapists and educational specialists, can be viewed as working together in an interdisciplinary team. The physician also can increase his or her effectiveness by understanding what role the medical evaluation plays in the evaluation and treatment of ADHD. Understanding what the physician can and should do and understanding the questions the physician can and should answer will improve the effectiveness of the other members of the team as well.

THE ROLE OF THE PHYSICIAN IN THE DIAGNOSTIC EVALUATION

The role of the physician in the diagnostic evaluation of children suspected of having ADHD can be presented as four questions to be answered.

1. Does the child's history or examination suggest the etiology of an underlying medically remediable problem contributing to the ADHD symptoms?
2. Are any medical diagnostic tests needed to determine the presence or absence of a remediable medical problem contributing to the ADHD symptoms?
3. What does the physical and neurological exam show?
4. Are any medical problems apparent from the history or exam that would indicate an increased risk from medication intervention?

This approach allows the parent and the referring clinician or nonmedical participant in the multidisciplinary team to understand the role of the medical evaluation of children with suspected ADHD. The greater understanding the nonmedical practitioner and parent have of the role of the medical evaluation, the more appropriate will be their expectations. The more clearly the medical practitioner understands the role of the medical evaluation of the child with ADHD, the more reasonable will be the medical practitioner's expectations and the more effective his or her participation in the evaluation.

Medically Remediable Problems

While there may be some controversy as to whether the symptoms of behavior disorder that occur as the result of medical illness should be a separate diagnostic categorization from ADHD (Wender, 1987; Cantwell & Baker, 1987), nevertheless medical evaluation is needed to be certain that the behavioral symptoms observed are not the result of a treatable medical illness. Cantwell and Baker (1987) mention specific illnesses that can cause abnormal behavior, including Sydenham's chorea, hyperthyroidism, infection with pinworms and sleep apnea. Essentially all medical illnesses have the potential to cause some ADHD symptoms. It is most uncommon, however, for the behavioral manifestations of medical illness to be the major symptoms. As a result, it is not likely that medical evaluation in a child who otherwise appears healthy to family and school personnel will uncover a specific medical etiology for the behavior problem. Some medical factors have been shown to be associated with ADHD. These include a history of fetal postmaturity, long labor, maternal toxemia, encephalitis or other brain injury, frequent ear infections or subclinical lead poisoning. However, a history of ADHD in other family members is often the only cause found. While some of these causes of ADHD are not remediable, thorough evaluation for these identifiable factors is an important part of the evaluation for a medical cause of ADHD.

The routine medical evaluation includes a history of the presenting problem; a past history with information about the pregnancy, labor and delivery and the child's development; and a review of systems. The physician should ask about symptoms of disease occurring in organ systems such as the central nervous system, gastrointestinal system, genitourinary system, cardiovascular system, hematopoietic system and skin. A review of the family history for medical as well as psychosocial problems should also be included. The family physician or pediatrician who has been familiar with the child for some time may be able to accomplish this evaluation for medical causes of behavioral abnormality quickly and simply. The ease of this evaluation for the medical practitioner and the likelihood of it being negative do not diminish its importance (American Academy of Pediatrics, 1987). The medical history should contain the results of completed and up-to-date tests of vision and hearing.

Medication needed for treatment of other disorders may produce behavioral change as a side effect. Phenobarbital and diphenylhydantoin, which are anticonvulsants used to treat generalized tonic/clonic seizures as well as partial complex seizures, have been implicated as a cause of ADHD symptoms (Pellock et al., 1988). A child taking phenobarbital who is also having difficulty with ADHD symptoms must be carefully evaluated. The decision whether to discontinue the phenobarbital or diphenylhydantoin, change to an alternate anticonvulsant or proceed with evaluation and treatment of ADHD symptoms without changing the medications must be based upon medical evaluation of the need for the anticonvulsant, alternatives and previous response to medications. Phenobarbital is present in many medications. If the child is taking medication on a regular basis, it must be determined whether this medication is contributing to the ADHD symptoms.

Medical evaluation must also determine the child's growth pattern. The child's present height and weight are documented and history of growth pattern obtained. Baseline measures of blood pressure and heart rate and signs or symptoms of cardiovascular disease are documented.

Medical Diagnostic Studies

Medical diagnostic studies are often undertaken in order to determine whether a medical illness is present. An important part of the medical evaluation for ADHD is the determination of the need for medical diagnostic studies. Clinical evaluation alone may not be sufficient to exclude medical illnesses as the underlying cause of ADHD symptoms. The need for medical diagnostic testing to uncover a possible remediable disorder causing the behavior symptoms is the second determination made by the medical evaluation.

EEG

The electroencephalogram (EEG) can help establish the diagnosis of epilepsy as the remediable cause of ADHD symptoms. An EEG is obtained by placing wires on the skin over the brain and measuring the voltage differences between them. Changes in voltage occurring over time are plotted on paper. The ups and downs of the voltage measurement produce a pattern of electrical change. Many patients with epilepsy have a characteristic pattern of abnormality on the electroencephalogram. While problems such as brain tumor and abscess, subdural and intracranial hemorrhage and metabolic abnormalities also produce changes in the characteristic pattern of the EEG recording, other diagnostic studies have essentially replaced the usefulness of the EEG in the diagnosis of all disorders except epilepsy.

Primary generalized absence epilepsy, which has been called petit mal seizures in the past, is characterized by clinical symptoms of brief episodes of abrupt inattention associated often with eye fluttering and sometimes with jerky movements of the hands or additional body movements. The appearance of a child and his EEG before and during a generalized absence seizure is represented in Figure 3.1. These seizures may occur frequently during the day. Clinically observed spells lasting a few seconds, may occur as often as four to five times an hour. The sudden loss of attention resulting from generalized absence seizures is usually associated with eye blinking. These symptoms are rarely confused with ADHD. When a child with ADHD has unusual sudden episodes of inattentiveness or when a child with previously diagnosed generalized absence seizures has inattentive episodes with eye blinking or other movements, the possibility of epilepsy may be raised as the cause of the inattentive episodes. Primary generalized absence seizures are spells that are associated with a characteristic three-cycle-per-second spike-wave pattern on the EEG. When the characteristic pattern of generalized absence epilepsy is seen on the EEG along with appropriate clinical symptoms, the clinical diag-

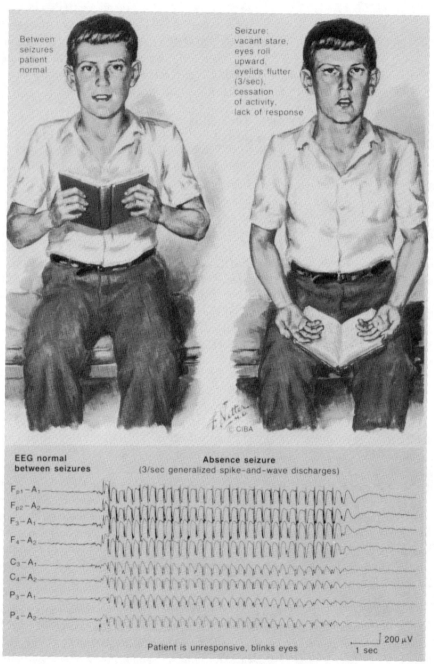

Between
seizures
patient
normal

Seizure:
vacant stare,
eyes roll
upward,
eyelids flutter
(3/sec),
cessation
of activity,
lack of response

F. Netter
© CIBA

**EEG normal
between seizures**

Absence seizure
(3/sec generalized spike-and-wave discharges)

$F_{p1}-A_1$

$F_{p2}-A_2$

F_3-A_1

F_4-A_2

C_3-A_1

C_4-A_2

P_3-A_1

P_4-A_2

$200 \mu V$

Patient is unresponsive, blinks eyes

1 sec

Figure 3.1 EEG before and during generalized absence seizure. From *CIBA Collection of Medical Illustrations* by Frank H. Netter, M.D. All rights reserved. Copyright 1986 by CIBA-GEIGY Corporation. Used by permission of the publisher.

nosis of absence epilepsy can be established. Most children with ADHD symptoms do not have paroxysmal episodes of loss of attention and eye blinking. However, some children seen for evaluation of possible ADHD have staring spells as a major symptom. If the possibility of primary generalized absence seizures (petit mal) still remains after evaluation, including history and exam, an EEG can be obtained to help differentiate ADHD from generalized absence epilepsy.

EEG AND ADHD SYMPTOMS.   The electroencephalogram is useful in the diagnosis of primary generalized absence epilepsy (petit mal). The EEG is needed in children whose paroxysmal staring spells raises the possibility of seizures. The EEG has also been studied in relation to its ability to diagnose learning and behavior problems. There have been several attempts to judge the effectiveness of medication using an EEG (Epstein, Lasgna, Conners & Rodriguez, 1968; Steinberg, Troshinsky & Steinberg, 1971; Satterfield, Cantwell, Saul, Lesser & Podosin, 1973; Shekim, Dekirmenjian, Chapel, Javaid & Davis, 1979). A report by Halperin, Gittelman, Katz and Struve (1986) is representative of these studies. The authors rated a group of 80 children with ADD defined by clinical exam and Conners rating scales. Baseline as well as placebo controlled trials of drug adjustment were used to determine the usefulness of EEG recordings. No relationship was found between EEG abnormalities and the severity of symptoms or responsiveness to methylphenidate treatment. Caresia, Pugnetti, Besana, Barteselli, Cazzullo, Musetti and Scarone (1984) studied EEG recordings and power spectral analysis in an attempt to predict responders to pemoline. They found that the power spectrum of the EEG was not helpful in predicting the outcome of trials of pemoline in children. They found what they described as a paradoxical calming effect of pemoline on the EEG of adult patients who would eventually show a clinical response to pemoline. Studies of EEG and various behavioral conditions have shown a great number of abnormalities in many children who have ADHD and other behavioral symptoms. However, the nonspecific nature of the abnormality and the finding that similar abnormalities are seen in some asymptomatic children result in the finding that an EEG cannot be used to help make the diagnosis of ADHD. A negative EEG will not exclude ADHD, and changes in the EEG do not determine whether ADHD is improving, worsening or responding to medications. While the EEG is a very helpful test in determining the presence or absence of epilepsy as a cause of sudden spells of inattention, most children with ADHD symptoms do not have the clinical features that suggest absence epilepsy. EEG testing, therefore, is needed for only a small percentage of children suspected to have ADHD.

TOPOGRAPHIC EEG MAPPING.   The EEG can be recorded as a topographic picture of the head that in some respects resembles the slices seen on CT or MRI images. That dyslexia could be diagnosed by this process, referred to as "BEAM," has been suggested by Duffy, Denckla, Bartels, Sandini and Kiessling (1980). Among a group of dyslexic readers, a significant decrease in the amplitude of the P300 wave using topographic mapping was reported by Trommer, Bernstein, Rosenberg and Armstrong (1988). However, these authors concluded that the topographic mapping of evoked potentials alone was not sufficient for diagnosis of dyslexia. EEG mapping has also been suggested as a potentially useful diagnostic tool for ADHD (Senf, 1988). Although these reports are positive and optimistic, the technique of EEG mapping has not been widely enough studied to be considered more than experimental. Since the mapping of EEG changes the display but not the information contained in a routine EEG, one might suspect that the initial positive reports will not be confirmed in subsequent studies.

EVOKED POTENTIALS AND REMEDIABLE MEDICAL ETIOLOGY.   Evoked potentials begin with a visual event such as the flashing of a particular pattern on a TV screen or an auditory event such as the occurrence of a click or sound. These events produce a very slight change in the pattern of the electroencephalogram. This occurs in all normal subjects. The very tiny change associated with the visual or auditory event is of much smaller magnitude than the normal changes in voltage seen in the routine electroencephalogram and therefore cannot ordinarily be seen. If the click or pattern is repeated a second time, the two recordings will have the same click response pattern, but the EEG pattern unrelated to the click will change randomly. If repeated EEG tracings are averaged, eventually all of the ordinary EEG signal becomes a flat line. The repeated visual or auditory stimulus (click) produces a repetitive signal that becomes relatively larger as the signals are averaged. Evoked-potential testing may show a characteristic pattern for some types of brain tumors, multiple sclerosis and some other disorders. Ordinarily these disorders would not be within the differential diagnosis of children presenting with behavior and learning problems, and standard evoked-potential testing usually is not part of the evaluation of possible medical causes for ADHD symptoms.

Some studies, however, have found evoked potentials helpful in the diagnosis and follow-up of children with ADHD and other behavioral symptoms. Klorman, Salzman, Borgstedt and Dainer (1981) reported on the late positive component of the evoked potential performed during a continuous performance task involving letter ordering. In this report evoked potentials were studied in relation to methylphenidate. In comparison with normal children, subjects diagnosed with attention deficit had lower amplitude of the late component (P300). The children treated with methylphenidate then had an enhancement of this depressed component.

Dainer, Klorman, Salzman, Hess, Davidson and Michael (1981) studied evoked potentials of 19 learning-disordered and 19 normally achieving children with a continuous performance test and showed a difference in late positive components of evoked potential in relation to "critical stimuli" in the task. Prichep, Sutton and Hakerm (1976) and Klorman, Salzman, Pass, Borgstedt and Dainer (1979) showed that during tasks requiring focused attention, hyperkinetic children with learning problems exhibited smaller evoked response than did normal children. Satterfield, Schell and Backs (1987) studied auditory evoked response potentials and EEG recordings from childhood through adolescence in a longitudinal study of 34 nondelinquent normals, 25 nondelinquent hyperactives and 9 delinquent hyperactives. The results showed abnormal maturational changes in the nondelinquent hyperactive subjects and were more likely to be normal in the delinquent hyperactive subjects.

Logan, Farrell, Malone and Taylor (1988) studied P300 response on the event-related potential using an oddball paradigm to determine whether this test could be used to predict medication response. Twelve out of 14 children with ADHD responded to medication according to psychological measures and behavioral observations. These 12 also responded with P300 increase in amplitude and more clearly delineated P300 response. They concluded "that the use of VRP appears to be an effective and perhaps a more objective method for evaluation of stimulant medication effect in patients with *Attention deficit disorder*. It also appears to be sufficiently sensitive to predict optimal medication dosage in patients who respond favorably to stimulant drug therapy" (p. 72). Another explanation, however, is that since attention is required for a normal P300 response, the response of P300 to medication is the secondary result of the child's improved concentration and attention rather than a measure of the underlying process.

Other studies of evoked potentials have shown no correlation with the diagnosis and treatment of ADHD. Conners and Wells (1986) find the results of a number of studies difficult to correlate with otherwise known theories of attention deficit. Some authors have not found a relationship between abnormal evoked potentials and ADHD symptoms. Evoked potentials were evaluated in relation to attention and reading retardation by Lovrich and Stamm (1983). As the subjects counted signals in one ear, event-related potentials were recorded. Different wave forms were noted with children who were reading retarded. Evoked potentials related to attention, however, appeared to be normal in comparison with controls.

In order to achieve an evoked potential response in ADHD children, authors often utilize unique clinical situations and unique experimental designs. There is wide variability from one laboratory to another. Evoked-response information suggests a physiological basis to the behavior abnormalities that are the ADHD syndrome. However, the usefulness of evoked-potential studies in the diagnosis and treatment of ADHD symptoms remains uncertain.

Computed Tomography and Magnetic Resonance Imaging (CT & MRI)

Computed tomography (CT) and magnetic resonance imaging (MRI) provide a picture of the structure of the brain. Figure 3.2 is an example of a CT image in a normal child. Figure 3.3 is an example of an MRI image in a normal child. Remediable medical conditions that alter brain structure, such as brain abnormalities, hydrocephalus, hemorrhage and others, can be diagnosed using these imaging techniques. Figure 3.4 is an example of a CT image in a child with a brain injury. Figure 3.5 is an example of an MRI image of a child with a brain tumor.

Computed tomography (CT) employs a thin beam of x-ray. After passing through the patient, the x-ray beam not absorbed is measured by an electronic sensor. In ordinary x-ray the beam not absorbed by the patient is recorded directly on x-ray film. For CT, the pattern of x-ray absorption measured by the electronic sensor is converted by a computer into a picture, or slice. This allows direct information about the brain structure to be obtained. Conditions that result in an alteration of the x-ray density within the brain produce an abnormal appearance on the CT scan.

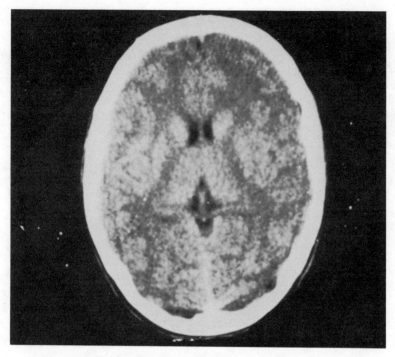

Figure 3.2 Normal mid-cerebral axial CT section.

Tumor, hydrocephalus, abscess, hemorrhage and malformations of the brain are particularly well visualized by CT.

Magnetic resonance imaging (MRI) produces images of brain structure displayed in slices that have some similarities with CT. Unlike CT, MRI utilizes the radio waves emitted by molecules within the body in response to a radio frequency pulse in a strong magnetic field. Although the advent of CT scanning resulted in a revolution of improved imaging of the brain, within 15 years of the introduction of CT, magnetic resonance imaging had replaced it for many applications. MRI produces more detailed pictures of brain anatomy, allowing a diagnosis of some abnormalities that could not be seen as well on CT. CT, however, is less expensive and faster than MRI. It can be used in the presence of electronic pacemakers and visualizes calcium better than MRI. In situations where these features are important, CT may be preferable to MRI.

On occasion, a child evaluated for ADHD will have signs or symptoms suggesting a disorder such as hydrocephalus, brain tumor, hemorrhage or abscess that requires specific medical or surgical treatment. A CT or MRI scan may be needed to uncover this problem so that appropriate surgical or medical intervention can be undertaken. The medical evaluation outlined earlier should include evaluation of the history and physical findings to determine whether a CT or MRI scan is needed to diagnose a medically or surgically remediable disorder.

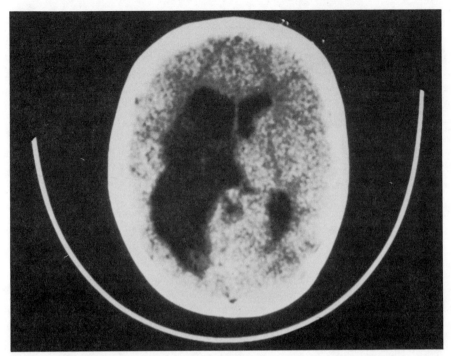

Figure 3.3 Mid-cerebral axial CT section showing a large atrophic lesion.

CT AND MRI IMAGING AND ADHD SYMPTOMS.   Studies using CT scans have been disappointing in the search for a medical test that can diagnose ADHD. A report by Thompson, Ross and Horwitz (1980) and an additional study reported by Denckla, LeMay and Chapman (1985) found that even in children with minor neurological abnormality, the CT images were not helpful in making the diagnosis or following the progress of behavioral symptoms. Harcherik, Cohen, Ort, Paul, Shaywitz, Volkmar, Rothman and Leckman (1985) studied CT scans in ADHD as well as other psychiatric syndromes and measured ventricular volume and brain density by quantitative computer-based methods. There were no significant differences between neuropsychiatric patients and medical control patients in total ventricular volume, right-left ventricular volume ratios, ventricular asymmetries, ventricle-brain ratios or brain density.

While CT studies in ADHD children have been disappointing, there has been a suggestion that groups of children with similar problems may be differentiated by CT scans. Hier, LeMay, Rosenberger and Perlo (1978) studied the CT brain scans of 24 dyslexics between the ages of 14 and 47 and found an increased number of individuals with a reversal of the usual posterior hemispheral asymmetry present in the majority of normal individuals. This brain asymmetry reversal serves as evidence that a group of children with dyslexia are physically different from those

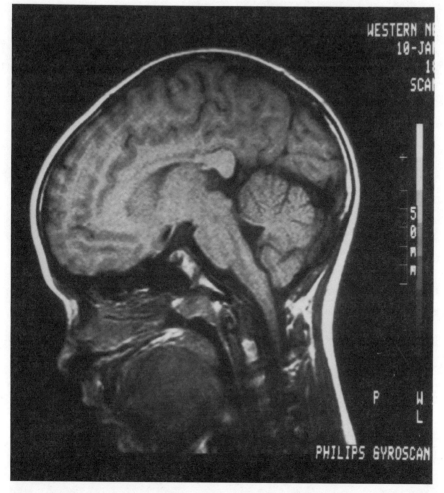

Figure 3.4 Midsagittal T. Weighted MRI section brain stem, cerebellum and medial cerebral hemisphere in a normal child.

without dyslexia. While this asymmetry differentiated a group of dyslexic children, in individual children this finding may or may not be present, and it may be present in many normal children. As a result, even in this group the reversal of brain asymmetry seen on CT scans could not be used to diagnose the problem in an individual child or predict the outcome of intervention.

A CT or MRI scan is needed in a child with ADHD symptoms only when other signs or symptoms are present to suggest one of the conditions that would call for such diagnostic studies in children without inattention and hyperactive symptoms (Behar, Rapoport, Berg, Denckla, Mann, Cox, Fedio, Zahn & Wolfman, 1984).

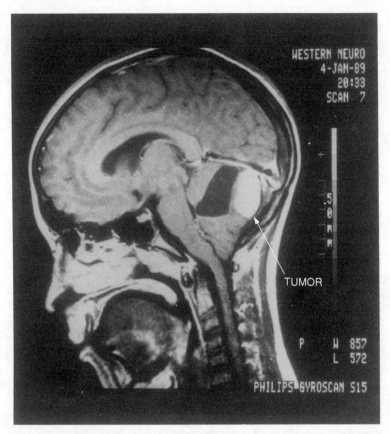

Figure 3.5 Midsagittal T. Weighted MRI section with pilocystic astrocytoma.

Other Medical Diagnostic Testing

Blood tests and other common medical tests are sometimes needed for children suspected to have ADHD. For example, if symptoms such as heat intolerance, smooth/moist skin, rapid pulse and tremor are noted, blood studies to measure the thyroid status of the child may be needed. Pallor, poor dietary ingestion of iron or other suggestion of anemia may lead the medical practitioner to obtain a blood count to determine the presence or absence of anemia. Other findings in the history or exam may suggest the need to obtain a blood chemistry evaluation to check on the status of glucose metabolism, sodium or potassium balance, liver function, or kidney function. Exercise intolerance by history or the findings of a heart murmur, cyanosis or other findings suggesting cardiovascular abnormality may prompt the medical practitioner to obtain a chest x-ray or electrocardiogram to further evaluate the cardiac status. Blood studies to rule out mononucleosis or other chronic infection, appropriate testing to determine the presence of pinworms, or a sinus x-ray to determine the presence of sinusitis are just a few more of the medical diagnostic tests used to uncover common medical problems that could indirectly be responsible for behavior abnormality. Usually, the history and exam are sufficient to exclude the illnesses mentioned above, and these additional diagnostic tests are rarely needed.

Physical and Neurological Exam: Soft Signs and Minor Physical Anomalies

Can a diagnosis of ADHD be made on physical exam?   Mikkelsen, Brown, Minichiello, Millican and Rapoport (1982) credit Bender (1956) as being one of the first to introduce the term "soft signs." McMahon and Greenberg (1977) credit Larsen (1964) and Werry, Minde, Guzman, Weiss, Dogan and Hoy (1972) for linking soft neurological signs with hyperactivity and showing that hyperactive subjects display these signs with greater frequency. In referring to symptoms of inattention and hyperactivity, the American Academy of Pediatrics (1987) has recommended that to establish an accurate diagnosis, a physical, neurological and neuromaturational examination should be performed.

Soft Signs

There are several factors contributing to the controversy and confusion over the presence and value of abnormalities on physical examination in ADHD children. Two different groups of soft signs are described by Mikkelson et al. (1982). The first group of soft signs, such as clumsiness, overflow and speed of movements, may be reliably reproduced from one day to the next and one examiner to the next but are considered "soft" because they are not clearly associated with a dysfunction in a specific area of the brain. These signs might also be called nonlocalizing neurological abnormality.

The second group includes traditional neurological signs such as reflex or tone asymmetries, but of mild degree or poor reliability and reproducibility. The combination of right-side weakness, increased reflexes, Babinski's sign and increased tone in the right arm and leg would be considered "hard" neurological signs and suggest a specific area of brain dysfunction. A normal child may have a slightly increased deep-tendon reflex, a slight degree of increased tone, or a mild degree of incoordination in one arm. These asymmetries might even vary from one day to the next so that an increase in the right-biceps reflex on one day might be followed by an increase in the left-biceps reflex on the next day.

These minor asymmetries would be considered of uncertain significance because of their uncertain reliability and reproducibility. In a child with a minor degree of increased reflexes and tone in the right arm and leg and decreased strength, there would be a much lower likelihood of uncovering a specific abnormality within the left hemisphere. These signs, then, are considered soft because of the unreliability, variability and minor degree of the abnormality.

Different studies have chosen different signs to evaluate. For example, McMahon and Greenberg (1977) chose to study three signs. One was posturing of the upper extremities by flexion at the elbows and hyperextension at the wrists when a subject was asked to walk ten paces on his heels. The second was posturing of the upper extremities with extension of the elbows and palmar flexion of the wrists when the subject was asked to walk ten paces on tiptoe. The third was dysrhythmic or dysynchronous movements or posturing of the hands or fingers when a subject alternately supinated and pronated the forearms. McMahon and Greenberg's study found that there was a high degree of variability of response within individuals and no evidence of interaction between treatment and subject responses. They concluded that "the value of these signs for purposes of diagnosis or assessment of therapy is doubtful" (p. 584). They further concluded that "these observations raised serious doubt whether testing for these soft neurological signs has any justification in a clinical setting" (p. 587).

Halperin and Gittelman (1986) used a 130-item test for soft signs (Clements & Peters, 1962) to study a group of 80 children with ADD as defined by clinical exam and Conners rating scales. Using a placebo controlled trial of medication, soft signs of the group of responders were not different from those of the group who did not respond to medication. The authors concluded that "in view of the findings that these neurological measures are not related to either treatment responsivity nor the severity of behavioral disorder, the need for a determination of neurological status prior to the initiation of stimulant treatment in hyperactive children seems unwarranted unless the presence of specific neurological disorder is suspected" (p. 824). Sleator, Ullmann and von Neumann (1982) propose that a physician can make the diagnosis of hyperactivity based upon an interview with the parents and the teacher questionnaire. They argue against the use of complex diagnostic instruments and suggest that most psychiatric and neurological examination of the child is of little value in the evaluation for inattention and hyperactivity.

Denckla and Rudel (1978) assessed scores for timed right- and left-sided performance on eight different movements, overflow movements and other changes such as "sticky turns." They found that "overflow movements differentiated hyperactive boys from control boys at all ages" (p. 233). The authors further concluded that "these associated (overflow) movements appear to be the stigmata of deficient motor inhibition/control which has been suggested as being central to the hyperactive syndrome" (p. 233). Denckla, Rudel, Chapman and Krieger (1985) used six motor tasks, measuring time to do the task as well as observations of overflow. Using these signs, a group of children with dyslexia but no ADD symptoms was differentiated from a group of children with dyslexia who, although they had not been screened for ADD, showed signs of ADD as well as dyslexia. Figure 3.6 from Denckla et al. (1985) illustrates in graphic terms the separation of the discriminant scores of the groups of hyperactive dyslexic boys screened for ADD and those not screened. One can also see the overlap between the groups. Denckla et al. (1985) devised a detailed neurological examination recommended for children with ADD as well as other possible behavior disorders. The neurological abnormalities are now called "subtle signs", and the exam that had been used by Mikkelson et al. (1982), among others, has been revised. Unreliable or seldom scored signs have been dropped, and some signs previously not used have been added. This revision

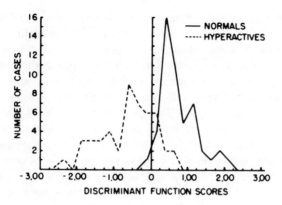

Figure 3.6 Discriminant function scores. From Denckla, M.B. and Rudel, R.G. Anomalies of Motor Development in Hyperactive Boys. Copyright 1978 by *Annals of Neurology*. Used by permission of the publisher.

has the potential advantage of standardizing the soft signs, now called the subtle-signs, exam (presuming that other authors will adopt this exam). The change in exam, however, has the disadvantage of making it even more difficult to compare studies that utilize the new exam with older studies that employed a different exam.

The value of neurological examination for prediction of medication response in ADHD children is supported by Urion (1988) in a preliminary report. Three groups of 50 children with the diagnosis of ADHD based upon DSM-III-R criteria, including Conners Parent's and Teacher's Questionnaire scores in excess of 15 (mean = 18) were studied. The group of 50 that had essentially no abnormalities on classic and extended neurological examination responded well to methylphenidate. Of these 50 children, 43 responded favorably, as defined by a Conners parent and teacher hyperkinesis score that decreased at least seven points in addition to parental and school impressions of improved attention. But the remaining 100 children had difficulties on at least 10 of 12 measures of the Denckla Timed Motor Performance Tasks or performed poorly on the Rey Osterrieth Complex Figure Test. Despite meeting the criteria for the DSM-III-R diagnosis of ADHD, only 18 of these 100 children responded positively to methylphenidate. This preliminary result supports use of the extended neurological exam to help predict medication response. The overall response rate of 41 percent for all 150 children in this study is quite low. It is not clear why this group of children had such a low response rate. In addition, the 18 percent response rate of the group with the abnormal extended neurological exam is lower than the response rate found for placebo in most studies. Considering these unusual features, one must be hesitant to draw conclusions about other groups based on this study.

The findings of Denckla (1985) and others showing that certain soft signs can distinguish groups of ADD from normal or dyslexic children are important. These studies demonstrate a physical difference that distinguished children with learning and attention problems. There is now evidence that a group defined by clinical and psychological testing is physically as well as behaviorally different from other children. The body of work concerning soft signs has a great significance in our understanding that there is a physical basis for learning and attention problems.

In a review of 45 studies of the relationship of neurological soft signs and hyperactivity, Reeves and Werry (1987) relate the difficulty of drawing conclusions to the variability of signs described. They believe the majority of studies have found an increased number of soft signs in hyperactive as compared to normal children. However, they state that "in view of the uncertain etiologic, diagnostic, prognostic and pharmacotherapeutic value of soft signs in hyperactivity, it seems only right to conclude that apart possibly from pinpointing specific problems (e.g., dyspraxia) not peculiar in any way to hyperactivity, soft signs have yet to demonstrate any clear clinical utility in hyperactivity (ADD)" (p. 241).

It is recommended that some tests of coordination be performed as part of the search for signs of an underlying medically remediable neurological disorder. Observations for nonspecific or nonlocalized neurological abnormalities are listed below.

1. *Eye Movements.*   Ask the child to follow an object such as the examiner's finger through full horizontal and vertical range of movement. Watch the smoothness of pursuit movements. Some ADHD children will lose concentration during the exam and look at the wall or other objects in the room momentarily and then look back at the examiner's finger. These lapses of attention are readily apparent and may provide an insight into the child's variable focus of attention.

2. *Finger Sequencing.*   Ask the child to sequentially touch the second, third, fourth and then fifth fingers to the thumb and repeat the sequence several times. Watch for slowness and overflow of movements to other parts of the body, including the other hand, legs, tongue, face, arms and shoulders. It often appears that the ADHD child has difficulty focusing and directing effort to one part of the body.

3. *Tandem Gait.*   Ask the child to walk with one foot placed directly in front of the other. Watch to see how the child translates verbal direction into physical activity. Many ADHD children require repeated demonstration because they cannot observe or listen to the examiner or they impulsively start a task before directions are completed.

4. *Choreiform Movements.*   Ask the child to hold arms outstretched with palms facing forward and eyes closed. Watch to see whether the fingers wiggle in piano-playing movements (chorea). Watch to see whether other parts of the body, such as the tongue, legs and trunk, begin to wiggle.

Remember, younger children have more of these signs than older children.

Several more formal and quantitative soft-sign exams are available. One of the most comprehensive is the Physical and Neurological Examination for Soft Signs (PANESS). The reader is referred to Guy (1976, p. 383–406) for this exam.

Is the soft-signs exam useful in determining the presence or absence of attention and learning problems? The American Academy of Pediatrics (1987) recommended a physical, neurological and neuromaturational examination, without specifying what exam should be done or how this information might be used. Studies that show statistically significant differences between groups of children based upon soft signs also include the fact that many children with a normal soft-signs exam have learning and attention problems and many children with an abnormal soft-signs exam do not have attention deficit (Denckla, 1985). For this reason, soft signs alone cannot be used to rule out attention deficit or diagnose it. If a random sampling of children is tested, more will have soft signs than have attention deficit. Therefore, a child with a positive soft-signs examination may have either normal attention skills or ADHD. The presence or absence of soft signs may be of interest but cannot be used to establish the diagnosis. Furthermore, other studies have shown that the change of soft signs is not an adequate indicator of medication response. Follow-up soft-signs examination cannot be used to determine the success or failure of treatment. It is important to understand that the concept of soft signs has been useful in adding to our research knowledge and understanding of ADHD and has indicated that there is a biological and physical basis for attention deficit. A soft-signs exam, however, cannot be used either to establish or rule out the diagnosis of attention deficit and cannot be used to determine the effectiveness of treatment.

Minor Physical Anomalies and ADHD

Can minor physical anomalies (MPA) such as narrow or widely separated eyes, low-set ears, abnormal position of facial features, shape or space between fingers or toes or unusual creases in the palm indicate ADHD? Some reports suggest that minor physical anomalies can be associated with ADHD symptoms. Pomeroy, Sprafkin and Gadow (1988) reviewed studies of normal populations including more than 1500 children in ten studies. There were 933 newborns included in the studies reviewed. These studies found that the group of children within the normal population scoring highest for minor physical anomalies also had abnormal behavior. The children with high anomaly scores had inability to delay gratification, oppositionalism and perseveration. They also had high teacher ratings of hyperactivity for boys, peer nomination of "mean-noisy" for boys and girls, sleep problems and parental reports of hyperactive, impulsive behavior at two years. In boys, high anomaly scores correlated with distractibility, gross motor incoordination, hyperactivity and restlessness. Some studies, however, found no correlation with severity of hyperactivity.

Pomeroy et al. (1988) studied a group of 193 children with Down's syndrome (Trisomy 21) and compared them to 154 mentally retarded children without Down's syndrome. Despite the much higher incidence of minor congenital anomalies in the Down's syndrome group, the incidence of conduct disorder (10 percent) was the same in both samples and the hyperkinetic syndrome was only slightly more common in the Down's syndrome group (9 percent vs. 7 percent) Pomeroy et al. (1988) concluded from this data that "it is apparent, therefore, that even in this grossly deviant group of children with known chromosomal abnormality and high prevalence of minor physical anomalies, the manifestation of psychiatric

TABLE 3.1. Exam for Minor Physical Anomalies

Anomaly	Scoring Weights
Head	
Head circumference	
> 1.5 S.D.	2
1 >< 1.5 S.D.	1
'Electric' hair	
very fine hair that won't comb down	2
fine hair that is soon awry after combing	1
Two or more whorls	0
Eyes	
Epicanthus	
where upper and lower lids join at the nose,	
point of union is: deeply covered	2
partly covered	1
Hypertelorism	
approximate distance between tear ducts:	
> 1.5 S.D.	2
1.25 to 1.5 S.D.	1
Ears	
Low-set	
Bottom of ears in line with:	
mouth (or lower)	2
area between mouth and nose	1
Adherent lobes	
lower edges of ears extend:	
upward and back toward crown of head	−2
straight back toward rear of neck	1
Malformed	1
Asymmetrical	1
Soft and pliable	0
Mouth	
High palate	
roof of mouth steepled	2
roof of mouth moderately high	1
Furrowed tongue	1
Smooth-rough spots on tongue	0
Hands	
Fifth finger	
markedly curved inward toward other fingers	2
slightly curved inward toward other fingers	1
Single transverse palmar crease	1
Index finger longer than middle finger	1

TABLE 3.1.   (Continued)

Anomaly	Scoring Weights
Foot	
Third toe	
definitely longer than second toe	2
appears equal in length to second toe	1
Partial syndactyly of two middle toes	1
Gap between first and second toe (approximately 1/4 inch)	1

Quinn, P. O. and Rapoport, J. L. "Minor Physical Anomalies and Neurologic Status in Hyperactive Boys". Copyright 1974 by *Pediatrics*. Reprinted with permission of the publisher and authors.

and behavioral disturbance was (a) non-universal, (b) diagnostically non-specific and (c) probably a factor of mental retardation and not the Down's Syndrome" (p. 467).

A study of 100 emotionally disturbed children by Pomeroy et al. (1988) concluded that higher MPA scores were found at a frequency "which is greater than expected in a random population. The clinical features of the children with higher MPA scores were inattention, speech delay and clumsiness" (p. 472). In the final analysis the authors concluded that "the findings of the present study for school-labeled, emotionally disturbed children do not support the measurement of minor physical anomalies as a routine procedure for identifying children at risk because many other straightforward, historical, developmental and performance measures help define these children's educational and clinical needs" (p. 472).

The search for congenital anomalies, as illustrated in Table 3.1, is part of the general physical examination. Eyes that are too close together or too far apart, ears that lie too low on the skull, abnormal finger or palm creases, and abnormal distance between the first or second toes are findings that are associated with certain genetic defects. Most children, however, who have minor anomalies do not have a specific genetic abnormality. Some children with minor congenital abnormalities may have ADHD. However, like the soft-signs exam, the diagnosis of learning or attention problems can be neither made nor excluded on the basis of presence or absence of minor congenital anomalies.

Contraindication to Medication Intervention

The fourth aspect of the medical evaluation involves evaluation for medication intervention. The decision whether to undertake medication intervention and if so, which medication to use and which dosages, treatment schedule and reevaluation program are needed is the subject of another chapter in this volume.

The initial medical evaluation should obtain information concerning possible contraindications to medication intervention. Medical history should include inquiry into possible previous episodes of overanxious or psychotic behavior as these may be exaggerated by some medications used for the treatment of ADHD symptoms. History of abnormal movements and/or multiple habit spasms or tics, especially with vocalization, would raise a caution concerning the use of stimulant medication because of the possibility of exaggerating symptoms of Tourette's syndrome. Poor dietary history might suggest concern for the possible anorexic effects of medication. A history of previous treatments, especially medications, such as stimulants, tranquilizers or antidepressants, should be obtained. A history of medication ingestion for other illnesses is needed to determine if these might interact with medication for ADHD. Ability and willingness of the family to participate in nonmedication intervention programs and follow through with reevaluation programs will contribute to reducing the risk of medication intervention. Finally, findings on exam that might include increased risk of medication include the age of the patient, cardiovascular status (e.g., pulse rate, blood pressure), presence of psychosis, or overanxiousness or tenseness.

SUMMARY

The physician's role includes directing the search for remediable medical causes of ADHD, participating in the multidisciplinary diagnostic evaluation and when medication is indicated, supervising the medication intervention program. Medical evaluation includes:

1. Searching for a medically remediable cause for ADHD symptoms such as hyperthyroidism, pinworms, sleep apnea, iron-deficiency anemia, or medications such as phenobarbital. Disorders that are correlated directly with ADHD but not remediable include perinatal factors, previous ear infection, brain injury or encephalitis, previous lead poisoning and, most commonly, heredity.

2. A decision concerning the need for medical diagnostic testing. Medical diagnostic testing ranges from a blood count to an MRI scan. Each test is helpful to exclude specific medical illness that can occasionally masquerade as ADHD. These tests do not help make or confirm the diagnosis of ADHD, and unless specific indications of other disorders are present these tests are usually not needed.

3. An appropriate physical and neurological examination. Research studies using examinations for anomalies and soft signs have given us valuable information suggesting that there is a physiological basis to the cluster of clinical symptoms comprising ADHD. These findings are less helpful than other tests for the diagnosis or exclusion of ADHD because these findings are often present in normal children and often absent in children with ADHD. A limited soft-signs exam as presented is recommended.

4. Baseline evaluation to determine any contraindication to medication intervention and to serve as a comparison at subsequent reevaluation. While the decision to use medication is part of medication treatment rather than

diagnostic evaluation, gathering information on risks of possible medication intervention is part of the physician's initial diagnostic evaluation. A family medical and social history may contain clues to psychosis or Tourette's syndrome; other family members may have had positive or negative response to medications for ADHD; and the family may have a good or poor history of following through with treatment programs. The child's medical history may show symptoms such as previous reactions to medications, psychosis, growth problems or cardiovascular problems suggesting increased medication risk. During physical exam, clues to increased medication risk may be found, including the child's age; abnormalities of height, weight or blood pressure; signs of tics, psychosis or depression; or abnormalities suggesting disorders of other organ systems.

An understanding of the medical evaluation by the patient, family, teacher, psychologist, social worker or other school/community nonmedical personnel of what the medical evaluation can and cannot accomplish will lead to more effective utilization of medical services. The medical practitioner must also understand what the medical evaluation can accomplish. Medical evaluation is a part of the multidisciplinary evaluation for ADHD. Additional qualitative or quantitative information by direct observation as well as reports from other observers such as parents and teachers will be needed to establish the diagnosis of ADHD. This additional information can be obtained by the medical practitioners who performed the medical evaluation if they have appropriate training and expertise. In a multidisciplinary team, nonmedical practitioners may perform the other parts of the evaluation.

CHAPTER 4

The Evaluation of School Functioning

Attention-disordered children present an unpredictable variety of school problems. For a significant percentage, problems are observed in the preschool setting and future problems are then anticipated (Schleifer, Weiss, Cohen, Elman, Cvejic & Kruger, 1975; Campbell et al., 1977). In higher grades, continued attention and arousal problems combine with a history of negative experiences to exert a cumulative, negative impact on behavior and achievement. With older children, a careful school history concerning experiences in the early grades, as well as the apparent progression of problems, must be carefully documented by the practitioner.

Parental history, report cards and yearly group achievement tests are usually the best sources of this data. In the earlier grades, it is the child's restless, fidgeting behavior that is most apparent to the classroom teacher. It is not surprising that the greatest percentage of hyperactive attention-disordered children are identified in the lower grades. The nonhyperactive attention-disordered child may be misidentified as poorly motivated or learning impaired. The second most frequent problem that disturbs teachers throughout the ADHD child's academic history is a lack of work completion. Teachers report an apparent lack of congruence between the child's observed capabilities or achievement test scores and day-to-day classroom performance.

Based upon the demands and structure of our present educational system, attention-related problems frequently have a significant negative impact on a child's functioning. It is essential that school data concerning the child's behavior, work completion, achievement and social interaction be obtained as an integral part of the assessment process. Since teachers usually spend significantly more structured and unstructured time with a student than any other adult in the child's life for a period of a year, they are often of great assistance in helping the practitioner understand the nature of the child's behavior and the impact that behavior has on the child's functioning. It has been suggested that a diagnosis of attention disorder should not be made for a child capable of functioning effectively in the school system (Ullman et al., 1985).

It is important to obtain a description of the child's behavior in various school situations. It is uncommon for an ADHD child to have equal behavioral difficulty across all school activities and situational contexts. Obtaining behavioral/situational data helps the practitioner to gain an understanding of possible compensatory strategies the ADHD child may use to function better in some situations than in others. This type of data also allows the practitioner to develop an understanding of the classroom environment and specific teacher factors that may minimize or escalate the ADHD child's problems.

It is also essential for the practitioner to obtain a description of the ADHD child's social and problem-solving skills as they relate to various social settings. It is not uncommon for an ADHD child to function well with a single playmate but to struggle in a group setting.

Finally, the practitioner must obtain data concerning the child's academic achievement and estimates of the child's classroom performance on a daily basis. Frequently, ADHD children have better achievement than they are able to demonstrate during classroom activities. This is not surprising given the fact that inability to pay attention or persist on task often results in a performance level below an individual's capabilities. It is important for the practitioner to keep in mind that the ADHD child's behavioral description, achievement and social skills constitute important data, but this data is even more important to evaluate in the context of the situations in which it is observed. Situational data provides a measure of the effect these factors have on the child's day-in and day-out school functioning.

It is important for the practitioner to be aware that attention problems within the school setting are often inferred, usually from an inadequate work product. Such problems, however, could also be caused by lack of interest, inappropriate reinforcement or cognitive or learning impairments (Shaffer & Schonfeld, 1984). Figure 4.1 contains an overview of the type of school data the practitioner must collect, as well as specific methods and instruments that can be used to collect this data. The remainder of this chapter will be devoted to a review of these methods and instruments.

TEACHER REPORT QUESTIONNAIRES

Conners Teacher's Rating Scale

The original 39-item Conners Teacher's Rating Scale (Conners, 1969; 1970; 1973) was revised and shortened to 28 items (Goyette, Conners & Ulrich 1978; Conners, 1982). The shortened rating scale, which appears in Figure 4.2, contains many of the characteristics of the original scale. Items that did not load in previous factor analytic studies were omitted and similar or redundant items were combined into single items (Ross & Ross, 1982). Trites, Blouin and Laprade (1982) conducted a factor analysis of the Conners Teacher's Rating Scale using a stratified sample of almost 1000 school children. Their research suggests that a primary hyperkinesis factor is present, and use of the Connors Teacher's Scale as an assessment device for attention deficit and hyperactivity is a valid procedure. Conners (1987) revised their data and provided standard scores for the Teacher's Rating Scale for children from ages 4 through 12 years.

The Conners Teacher's Rating Scale is the most widely used research and applied questionnaire for teacher rating of attention and activity-related problems.

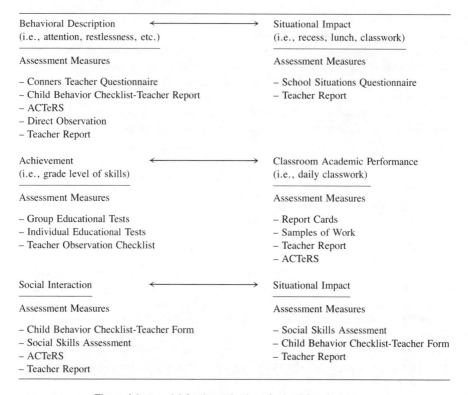

Behavioral Description ⟵⟶	Situational Impact
(i.e., attention, restlessness, etc.)	(i.e., recess, lunch, classwork)

Assessment Measures	Assessment Measures
– Conners Teacher Questionnaire	– School Situations Questionnaire
– Child Behavior Checklist-Teacher Report	– Teacher Report
– ACTeRS	
– Direct Observation	
– Teacher Report	

Achievement ⟵⟶	Classroom Academic Performance
(i.e., grade level of skills)	(i.e., daily classwork)

Assessment Measures	Assessment Measures
– Group Educational Tests	– Report Cards
– Individual Educational Tests	– Samples of Work
– Teacher Observation Checklist	– Teacher Report
	– ACTeRS

Social Interaction ⟵⟶	Situational Impact

Assessment Measures	Assessment Measures
– Child Behavior Checklist-Teacher Form	– Social Skills Assessment
– Social Skills Assessment	– Child Behavior Checklist-Teacher Form
– ACTeRS	– Teacher Report
– Teacher Report	

Figure 4.1 A model for the evaluation of school functioning.

It is fairly simple for a classroom teacher to complete. The 28 items are scored on a factor basis, yielding three factors titled conduct problem, hyperactivity and inattentive-passive. The scale is also scored for a ten-item hyperkinesis index that contains the ten items Conners included in an abbreviated parent-teacher questionnaire (Conners, 1973). Each item is scored on a four-point scale according to the following ratings of severity: Not at all (score = 0); Just a little (score = 1); Pretty much (score = 2); and Very much (score = 3).

The hyperkinesis index is considered to be a sensitive measure of attention-disordered behavior in the classroom, as well as an excellent measure of a child's response to treatment interventions, specifically medication. Items on the hyperkinesis index include descriptors referring to restlessness, temper outbursts, unpredictable behavior, distractibility, poor attention span, excitability, impulsivity, failing to finish things and being easily frustrated in efforts. The hyperkinesis index is computed by adding the scores of the ten critical items and dividing by ten, then comparing the child's score to factor norms (Goyette et al., 1978). Although Dr. Conners has allowed this questionnaire to be reproduced and widely used over the past 20 years, it has recently been copyrighted. A redesigned questionnaire, scoring sheet and administration manual is now available from Multi-Health Systems, Inc., 908 Niagara Falls Blvd., North Tonawanda, New York 14120.

Child Name:_____ Child Age:____ Child Sex:_____ Teacher:_____

Instructions: Read each item below carefully, and decide how much you think the child has been bothered by this problem during the past month.

Not at All	Just a Little	Pretty Much	Very Much	CTRS-28
0	1	2	3	1. Restless in the "squirmy" sense
0	1	2	3	2. Makes inappropriate noises when s/he shouldn't
0	1	2	3	3. Demands must be met immediately
0	1	2	3	4. Acts "smart" (impudent or sassy)
0	1	2	3	5. Temper outbursts and unpredictable behavior
0	1	2	3	6. Overly sensitive to criticism
0	1	2	3	7. Distractibility or attention span a problem
0	1	2	3	8. Disturbs other children
0	1	2	3	9. Daydreams
0	1	2	3	10. Pouts and sulks
0	1	2	3	11. Mood changes quickly and drastically
0	1	2	3	12. Quarrelsome
0	1	2	3	13. Submissive attitude toward authority
0	1	2	3	14. Restless, always up and on the go
0	1	2	3	15. Excitable, impulsive
0	1	2	3	16. Excessive demands for teacher's attention
0	1	2	3	17. Appears to be unaccepted by group
0	1	2	3	18. Appears to be easily led by other children
0	1	2	3	19. No sense of fair play
0	1	2	3	20. Appears to lack leadership
0	1	2	3	21. Fails to finish things that s/he starts
0	1	2	3	22. Childish and immature
0	1	2	3	23. Denies mistakes or blames others
0	1	2	3	24. Does not get along well with other children
0	1	2	3	25. Uncooperative with classmates
0	1	2	3	26. Easily frustrated in efforts
0	1	2	3	27. Uncooperative with teacher
0	1	2	3	28. Difficulty in learning
Not at All	Just a Little	Pretty Much	Very Much	

Figure 4.2 Conners Teacher's Questionnaire, by C. K. Conners. Copyright 1988 by Multi-Health Systems, Inc. Used with permission of the author and publisher.

Although in the past a cutoff score for the hyperkinesis index of 1.5 was considered to reflect significant problems with attention difficulty, age-by-sex normative data has clearly demonstrated that this is an inefficient application of the hyperkinesis index. For example, females typically get lower scores than males, and the mean of the hyperkinesis index decreases with age. For example, a score of approximately 1.8 for a 3- to 5-year-old group of males is only one standard deviation above the average, but for a 15- to 17-year-old, an approximate score of 1.3 is two standard deviations above the average. Thus, an arbitrary cutoff score of 1.5 would result in false positives for younger children and false negatives for adolescents (Goyette et al., 1978). Based on a comparison of the child's score with the sex-by-age normative data, the practitioner can make a statistically relevant comparison of the child's attentional skills to a normative sample. A cutoff point of approximately two standard deviations higher than the mean would be considered a significant indicator of attentional problems in the classroom.

The practitioner must also be aware that children experiencing attention problems without concomitant difficulty with hyperactive, restless behavior may not present an equally elevated hyperkinesis index. Brown (1985) found that children with attention disorder and concomitant problems with hyperactivity were rated approximately 0.8 to 1.0 higher on the hyperkinesis index than attention-disordered children without concomitant hyperactive, restless behavior. The practitioner must also be aware that noncompliant children who are not inattentive temperamentally may also obtain elevated ratings on the hyperkinesis index because of their resistent behavior.

Loney and Milich (1981) modified the Conners Teacher's Rating Scale and developed a ten-item scale with five items tapping inattention-overactivity and five items tapping aggression. It has been suggested that this measure can be used to identify children with ADHD, children with aggressive problems and children with both (Langhorne & Loney, 1979).

ADD-H: Comprehensive Teacher Rating Scale (ACTeRS)

In response to statistical and definitional criticisms of the Conners Teacher's Rating Scale, Ullmann, Sleator and Sprague (1985) developed the ADD-H: Comprehensive Teacher Rating Scale (ACTeRS), which appears in Figure 4.3. The items on the ACTeRS are scored on a five-point scale, where "Almost Never" equals one and "Almost Always" equals five. Two of the categories (attention and social

ATTENTION	Amost Never				Almost Always
1. Works well independently	1	2	3	4	5
2. Persists with task for reasonable amount of time	1	2	3	4	5
HYPERACTIVITY					
7. Extremely overactive (out of seat, "on the go")	1	2	3	4	5
8. Overreacts	1	2	3	4	5
SOCIAL SKILLS					
12. Behaves positively with peers/classmates	1	2	3	4	5
13. Verbal communication clear and "connected"	1	2	3	4	5
OPPOSITIONAL					
19. Tries to get others into trouble	1	2	3	4	5
20. Starts fights over nothing	1	2	3	4	5

Figure 4.3 Sample questions from the ACTeRS. By R. K. Ullmann, E. K. Sleator and R. L. Sprague, ADD-H: Comprehensive Teacher's Rating Scale. Copyright 1986, 1988 by MetriTech, Inc. Used with permission of the publisher.

skills) are worded positively, and higher scores reflect more appropriate behavior; the remaining two categories (hyperactivity and oppositional behavior) are worded negatively, and a higher score indicates less desirable behavior. Normative data was collected for elementary school children, ranging from kindergarten through fifth grade. Boys and girls were found to differ considerably in all but social competence ratings. No significant normative differences were found within sex between different grades. A sample of male normative data is provided in Figure 4.4.

To obtain percentile scores, the practitioner must sum the numbers circled in each of the categories and place them on the profile sheet. On these normative profile sheets, for all subscales, the higher percentile score reflects more appropriate behavior. According to Ullmann et al. (1985), scoring at the tenth percentile or below reflects significant attention-related problems. Children scoring between the tenth and twentieth percentile are presenting with attention problems, and their behavioral severity on the other three scales must be taken into account when considering the child's attention difficulty within the classroom. The primary value of the ACTeRS is that it offers the practitioner separate ratings for attention and hyperactivity. This scale also provides a normative measure of social skills and the extent to which the child is experiencing difficulty with oppositional behavior towards authority. The last four items on the original scale are evaluated qualitatively and provide the practitioner with the teacher's observations concerning the child's integration and acceptance with classmates and the amount of additional teacher time the child is requiring. These items were eliminated from a recent revision of the ACTeRS. The ACTeRS is available from MetriTech, Inc., 111 North Market Street, Champaign, Illinois 61820.

Child Behavior Checklist—Teacher Form

This is a 113-item questionnaire with two pages provided for recording teacher observations of the child's academic progress and overall functioning within the classroom. It was originally developed in 1978 by Thomas Achenbach at the University of Connecticut as a parent report measure. Edelbrock and Achenbach (1984) constructed a parallel form to obtain teacher ratings of many of the same problems that parents rate. Because of the fact that parents and teachers rate somewhat different items and observe children in different contexts, it is not necessary for teachers and parents to agree in their ratings of similar children (Achenbach, 1984). The teacher, who is asked to rate problematic behaviors based on observations of a child, must have interacted with the child for at least a two-month period.

The Child Behavior Checklist—Teacher's Report Form appears in Figure 4.5. Parts I through IX consist of questions concerning the child's overall academic and classroom performance. The 113 items that comprise Part XII are divided into eight or nine behavioral scales depending on the child's age and sex. These scales

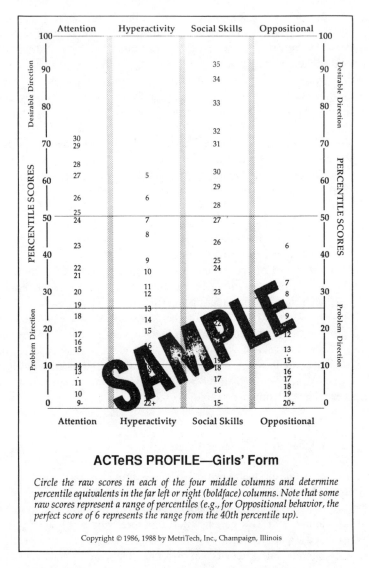

ACTeRS PROFILE—Girls' Form

Circle the raw scores in each of the four middle columns and determine percentile equivalents in the far left or right (boldface) columns. Note that some raw scores represent a range of percentiles (e.g., for Oppositional behavior, the perfect score of 6 represents the range from the 40th percentile up).

Figure 4.4 ACTeRS profile–girl's form, by R. K. Ullmann, E. K. Sleator and R. L. Sprague. ADD-H: Comprehensive Teacher Rating Scale. Copyright 1986, 1988 by MetriTech, Inc. Used with permission of the publisher.

deal with specific childhood diagnostic categories (Anxiety, Social Withdrawal, Depression, Immaturity, Self-Destruction, Inattention, Unpopular, Delinquent, Aggressive, Obsessive/Compulsive and Nervous/Overactive).

The 113 items on Part XII are rated as 0 (Not true, as far as you know), 1 (Somewhat or sometimes true) or 2 (Very true or often true). The score for each diagnostic category is obtained by summing the points for those items loading on each scale. The scores are plotted on profile sheets using percentiles or

CHILD BEHAVIOR CHECKLIST - TEACHER'S REPORT FORM

PUPIL'S AGE	PUPIL'S SEX ☐ Boy ☐ Girl	RACE	PUPIL'S NAME
GRADE	THIS FORM FILLED OUT BY ☐ Teacher (name) _____		
DATE	☐ Counselor (name) _____ ☐ Other (specify)_____ name:		SCHOOL

PARENTS' TYPE OF WORK (Please be specific – for example, auto mechanic, high school teacher, homemaker, laborer, lathe operator, shoe salesman, army sergeant.)

FATHER'S
TYPE OF WORK _____

MOTHER'S
TYPE OF WORK _____

I.   How long have you known this pupil?

II. How well do you know him/her?   ☐ Very Well   ☐ Moderately Well   ☐ Not Well

III. How much time does he/she spend in your class per week?

IV. What kind of class is it?   (Please be specific, e.g., regular 5th grade, 7th grade math, etc.)

V.   Has he/she ever been referred for special class placement, services, or tutoring?

☐ No   ☐ Don't Know   ☐ Yes – what kind and when?

VI. Has he/she ever repeated a grade?

☐ No   ☐ Don't Know   ☐ Yes – grade and reason

VII. Current school performance – list academic subjects and check appropriate column:

Academic subject	1. Far below grade	2. Somewhat below grade	3. At grade level	4. Somewhat above grade	5. Far above grade
1. _____	☐	☐	☐	☐	☐
2. _____	☐	☐	☐	☐	☐
3. _____	☐	☐	☐	☐	☐
4. _____	☐	☐	☐	☐	☐
5. _____	☐	☐	☐	☐	☐
6. _____	☐	☐	☐	☐	☐

Figure 4.5 Child Behavior Checklist–Teacher's Report Form. From T. M. Achenbach and C. Edelbrock, Child Behavior Checklist–Teacher's Report Form. Copyright 1980. Printed with permission of the authors and publisher.

VIII. Compared to typical pupils of the same age:	1. Much less	2. Somewhat less	3. Slightly less	4. About average	5. Slightly more	6. Somewhat more	7. Much more
1. How hard is he/she working?	☐	☐	☐	☐	☐	☐	☐
2. How appropriately is he/she behaving?	☐	☐	☐	☐	☐	☐	☐
3. How much is he/she learning?	☐	☐	☐	☐	☐	☐	☐
4. How happy is he/she?	☐	☐	☐	☐	☐	☐	☐

IX. **Most recent achievement test scores** (if available):

Name of test	Subject	Date	Percentile or grade level obtained

X. **IQ, readiness, or aptitude tests** (if available):

Name of test	Date	IQ or equivalent scores

XI. **Please feel free to write any comments about this pupil's work, behavior, or potential, using extra pages if necessary**

_____

_____

_____

Figure 4.5 (continued)

Below is a list of items that describe pupils. For each item that describes the pupil now or within the past 2 months, please circle the 2 if the item is **very true** or **often true** of the pupil. Circle the 1 if the item is **somewhat** or **sometimes true** of the pupil. If the item is **not true** of the pupil, circle the **0**. Please answer all items as well as you can, even if some do not seem to apply to this pupil.

0 = Not True (as far as you know)   1 = Somewhat or Sometimes True   2 = Very True or Often True

0 1 2	1. Acts too young for his/her age	0 1 2	31. Fears he/she might think or do something bad
0 1 2	2. Hums or makes other odd noises in class	0 1 2	32. Feels he/she has to be perfect
0 1 2	3. Argues a lot	0 1 2	33. Feels or complains that no one loves him/her
0 1 2	4. Fails to finish things he/she starts	0 1 2	34. Feels others are out to get him/her
0 1 2	5. Behaves like opposite sex	0 1 2	35. Feels worthless or inferior
0 1 2	6. Defiant, talks back to staff	0 1 2	36. Gets hurt a lot, accident-prone
0 1 2	7. Bragging, boasting	0 1 2	37. Gets in many fights
0 1 2	8. Can't concentrate, can't pay attention for long	0 1 2	38. Gets teased a lot
0 1 2	9. Can't get his/her mind off certain thoughts;	0 1 2	39. Hangs around with others who get in trouble
	obsessions (describe):_____	0 1 2	40. Hears things that aren't there (describe):
			_____
0 1 2	10. Can't sit still, restless, or hyperactive	0 1 2	41. Impulsive or acts without thinking
		0 1 2	42. Likes to be alone
0 1 2	11. Clings to adults or too dependent		
		0 1 2	43. Lying or cheating
0 1 2	12. Complains of loneliness	0 1 2	44. Bites fingernails
0 1 2	13. Confused or seems to be in a fog	0 1 2	45. Nervous, high-strung, or tense
0 1 2	14. Cries a lot	0 1 2	46. Nervous movements or twitching (describe):
0 1 2	15. Fidgets		_____
0 1 2	16. Cruelty, bullying, or meanness to others		
		0 1 2	47. Overconforms to rules
0 1 2	17. Daydreams or gets lost in his/her thoughts	0 1 2	48. Not liked by other pupils
0 1 2	18. Deliberately harms self or attempts suicide		
		0 1 2	49. Has difficulty learning
0 1 2	19. Demands a lot of attention	0 1 2	50. Too fearful or anxious
0 1 2	20. Destroys his/her own things		
		0 1 2	51. Feels dizzy
0 1 2	21. Destroys property belonging to others	0 1 2	52. Feels too guilty
0 1 2	22. Difficulty following directions		
		0 1 2	53. Talks out of turn
0 1 2	23. Disobedient at school	0 1 2	54. Overtired
0 1 2	24. Disturbs other pupils		
		0 1 2	55. Overweight
0 1 2	25. Doesn't get along with other pupils		56. Physical problems without known medical cause:
0 1 2	26. Doesn't seem to feel guilty after misbehaving	0 1 2	a. Aches or pains
		0 1 2	b. Headaches
0 1 2	27. Easily jealous	0 1 2	c. Nausea, feels sick
0 1 2	28. Eats or drinks things that are not food	0 1 2	d. Problems with eyes (describe): _____
	(describe): _____		
	_____		_____
		0 1 2	e. Rashes or other skin problems
		0 1 2	f. Stomachaches or cramps
0 1 2	29. Fears certain animals, situations, or places	0 1 2	g. Vomiting, throwing up
	other than school (describe): _____	0 1 2	h. Other (describe): _____
	_____		_____
0 1 2	30. Fears going to school		

Figure 4.5 (continued)

0 1 2   57. Physically attacks people

0 1 2   58. Picks nose, skin, or other parts of body (describe): _____

0 1 2   59. Sleeps in class

0 1 2   60. Apathetic or unmotivated

0 1 2   61. Poor school work

0 1 2   62. Poorly coordinated or clumsy

0 1 2   63. Prefers being with older children

0 1 2   64. Prefers being with younger children

0 1 2   65. Refuses to talk

0 1 2   66. Repeats certain acts over and over; compulsions (describe): _____

0 1 2   67. Disrupts class discipline

0 1 2   68. Screams a lot

0 1 2   69. Secretive, keeps things to self

0 1 2   70. Sees things that aren't there (describe): _____

0 1 2   71. Self-conscious or easily embarrassed

0 1 2   72. Messy work

0 1 2   73. Behaves irresponsibly (describe): _____

0 1 2   74. Showing off or clowning

0 1 2   75. Shy or timid

0 1 2   76. Explosive and unpredictable behavior

0 1 2   77. Demands must be met immediately, easily frustrated

0 1 2   78. Inattentive, easily distracted

0 1 2   79. Speech problem (describe): _____

0 1 2   80. Stares blankly

0 1 2   81. Feels hurt when criticized

0 1 2   82. Steals

0 1 2   83. Stores up things he/she doesn't need (describe): _____

0 1 2   84. Strange behavior (describe): _____

0 1 2   85. Strange ideas (describe): _____

0 1 2   86. Stubborn, sullen, or irritable

0 1 2   87. Sudden changes in mood or feelings

0 1 2   88. Sulks a lot

0 1 2   89. Suspicious

0 1 2   90. Swearing or obscene language

0 1 2   91. Talks about killing self

0 1 2   92. Underachieving, not working up to potential

0 1 2   93. Talks too much

0 1 2   94. Teases a lot

0 1 2   95. Temper tantrums or hot temper

0 1 2   96. Seems preoccupied with sex

0 1 2   97. Threatens people

0 1 2   98. Tardy to school or class

0 1 2   99. Too concerned with neatness or cleanliness

0 1 2   100. Fails to carry out assigned tasks

0 1 2   101. Truancy or unexplained absence

0 1 2   102. Underactive, slow moving, or lacks energy

0 1 2   103. Unhappy, sad, or depressed

0 1 2   104. Unusually loud

0 1 2   105. Uses alcohol or drugs (describe): _____

0 1 2   106. Overly anxious to please

0 1 2   107. Dislikes school

0 1 2   108. Is afraid of making mistakes

0 1 2   109. Whining

0 1 2   110. Unclean personal appearance

0 1 2   111. Withdrawn, doesn't get involved with others

0 1 2   112. Worrying

113. Please write in any problems the pupil has that were not listed above:

0 1 2   _____

0 1 2   _____

0 1 2   _____

Figure 4.5 (continued)

standard scores based on the normative sample. The scales were developed by factor analyzing responses for a large sample of children. Normative data was first obtained in 1978 with disturbed 6- to 11-year-old males (Achenbach, 1978). Separate scoring profiles have been standardized for each sex at ages 6 through 11 and 12 through 16 years. Age-graded normative data is essential since the prevalence and severity of many behaviors associated with ADHD decline with age (Achenbach & Edelbrock, 1981). The scoring profiles provide standard scores based on normative samples for teacher ratings of academic performance, adaptive behavior and behavior problems. Behavioral-problem scales are organized as either internalizing (i.e., anxiety, social withdrawal) or externalizing (i.e., inattentive, aggressive). Summary internalizing, externalizing and total problem scores can also be computed. Figure 4.6 contains a sample profile sheet for girls, ages 6 through 11 years.

Kirby and Horne (1986) note that the hyperactivity and aggression scales on the Achenbach Child Behavior Checklist look fairly similar for a population of attention-disordered children and a population of aggressive, out-of-control children. Background information about the two groups, however, was very different. The aggressive children more likely came from chaotic homes where physical punishment was employed and aggression was modeled. Additionally, Edelbrock et al., (1984) found that boys presenting attention disorder without hyperactivity obtained high scores on the inattentive scale while boys experiencing attention disorder with hyperactivity also scored high on the nervous-overactive scale. The teacher and parent forms of the Achenbach Child Behavior Checklist are available from University Associates in Psychiatry, 1 South Prospect Street, Burlington, VT. 05401.

Teacher Observation Checklist

The Teacher Observation Checklist (Figure 4.7) was developed by Goldstein (1988b) as a brief teacher respondent checklist. When used in conjunction with the Conners Teacher's Rating Scale, Comprehensive Teacher Rating Scale or Child Behavior Checklist, the Teacher Observation Checklist provides additional descriptive data concerning the child's classroom functioning. The teacher's responses to this checklist are evaluated qualitatively.

Social Skills Assessment

The Social Skills Assessment Teacher Form (Goldstein, 1988a) (Figure 4.8) was developed to help provide an organized description of a child's social interaction with classmates. The form is evaluated qualitatively and no normative data has been collected by the author. Teacher responses to the questionnaire descriptors can also be helpful in assisting the practitioner in making specific treatment recommendations for the development of deficient social skills.

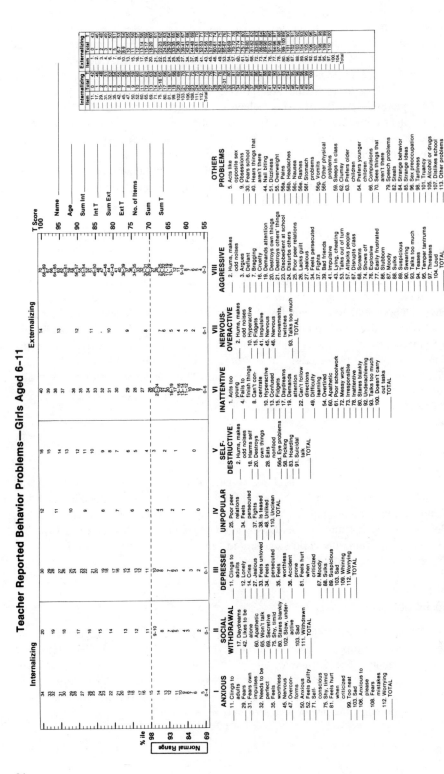

Figure 4.6 Teacher-reported behavior problems—girls aged 6–11. From T. M. Achenbach and C. Edelbrock, 1982. Child Behavior Checklist-Teacher's Report Form. Copyright 1982. Printed with permission of the authors and publisher.

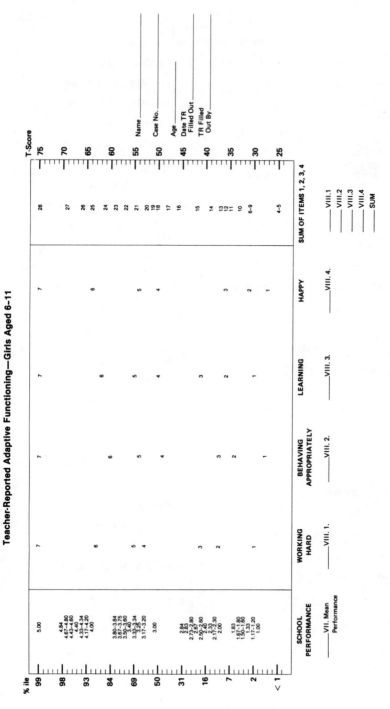

Figure 4.6 (continued)

85

NAME_____ GRADE_____ TEACHER_____ DATE_____

TEACHER OBSERVATION CHECKLIST

Please check the phrase in each section that best describes this student.

1. SELF-CONCEPT

☐ Appears to feel inadequate, self-critical

☐ Appears to have mild feelings of inadequacy

☐ Appears self-confident in most situations

☐ Confident in all areas, good concept of ability

☐ Over-confident, unrealistic

2. MOTIVATION

☐ Low interest, never initiates activity

☐ Little interest, limited and narrow

☐ Some enthusiasm

☐ Above-average, initiates some

☐ Enthusiastic interest

3. ADAPTABILITY TO NEW SITUATIONS

☐ Dependent, lost in new situations

☐ Difficult adjustment as a rule

☐ Usually adapts

☐ Adapts easily, confident in new areas

☐ Excellent adaptation

4. ATTENTION-SEEKING

☐ Constantly seeking attention

☐ Often seeks attention

☐ Moderately seeks attention

☐ Usually does not seek extra attention

☐ Does not seek extra attention

5. APPROACH TO A PROBLEM

☐ Slovenly, unorganized

☐ Inexact, careless

☐ Moderately careful

☐ Consistent and logical

☐ Precise organized approach

6. LISTENING TO INSTRUCTIONS

☐ Unable to follow instructions; always confused

☐ Usually follows simple instructions but often needs individual help

☐ Follows instructions that are familiar and not complex

☐ Remembers and follows extended instructions

☐ Usually skillful in remembering and following instructions

7. LEARNING RATE

☐ Learns very slowly

☐ Learns slowly

☐ Learns at an average rate

☐ Learns at above-average rate

☐ Learns quickly

8. WORK RATE

☐ Works very slowly

☐ Works slowly

☐ Works at an average rate

☐ Works at above-average rate

☐ Works quickly

Figure 4.7 Teacher Observation Checklist. By S. Goldstein. Copyright applied for 1988. Reprinted with permission of the author.

Please check the phrase in each section that best describes this student.

9. **FRUSTRATION — TOLERANCE**

☐ Gives up easily, cries

☐ Shows some ability to tolerate frustration

☐ Average degree of tolerance

☐ Above-average degree of tolerance

☐ Perseveres, handles frustration well

10. **COOPERATION**

☐ Continually disrupts classroom; poor impulse control

☐ Frequently demands attention; often speaks out of turn

☐ Waits his turn; average for age and grade

☐ Above-average; cooperates well

☐ Excellent ability; cooperates without adult encouragement

11. **VOCABULARY**

☐ Always uses immature, poor vocabulary

☐ Limited vocabulary, primarily simple nouns; few precise descriptive words

☐ Adequate vocabulary for age and grade

☐ Above-average vocabulary; uses numerous precise, descriptive words

☐ High level vocabulary; always uses precise words; conveys abstractions

12. **LANGUAGE USAGE**

☐ Always uses incomplete sentences with grammatical errors

☐ Frequently uses incomplete sentences; numerous grammatical errors

☐ Uses correct grammar; few errors in the use of prepositions, etc.

☐ Above-average oral language; rarely makes grammatical errors

☐ Always speaks in grammatically correct sentences

13. **FINE-MOTOR COORDINATION**

☐ Considerable difficulty using a pencil, cutting, tying

☐ Below average skills in writing/poor finger dexterity

☐ Average fine-motor skills

☐ Above-average ability to draw, print, or do cursive writing

☐ Excellent ability in drawing, coloring, cutting and writing

14. **GROSS MOTOR COORDINATION**

☐ Very poorly coordinated; clumsy

☐ Below average; awkward

☐ Average for age

☐ Above-average; does well in motor activities

☐ Excels in coordination; graceful

15. **VISUAL PERCEPTION**

☐ Much difficulty with reversals, directionality and illegible writing

☐ Below average written work and copying skills

☐ Average visual-perception of written material

☐ Above-average printing or writing

☐ Excellent, well organized, clearly legible written assignments

Figure 4.7 (continued)

SOCIAL SKILLS ASSESSMENT
(Teacher Form)

Student's Name _____ Date _____

Individual Completing this Form _____ Grade _____

Description of Child: Please check any statements which you feel describe this student
in interaction with peers. If parts of these statements apply
to this student, please qualify your response by specifically
underlining those parts.

Not True	Sometimes True	Frequently True	This Student:
____	____	____	appears socially isolated. A large proportion of school time is spent in solitary activities. isolation appears to result from the student's withdrawal as opposed to rejection by classmates.
____	____	____	interacts less with classmates due to shyness or timidity.
____	____	____	appears anxious in interactions with classmates and adults.
____	____	____	spends less time involved in activities with classmates due to a lack of social skills and/or appropriate social judgment.
____	____	____	appears to have fewer friends than most due to negative, bossy or annoying behaviors which alienates classmates.
____	____	____	appears to spend less time with classmates due to awkward or bizzare behaviors.
____	____	____	disturbs classmates by teasing, provoking, fighting or interrupting.
____	____	____	will openly strike back with angry behavior if teased by classmates.
____	____	____	is argumentative with adults and classmates. This student must have the last word in verbal exchange.
____	____	____	displays physical aggression towards objects or persons.

-over-

Figure 4.8 Social Skills Assessment–Teacher Form, by S. Goldstein. Copyright 1988. Used with the author's permission.

School Situations Questionnaires

The School Situations Questionnaire (Figure 4.9) was developed by Russell Barkley (1981a) as a means of assessing the impact of the child's attention and related deficits in specific school situations. Information from this questionnaire allows the practitioner to make the important connection between the child's attentional difficulties and the situations in which those difficulties cause problems. This form additionally enables the practitioner to develop an understanding of the child's compensatory skills, which in specific situations may reduce the negative impact of these attentional problems. The School Situations Questionnaire also allows the practitioner to understand teacher behaviors that in specific situations may minimize the negative impact of the child's attentional problems.

Barkley's original School Situations Questionnaire appears best for elementary school children. It has been revised by Goldstein (1987) into an adolescent form,

Figure 4.8 (continued)
Social Skills Assessment:

Not True	Sometimes True	Frequently True	This Student:
___	___	___	will use coercive tactics to force the submission of classmates. This student will manipulate or threaten.
___	___	___	speaks to others in an impatient or cranky tone of voice.
___	___	___	will say uncomplimentary things to others, including engaging in name calling, ridicule or verbal derogation.
___	___	___	will respond when a classmate initiates conversation.
___	___	___	engages in long conversations.
___	___	___	will share laughter with classmates.
___	___	___	will spontaneously contribute during a group discussion.
___	___	___	will volunteer in class and freely take a leadership role.
___	___	___	will spontaneoussly work with classmates during classroom activities.
___	___	___	will spontaneously join a group of classmates during recess.
___	___	___	will verbally initiate with classmates.

Additional Comments: _____

_____

_____

_____

_____

Figure 4.8 (continued)

which appears in Figure 4.10. Barkley developed his questionnaire primarily to provide the practitioner with qualitative information. From his research, Barkley noted that ADD children present with problems in at least 50% of the most frequently encountered school situations (Barkley, 1981a). Breen (1986), based on a sample of almost 600 children, developed normative data for the School Situations Questionnaire for children ranging in age from 6 to 11 years. The data is presented in Table 4.1.

Additional Teacher Report Questionnaires

There are other questionnaires that practitioners may find useful. Prinz, Connor and Wilson (1981) developed a Daily Behavior Checklist in an attempt to differentiate between hyperactive and aggressive behavioral problems within the school setting. The overlap between inattentive, overactive behaviors and aggressive, oppositional behaviors, especially within the school setting, is frequently a diagnostic thorn when attempting to make a diagnosis of attention disorder. The checklist provides

ELEMENTARY SCHOOL SITUATIONS QUESTIONNAIRE

Name of Child _____

Name of person completing this form _____

Does this child present problems for you in any of these situations.   If
so, indicate their severity and a brief description if possible.

Situation	Yes/No (Circle One)		If yes, how severe (Circle one) Mild Severe
While arriving at school	Yes	No	1 2 3 4 5 6 7 8 9
During individual task work	Yes	No	1 2 3 4 5 6 7 8 9
During small group activities	Yes	No	1 2 3 4 5 6 7 8 9
During free-play time in class	Yes	No	1 2 3 4 5 6 7 8 9
During lectures to the class	Yes	No	1 2 3 4 5 6 7 8 9
During recess	Yes	No	1 2 3 4 5 6 7 8 9
During lunch	Yes	No	1 2 3 4 5 6 7 8 9
While in the hallways	Yes	No	1 2 3 4 5 6 7 8 9
While in the bathroom	Yes	No	1 2 3 4 5 6 7 8 9
During field trips	Yes	No	1 2 3 4 5 6 7 8 9
During special assemblies	Yes	No	1 2 3 4 5 6 7 8 9
While on the bus	Yes	No	1 2 3 4 5 6 7 8 9

Figure 4.9 Elementary School Situations Questionnaire. From R. Barkley, *Hyperactive Children*. Copyright 1981 by Guilford Press. Used with permission of the author and publisher.

operational descriptions along with criteria for purposeful versus nonpurposeful behavior. Attention-disordered children typically exhibit impulsive, unplanned acts of aggression without a strong emotional basis, while a conduct-disordered child is typically much more angry and purposeful in his aggressive acts.

Kendall and Wilcox (1979) developed a 33-item Self-Control Rating Scale. The items of the scale primarily relate to issues of self-control and impulsivity. The scale is sensitive to classroom behavioral problems and, given the specificity of scale items, can be useful in identifying specific target behaviors for treatment intervention.

Davids (1971) developed a seven-characteristic rating scale to be completed by either parents or teachers. The scale covers school performance and hyperactivity symptoms. Each item is rated on a six-point scale, comparing the target child to other children. Although the scale has been the subject of research and may be sensitive to drug effects (Denhoff, Davids & Hawkins, 1971), it has found only limited clinical utility.

ADOLESCENT SCHOOL SITUATIONS QUESTIONNAIRE

Name of Adolescent _____

Name of person completing this form _____

Does this adolescent present problems for you in any of these situations?
If so, indicate their severity and a brief description if possible.

Situation	Yes/No (Circle One)	If yes, how severe (Circle one) Mild Severe
During individual task work	Yes No	1 2 3 4 5 6 7 8 9
During small group activities	Yes No	1 2 3 4 5 6 7 8 9
During free time in class	Yes No	1 2 3 4 5 6 7 8 9
During lectures in class	Yes No	1 2 3 4 5 6 7 8 9
During lunch	Yes No	1 2 3 4 5 6 7 8 9
While in the hallways	Yes No	1 2 3 4 5 6 7 8 9
While in the bathroom	Yes No	1 2 3 4 5 6 7 8 9
During special assemblies	Yes No	1 2 3 4 5 6 7 8 9
While on the bus	Yes No	1 2 3 4 5 6 7 8 9

Figure 4.10 Adolescent School Situations Questionnaire, by S. Goldstein, (1987). Used with the author's permission.

The Spring's Hyperactivity Rating Scale is a 33-item scale used to obtain ratings of children's behavior in the classroom (Spring, Blunden, Greenberg & Yellin, 1977). Teachers rate the items, which are organized into eleven categories, on a one-to-five Likert Scale. Normative data was collected for boys and girls, kindergarten through fourth grade. ADHD children score high on the categories containing items dealing with restlessness, distractibility and impulsivity. This

TABLE 4.1.   Norms for the Elementary School Situations Questionnaire

Age	n	# Problem Settings	Mean Severity
Boys:			
6–8	170	2.4 (3.3)*	1.5 (2.0)
9–11	123	2.8 (3.2)	1.9 (2.1)
Girls:			
6–8	180	1.0 (2.0)	0.8 (1.5)
9–11	126	1.3 (2.1)	0.8 (1.2)

*Note: These entries are means with standard deviations in parentheses.

Breen, M. J. "Normative Data on the Home Situations and School Situations Questionnaires," Copyright 1986. *ADD/H Newsletter*. Used by permission of the publisher.

scale, too, has not found much clinical utility but is used by some practitioners evaluating younger children.

Behar (1977) developed the Preschool Behavior Questionnaire. It is one of the few behavior rating scales designed for younger children, specifically ages three through six years. The scale is made up of 30 items, and teachers respond to each item on a three-point Likert Scale. The questionnaire can also be scored for three factor-based scales dealing with aggression, anxiety and hyperactivity. Campbell et al. (1982) demonstrated that this questionnaire can be used clinically to identify hyperactive toddlers.

Suggested Combination of Questionnaires

In situations where teachers have a limited amount of time, it is suggested that, at the very least, each of the child's teachers complete either the Conners or ACTeRS in addition to a measure of social skills and situational problems. In optimal situations, it is recommended that teachers complete these questionnaires, the Child Behavior Checklist and the Teacher Observation Checklist.

In secondary school settings it is frequently beneficial to obtain ratings by all of the adolescent's teachers. This enables the practitioner to be aware of patterns of consistency or discrepancy in the adolescent's problems throughout the school day. Additionally, classes in which the ADHD adolescent's attentional problems would be expected to cause less difficulty, such as physical education or shop classes, frequently provide useful data to assist the practitioner in making the distinction between skill deficit and purposeful misbehavior. It is not uncommon for ADHD adolescents to function significantly better in classes allowing more movement and requiring less sustained attention.

DIRECT OBSERVATION

It is recommended that the practitioner obtain observational data of the ADHD child's behavior in the school environment. This data can be used to check the accuracy of teacher observations on the questionnaires and provide insight into the role the teacher may play in the child's behavior. Direct observation can also provide insight for the practitioner into the myriad of social and nonsocial factors that may elicit problematic behavior. The School Situations Questionnaire can assist the practitioner in choosing an appropriate classroom or related school situation to observe. The practitioner may choose to observe either a single behavior or many. In either case, each behavior must be operationally defined, and the practitioner must determine the type of behavioral report that would be most beneficial.

The practitioner may wish to determine the frequency of a particular behavior during a rating period, the duration of that behavior or simply whether or not the behavior occurs at least once in a given interval of time. For example, if the target behavior is being out of seat, in some situations the number of times the child gets out of his seat would be important. In others, the amount of time the child spends out of his seat would be more critical, while in a third type of situation the progression and time of occurrence for out-of-seat behavior would be of interest. In the last case for example, the child may remain seated during the first 15 minutes of a half-hour work period but be out of his seat repeatedly during the last 15 minutes. This would be important data in structuring an intervention plan. Special educators and school psychologists are often helpful in collecting observational data for the community-based practitioner.

Specific normative data for classroom observation is usually not available. The majority of practitioners do not have the time to obtain normative data concerning the behaviors they are going to observe. It is additionally difficult to obtain normative data since the classroom level of acceptable behavior, such as talking and being out of seat, varies depending on a particular teacher's expectations and tolerance. A fairly simple but unscientific method of comparison involves simultaneously gathering data on another child in the classroom whom the teacher views as average in regard to the behavior to be observed (Deno, 1980). In this way, the practitioner can compare the target child's behavior to the behavioral norm within the child's classroom. The TOAD System described below is a simple four-behavior observational model that can be utilized in a classroom setting.

The TOAD System

The TOAD System allows the practitioner to collect interval data on four classroom behaviors that are frequently problematic for ADHD children. The four behaviors are talking out, out of seat, attention problems and disruption. Data is usually observed at 15-second intervals. All four behaviors are observed simultaneously. If any of the behaviors occur, whether once or more than once, a single notation is made for the interval period. Table 4.2 contains suggested operational definitions for the four behaviors. Figure 4.11 presents a sample coding sheet for the TOAD System.

TABLE 4.2. Operational Definitions of Behaviors in the TOAD System

1. Talking Out: Spoken words, either friendly, neutral, or negative in content, directed at either the teacher without first obtaining permission to speak or unsolicited at classmates during inappropriate times or during work periods.

2. Out of Seat: The child is not supporting his weight with the chair. Upon knees does not count as out of seat behavior.

3. Attention Problem: The child is not attending either to independent work or to a group activity. The child is therefore engaged in an activity other than that which has been directed and is clearly different from what the other children are doing at the time. This includes the child not following teacher directions.

4. Disruption: The child's actions result in consequences that appear to be interrupting other children's work. These behaviors might include noises or physical contact. They may be intentional or unintentional.

CHILD: _____   DATE: _____

TEACHER: _____   TIME BEGIN: _____ TIME END: _____

ACTIVITY: _____   LOCATION: _____

OBSERVER: _____   INTERVAL: ☐ 15 seconds ☐ 30 seconds

☐ 45 seconds ☐ 60 seconds

Interval	T	O	A	D		Interval	T	O	A	D		Interval	T	O	A	D		Interval	T	O	A	D
1.						33.						65.						97.				
32.						64.						96.						128.				

Figure 4.11 TOAD System.

Once the observation has been completed, the practitioner totals the number of affirmative observations in each category and divides this by the total number of observation points to obtain a percentage of negative behavior for each category. For example, if the child was observed for 100 intervals and was marked affirmatively for talking out in 50 of those intervals, talking out behavior would be 50%. This is considered a high percentage as it would be expected that the majority of children rarely talk out of turn in class. If the TOAD System is to be used extensively, it may be beneficial for the practitioner to collect normative data in the local school setting.

It is infrequent in the typical school evaluation of an ADHD child that the practitioner needs to obtain classroom observational data that codes all possible behaviors exhibited by the child during the observation time. All-encompassing observation systems are frequently complex, requiring multiple operational definitions and in-depth coding manuals for utilization. For example, the Stoneybrook Code (Abikoff, Gittelman-Klein & Klein, 1977) contains 14 observable behaviors. The Classroom Observation System (Whalen et al., 1978) contains 21 behaviors to be rated. Again, as with simpler rating systems, these systems require the collection of local normative data in order to compare the differences between the target child's behavior and the behavior of other children.

TEACHER COMMUNICATION

During the course of the school year, teachers may spend as much, if not more, structured and unstructured time with the child than any other adult. Once observational and questionnaire data has been obtained, it is frequently helpful to speak directly with the classroom teacher to clarify the teacher's comments and responses to the questionnaires. This will also assist in the interpretation of the observational data. Prior to the teacher conversation, it is suggested that the practitioner make note of any extreme responses on the questionnaires, including situations in which the child exhibits specific behaviors or extremes of behavior. The teacher can then be asked to clarify and expand on questionnaire responses. It is frequently helpful to attempt to identify social and nonsocial factors that may elicit difficulty within the school setting. Although the questionnaires are most helpful in obtaining data concerning the child's behavior, they do not provide very much insight into the chain of events that may precipitate problems. In complex situations, it may also be helpful, if the teacher has time, to request that a brief diary of the child's daily behavior be kept for one week.

ADDITIONAL SCHOOL DATA

The majority of parents save their children's report cards. Report cards provide the practitioner with an invaluable time line of the child's functioning as he has progressed through school. It is not uncommon for parents to be uncertain when problems began and specifically which problems came first. Report cards are often helpful in providing this pattern of data. Report cards are also useful in developing a general overview of the child's classroom performance since they typically reflect the quality of day-in and day-out work completion as opposed to acquired knowledge or academic achievement.

All school children complete a battery of achievement tests, usually on an annual or biannual basis. The most common batteries are the California Achievement Test, Stanford Achievement Test, Iowa Test of Basic Skills, Metropolitan Achievement Test and Sequential Tests of Educational Progress. They are often fairly extensive batteries that provide an in-depth analysis of the child's academic skills. The practitioner must keep in mind that these are group tests requiring a lengthy amount of time to complete. Often they are as much a measure of the attention-disordered child's lack of task persistence as a measure of achievement. Nevertheless, group tests provide valuable data that allows the practitioner to compare the child's achievement with day-in and day-out school performance.

The majority of ADHD children are not referred for special education services, and thus academic achievement data from individually administered tests is usually not available. When such data is available, it should be obtained and reviewed. Assessment instruments, including the Woodcock-Johnson Psycho-Educational Battery (Woodcock & Johnson, 1977), Woodcock Reading Mastery Tests (Woodcock, 1973), Peabody Individual Achievement Test (Dunn & Markwardt, 1970) and Key Math Diagnostic Inventory (Connoloy, Nachtman & Pritchett, 1976), can provide accurate in-depth measures of the child's academic achievement. Although many ADHD children present with some degree of achievement difficulty (Holborow & Berry, 1986), it is the practitioner's job to initially rule out learning problems as the primary etiological factor contributing to the child's attention and activity-level problems. Clinical evaluation procedures described in Chapter 6 will present an overview and specific approaches for both differential diagnosis and the identification of learning problems.

NECESSARY DATA FOR CONFIRMING ADHD AT SCHOOL

In making the diagnosis of ADHD within the school setting, it is recommended that a child either falls below the tenth percentile on the ACTeRS or is approximately two standard deviations higher than the same sex-and-age normative group for the hyperkinesis index on the Conners Teacher's Rating Scale. It is additionally suggested that these problems must cause the child difficulty in at least 50% of school situations. The collection of additional social, cognitive, academic, and situational data assists the practitioner in making a differential diagnosis (e.g., attentional problems secondary to learning disability) and clearly defining the unique aspects of the child's strengths and weaknesses within the school setting. This process facilitates the development of a treatment plan.

SUMMARY

This chapter provided a model for the collection of school data, involving the clarification and definition of situational behavior, social skills, scholastic achievement and classroom performance. Teacher report questionnaires and direct observational measures are invaluable in the collection of behavioral and social data from a variety of situations. Individual and group achievement tests, as well as report cards, provide essential educational data. Teacher observations elicited through a direct interview provide data concerning the child's classroom performance and insight into the social and nonsocial factors that may be contributing to the child's school functioning.

CHAPTER 5

Home Evaluation of Attention Disorder

The majority of children experiencing ADHD present attention and arousal-related problems early in life. The child's history within the home and community setting is an essential component of the practitioner's evaluation. The home evaluation typically involves collection of data concerning the child's behavioral and developmental history as well as current behavioral and social functioning. Parents can be extremely helpful in providing developmental data, anecdotal behavioral history and impressions of the progression of their child's problems.

The practitioner may use the parent interview/history session as an opportunity to provide the ADHD child's parents with an understanding of the causes and complexity of ADHD problems. The interview/history session is usually the practitioner's first lengthy interaction with the ADHD child's parents. The session also affords the practitioner the opportunity to develop hypotheses about the parent's skills and abilities and the role they may play in the child's problems. For the practitioner, the parent interview/history session is both an information-gathering and an information-giving event. Barkley (1981a) points out that the parental interview serves several purposes, including establishing rapport between the practitioner and parents, providing a source of descriptive information about the child and family, revealing the parents' view of problems, allowing the practitioner to narrow the focus of the evaluation, assisting the parents to develop an understanding of the child's problems and beginning the diagnostic process.

Norm-referenced questionnaires allow the practitioner to obtain an assessment of the child's functioning within the home setting in comparison to a normative group. For children with histories of multiple behavioral and developmental problems, the home evaluation may also involve in-depth assessment of the parents' skills and their ability to manage the child effectively. The home evaluation in some situations may include direct observation of the parent and child interacting either in a natural setting or within a playroom. As with the school assessment, it is essential for the practitioner to relate behavioral problems to specific situations in which they occur. It is also important for the practitioner to form etiological hypotheses of the contribution that temperament, family dynamics, parental skill, and developmental problems such as language disability make toward the ADHD child's behavior.

CHILDHOOD HISTORY FORM FOR ATTENTION DISORDER

Appendix 1 contains the Childhood History Form for Attention Disorder (Goldstein & Goldstein, 1985). This history form was developed to gather developmental, behavioral, social and academic history with an emphasis on attention and arousal-related problems. It represents a restructuring and modification of a number of generic history forms. The format of this questionnaire is modeled on a questionnaire developed by Gardner (1979). The history form can be used as a general framework to conduct the parent interview. Data from the parent questionnaires can be integrated at appropriate points into the history-taking session.

THE PARENT INTERVIEW/HISTORY SESSION

The parent interview/history session usually begins with an overview of the parents' perceptions concerning their child's problems. This often leads to a discussion of the parents' history, specifically directed at determining if parents experienced similar problems when younger. Data is gathered on extended family members, especially nieces and nephews. It is suggested that the practitioner determine whether siblings of the ADHD child are currently having or have at some time experienced similar problems. The history then proceeds through pregnancy, infancy, toddler, preschool and school-age periods. At each point the examiner is seeking to identify data that might be related to the development, occurrence and progression of attention and arousal problems. For this reason, it is essential for the practitioner to possess a good understanding of the developmental course and specific developmental problems that attention-disordered children experience at various ages. The practitioner must be able to develop a chronology for the occurrence of problems and their progression. Frequently, attention and arousal-related problems may begin from temperamental etiology but very quickly progress in severity as the result of environmental response. Practitioners must seek to identify and differentiate environmental factors. When evaluating an adolescent, this process of differential diagnosis is an especially complex task. Frequently, the ADHD adolescent's attention difficulty may be overshadowed by secondary emotional and behavioral problems. With younger children the problem is also complex but for a different reason. For younger children, there is often very little data concerning the child's behavior away from parents or family members. The practitioner must rely heavily on parental report, increasing the likelihood of misinterpreting a parent-child interactive problem as a temperamental disorder.

It is suggested that the practitioner elicit and clarify disciplinary methods that parents have used in an attempt to manage the child's behavior. Typically, there will be differences in methods between mothers and fathers. It is also recommended that the practitioner attempt to engage parents in a conversation concerning the child's positive attributes and specifically what each parent likes about the child. Parents struggling to speak positively about their child will in all likelihood have great difficulty following through with treatment recommendations because the necessary foundation for positive parent-child interaction is not present. Often practitioners will have no difficulty identifying these parents. Parents with a positive attachment to their child will describe their child's attention-related problems as nonpurposeful and make an effort to convince the practitioner that theirs is a loving, caring, nice child despite behavioral problems. Conversely, parents who are angry, unhappy and poorly bonded to their child struggle to speak positively about the child.

As part of the history session, it is also important to become aware of which professionals may have been consulted previously and what attempts have been made to modify the child's problems. It is also helpful for the practitioner to identify the specific problem or problems that motivate parents to seek help at this time. Parents who do not perceive the child as having significant difficulty but are following through with recommendations for evaluation because of complaints by the school or community may be only minimally motivated to follow through with treatment recommendations. As part of the evaluation, this data can be used by the practitioner to determine prognosis.

Some practitioners have the child present during the parent history session. Although it may afford the practitioner the opportunity to observe how parents manage the child, the child's behavior can also be a distraction that does not allow parents to sit and speak at length with the practitioner. Adolescents typically function better as participants during the parent history session. Involving the ADHD adolescent during this initial meeting can be helpful in motivating the adolescent to become an active participant in the evaluative process.

At the close of the interview/history session, it is beneficial for the practitioner to summarize the session by briefly reviewing the problems that have been identified, the situations in which they occur and the severity of these problems in comparison to the experiences of other children. Summarizing may also help parents understand the practitioner's recommendations, which may range in some cases from simply following the child over the coming few months to a need for further assessment to the need for immediate psychiatric hospitalization. A sample summary statement by a practitioner for John, an eleven-year-old fifth grader, follows.

Based on what we have discussed today, it appears that very early in his life you were aware that in many ways John was different from his siblings. As an infant he had problems fitting routines, was more irritable, restless and had difficulty nursing. As soon as he was mobile he was constantly into things. It appeared very early on that he had difficulty benefiting from his experiences and you were exasperated in your attempts to discipline him and alter his behavior. This has clearly had an effect on your relationship with him and has affected his role as a family member. In preschool he was restless, inattentive and overactive. You anticipated that he would have problems in kindergarten and your perceptions were correct. His academic career has been marked by complaints of poor work completion, apparent lack of motivation, restlessness, inattention and behavioral problems which appear non-purposeful. Although he appears to value social contact, he seems incompetent socially and has had difficulty maintaining long term friendships. Within the home setting he creates more problems than his siblings and has in fact been identified by his siblings as the "family problem." All of these experiences have affected his self-image and over the past year you have observed an increasing pattern of helplessness and an unwillingness to attempt challenging activities. It is positive to note that he is not presenting as seriously depressed, sleeps and eats well, has not had serious medical problems and the majority of the time appears to be a happy child from whom you derive pleasure. It is also positive to note that despite his difficulty with work completion, individually administered achievement tests at school suggest that he is learning adequately. As we have discussed the core symptoms of Attention-deficit Hyperactivity Disorder, it certainly appears that John's history strongly raises the possibility that he is experiencing such a disorder. It may therefore be beneficial for us to pursue further evaluation, obtain additional school data and administer psychometric testing in an attempt to clearly identify and understand John's problems, and design a treatment plan to help him function more effectively.

OBSERVATION OF PARENT-CHILD INTERACTION

Rarely does the practitioner have the time or the opportunity to directly observe the child functioning within the home setting. Additionally, ADHD children respond well in new or novel situations, and the practitioner's visit to the home may not allow observation of typical ADHD problems. It is also unusual for the practitioner to directly observe the parent and child interacting on structured tasks during the evaluation. Most practitioners have neither the facility nor the behavioral observation system in place to conduct such interactional evaluations.

Because parents frequently do not have the opportunity to watch their child function at length in a structured situation, some practitioners allow parents to observe parts of the evaluation through a one-way mirror or sit directly in the testing room. In the latter situation, parents are directed to be passive participants and simply observe the child. At times, the parents' presence affords the practitioner the opportunity to observe the parents' ability to sit and attend for a one-hour period, as well as to gain insight concerning the manner in which the child chooses to interact with each parent in such a setting. For children under the age of five, parents are routinely allowed to participate directly in the evaluation. Between the ages of five and ten, the child may be asked if she would like parents present during the evaluation. Most children feel more comfortable with their parents initially participating in the testing room.

Allowing parents to observe the evaluation not only involves them intimately in the evaluation process but helps them during feedback sessions to understand the test data and gain insight into the child's behavior. If the child has not been present during the parent history session, then having the parent participate in part of the evaluative session is frequently helpful in engaging the parent and child in a discussion of their perceptions of current problems. The practitioner must be aware that adolescents attempting to establish a sense of identity separate from their families typically prefer to be evaluated in private. However, adolescents aware of their problems and actively seeking help will value the opportunity to participate with their parents during the disposition session when the practitioner's impressions are discussed and recommendations for intervention are made.

Barkley (1981a) believes strongly that when direct observation of the parent and child is feasible it should be an integral part of the evaluation. Barkley designed a playroom setting for a clinic, furnished similar to a den or living room. He developed multiple tasks in which the parent is sequentially directed to engage the child. Activities generally revolve around compliance, beginning with simple tasks such as standing up and progressing to more complex tasks such as directing the child to complete math problems or build a house out of Lego blocks. Since adolescents resist this type of playroom setting, Barkley suggests that a different set of activities be used with adolescents. He recommends that the parent and adolescent engage in a discussion of topics ranging from the adolescent's compliance in the home setting for completing chores and homework to the adolescent's use of free time, favorite music and friends.

PARENT REPORT QUESTIONNAIRES

Conners Parent's Rating Scale

Developed by C. Keith Conners, the Parent's Rating Scale is the most widely used rating scale of parental opinion concerning attention disorder (Barkley, 1981a). The original 93-item Parent Questionnaire (Conners, 1970) was revised and shortened to 48 items (Conners, 1982). The Parent's Rating Scale appears in Figure 5.1. As with the Teacher's Rating Scale, the shortened Parent's Rating Scale retains most of the important characteristics of the original 93-item scale. Factor analysis of the 48-item scale yielded factors in the areas of Conduct Problems, Learning Problems, Psychosomatic, Impulsivity-Hyperactivity and Anxiety. As with the Teacher's Rating Scale, a hyperkinesis index was also obtained. The Parent's Rating Scale is simple for parents to complete. The 48 items are scored on a four-point scale with the following ratings: Not at all (score = 0); Just a little (score = 1); Pretty much (score = 2); and Very much (score = 3).

Of the 48 items in the Parent's Rating Scale, 10 are used to compute the hyperkinesis index. Items on the hyperkinesis index for the Parent's Rating Scale include descriptors of excitability, impulsivity, excessive crying, restlessness, failing to finish things, distractibility, inattention, being frustrated in efforts, disturbing other children and wide or drastic mood changes. The hyperkinesis index is a sensitive measure of attention-disordered behavior within the home setting, as well as a measure of a child's response to treatment interventions, specifically medication. The hyperkinesis index is computed by adding the scores of the ten critical items, dividing by ten, and comparing the child's score to factor norms such as those developed by Goyette et al. (1978). As with the Teacher's Rating Scale, the Parent's Rating Scale has recently been copyrighted and is available from Multi-Health Systems, Inc.

As with the Teacher's Rating Scale, many past research studies on the Parent's Scale utilized a hyperkinesis index score of 1.5 as the cutoff score considered to reflect significant problems with attention. Age-by-sex normative data generated from parental responses to the Parent's Questionnaire has demonstrated that this is an inefficient application of the hyperkinesis index. Based upon a comparison of the child's score with the sex-by-age normative data, the practitioner can make a statistically relevant comparison of the child's attentional skills to a normative

Instructions: Read each item below carefully, and decide how much you think your child has been bothered by this problem during the past month.

Not at All	Just a Little	Pretty Much	Very Much	CPRS-48
0	1	2	3	1. Picks at things (nails, fingers, hair, clothing)
0	1	2	3	2. Sassy to grown-ups
0	1	2	3	3. Problems with making or keeping friends
0	1	2	3	4. Excitable, impulsive
0	1	2	3	5. Wants to run things
0	1	2	3	6. Sucks or chews (thumb, clothing, blankets)
0	1	2	3	7. Cries easily or often
0	1	2	3	8. Carries a chip on his/her shoulder
0	1	2	3	9. Daydreams
0	1	2	3	10. Difficulty in learning
0	1	2	3	11. Restless in the "squirmy" sense
0	1	2	3	12. Fearful (of new situations, new people or places, going to school)
0	1	2	3	13. Restless, always up and on the go
0	1	2	3	14. Destructive
0	1	2	3	15. Tells lies or stories that aren't true
0	1	2	3	16. Shy
0	1	2	3	17. Gets into more trouble than others same age
0	1	2	3	18. Speaks differently from others same age (baby talk, stuttering, hard to understand)
0	1	2	3	19. Denies mistakes or blames others
0	1	2	3	20. Quarrelsome
0	1	2	3	21. Pouts and sulks
0	1	2	3	22. Steals
0	1	2	3	23. Disobedient or obeys but resentfully
0	1	2	3	24. Worries more than others (about being alone, illness or death)
0	1	2	3	25. Fails to finish things
0	1	2	3	26. Feelings easily hurt
0	1	2	3	27. Bullies others
0	1	2	3	28. Unable to stop a repetitive activity
0	1	2	3	29. Cruel
0	1	2	3	30. Childish or immature (wants help s/he shouldn't need, clings, needs constant reassurance)
0	1	2	3	31. Distractibility or attention span a problem
0	1	2	3	32. Headaches
0	1	2	3	33. Mood changes quickly and drastically
0	1	2	3	34. Doesn't like or doesn't follow rules or restrictions
0	1	2	3	35. Fights constantly
0	1	2	3	36. Doesn't get along well with brothers or sisters
0	1	2	3	37. Easily frustrated in efforts
0	1	2	3	38. Disturbs other children
0	1	2	3	39. Basically an unhappy child
0	1	2	3	40. Problems with eating (poor appetite, up between bites)
0	1	2	3	41. Stomach aches
0	1	2	3	42. Problems with sleep (can't fall asleep, up too early, up in the night)
0	1	2	3	43. Other aches and pains
0	1	2	3	44. Vomiting or nausea
0	1	2	3	45. Feels cheated in family circle
0	1	2	3	46. Boasts and brags
0	1	2	3	47. Lets self be pushed around
0	1	2	3	48. Bowel problems (frequently loose, irregular habits, constipation)
Not at All	Just a Little	Pretty Much	Very Much	

Figure 5.1 Conners Parent's Questionnaire, by C. K. Conners. Copyright 1988 by Multi-Health Systems, Inc. Used with permission of the author and publisher.

sample. A cutoff point of approximately two standard deviations higher than the mean would be considered to reflect significant attention-related problems in the home setting. On the average, females generally have lower hyperkinesis indices than males. Overall, the hyperkinesis index decreases with age. For 3- to 5-year-old females, for example, the mean plus two standard deviation cutoff is approximately 2.1, whereas the mean plus two standard deviations for the 15- to 17-year-old female group is approximately 1.1 (Goyette et al., 1978).

The practitioner must be aware that children with a pattern of noncompliant behavior within the home setting are at risk to obtain elevated hyperkinesis indices because of their inability or unwillingness to meet parental expectations and demands. Over time, this pattern of behavior can be greatly intensified by repeated negative child-parent interactions. The practitioner gathering data about the child's behavior in the home setting is frequently unaware of the long-term development of this pattern of behavior but is made aware only of the current level of problem. A long-standing pattern of child-parent conflict frequently results in the child presenting as highly excitable, easily frustrated, quick to cry, unable to finish things and excessively moody. All of these characteristics load as critical items on the hyperkinesis index. As with the Teacher's Rating Scale, another important point to consider is that children experiencing attention problems without concomitant difficulty with restless behavior will present with a lower hyperkinesis index than children with attention and hyperactivity problems.

Child Behavior Checklist—Parent Form

This questionnaire was designed to record behavioral problems and competencies of children aged 2 through 16, as observed by parents or adult caretakers. It was originally developed by Thomas M. Achenbach (1978). In 1982, Achenbach completed a revision of the scoring profile.

The Child Behavior Checklist contains a 113-item questionnaire in which possible behavioral descriptors for a child are rated 0 (Not true, as far as you know), 1 (Somewhat or sometimes true), or 2 (Very true or often true). The Child Behavior Checklist also contains two pages of questions concerning the child's social activities and social interaction. Information from these two pages yield scores for social competence scales. Parents are asked to rate their child's behavior as it has occurred over the previous six months. The scoring profile has separate normative data for each sex at ages 4 to 5, 6 to 11 and 12 to 16 years. A shorter, alternate questionnaire and slightly different scales are provided for each sex at ages two to three years. The Child Behavior Checklist—Parent Form appears in Figure 5.2.

Behavioral problem scales are organized as either internalizing (i.e., schizoid, depressed, uncommunicative, obsessive/compulsive and somatic complaints) or externalizing (i.e., hyperactive, aggressive and delinquent). Some of the scales (i.e., social withdrawal) are classified as intermittent, falling between the internalizing-externalizing dichotomy. The social competence scales are labeled activities, social and school on the basis of their content. Achenbach and Edelbrock (1983) developed names for the behavioral scales that appear to summarize the items that comprise each scale. They note, however, that the scales are not directly equivalent

CHILD BEHAVIOR CHECKLIST FOR AGES 4-16

For office use only
ID #

CHILD'S NAME

PARENT'S TYPE OF WORK (Please be specific—for example: auto mechanic, high school teacher, homemaker, laborer, lathe operator, shoe salesman, army sergeant, even if parent does not live with child.)

SEX	☐ Boy ☐ Girl	AGE		RACE	

FATHER'S TYPE OF WORK:_____

MOTHER'S TYPE OF WORK:_____

TODAY'S DATE

Mo. _____ Day _____ Yr. _____

CHILD'S BIRTHDATE

Mo. _____ Day _____ Yr. _____

THIS FORM FILLED OUT BY:

☐ Mother

☐ Father

☐ Other (Specify):

GRADE IN SCHOOL

I. Please list the sports your child most likes to take part in. For example: swimming, baseball, skating, skate boarding, bike riding, fishing, etc.

☐ None

Compared to other children of the same age, about how much time does he/she spend in each?

Compared to other children of the same age, how well does he/she do each one?

	Don't Know	Less Than Average	Average	More Than Average		Don't Know	Below Average	Average	Above Average
a. _____	☐	☐	☐	☐		☐	☐	☐	☐
b. _____	☐	☐	☐	☐		☐	☐	☐	☐
c. _____	☐	☐	☐	☐		☐	☐	☐	☐

II. Please list your child's favorite hobbies, activities, and games, other than sports. For example: stamps, dolls, books, piano, crafts, singing, etc. (Do not include T.V.)

☐ None

Compared to other children of the same age, about how much time does he/she spend in each?

Compared to other children of the same age, how well does he/she do each one?

	Don't Know	Less Than Average	Average	More Than Average		Don't Know	Below Average	Average	Above Average
a. _____	☐	☐	☐	☐		☐	☐	☐	☐
b. _____	☐	☐	☐	☐		☐	☐	☐	☐
c. _____	☐	☐	☐	☐		☐	☐	☐	☐

III. Please list any organizations, clubs, teams, or groups your child belongs to.

☐ None

Compared to other children of the same age, how active is he/she in each?

	Don't Know	Less Active	Average	More Active
a. _____	☐	☐	☐	☐
b. _____	☐	☐	☐	☐
c. _____	☐	☐	☐	☐

IV. Please list any jobs or chores your child has. For example: paper route, babysitting, making bed, etc.

☐ None

Compared to other children of the same age, how well does he/she carry them out?

	Don't Know	Below Average	Average	Above Average
a. _____	☐	☐	☐	☐
b. _____	☐	☐	☐	☐
c. _____	☐	☐	☐	☐

Figure 5.2 Child Behavior Checklist—Parent Form. From T. M. Achenbach. Child Behavior Checklist for Ages 4–12—Parent Form. Copyright 1981. Used by permission of the author and publisher.

to a clinical diagnosis. "A high score on a behavior problem scale should never be the sole basis for conferring a diagnostic label" (p. 18). The practitioner must be aware that the items on the Achenbach scales were generated through factor analysis. Titles of the scales were arbitrarily determined by the authors. A sample profile for boys ages 6 to 11 years appears in Figure 5.3.

V. 1. About how many close friends does your child have? ☐ None   ☐ 1   ☐ 2 or 3   ☐ 4 or more

    2. About how many times a week does your child do things with them?   ☐ less than 1   ☐ 1 or 2   ☐ 3 or more

VI. Compared to other children of his/her age, how well does your child:

		Worse	About the same	Better
a.	Get along with his/her brothers & sisters?	☐	☐	☐
b.	Get along with other children?	☐	☐	☐
c.	Behave with his/her parents?	☐	☐	☐
d.	Play and work by himself/herself?	☐	☐	☐

VII. 1. Current school performance—for children aged 6 and older:

☐ Does not go to school

	Failing	Below average	Average	Above average
a. Reading or English	☐	☐	☐	☐
b. Writing	☐	☐	☐	☐
c. Arithmetic or Math	☐	☐	☐	☐
d. Spelling	☐	☐	☐	☐
Other academic subjects—for example: history, science, foreign language, geography. e. _____	☐	☐	☐	☐
f. _____	☐	☐	☐	☐
g. _____	☐	☐	☐	☐

2. Is your child in a special class?

☐ No   ☐ Yes—what kind?

3. Has your child ever repeated a grade?

☐ No   ☐ Yes—grade and reason

4. Has your child had any academic or other problems in school?

☐ No   ☐ Yes—please describe

When did these problems start?

Have these problems ended?

☐ No   ☐ Yes—when?

PAGE 2

Figure 5.2 (continued)

Achenbach and Edelbrock (1983), in their taxonomy of profile patterns, present a pattern for attention-disordered children at various ages generally characterized by elevated externalizing scales. It has been difficult to provide a clear-cut profile for children experiencing attention and arousal-related problems. This is not surprising since this population of children frequently presents a heterogeneous group of

VIII. Below is a list of items that describe children. For each item that describes your child **now or within the past 6 months**, please circle the **2** if the item is **very true** or **often true** of your child. Circle the **1** if the item is **somewhat** or **sometimes true** of your child. If the item is **not true** of your child, circle the **0**. Please answer all items as well as you can, even if some do not seem to apply to your child.

0 = Not True (as far as you know)   1 = Somewhat or Sometimes True   2 = Very True or Often True

0 1 2	1.	Acts too young for his/her age 16	0 1 2	31.	Fears he/she might think or do something bad		
0 1 2	2.	Allergy (describe): _____					
			0 1 2	32.	Feels he/she has to be perfect		
			0 1 2	33.	Feels or complains that no one loves him/her		
0 1 2	3.	Argues a lot					
0 1 2	4.	Asthma	0 1 2	34.	Feels others are out to get him/her		
			0 1 2	35.	Feels worthless or inferior 50		
0 1 2	5.	Behaves like opposite sex 20					
0 1 2	6.	Bowel movements outside toilet	0 1 2	36.	Gets hurt a lot, accident-prone		
			0 1 2	37.	Gets in many fights		
0 1 2	7.	Bragging, boasting					
0 1 2	8.	Can't concentrate, can't pay attention for long	0 1 2	38.	Gets teased a lot		
			0 1 2	39.	Hangs around with children who get in trouble		
0 1 2	9.	Can't get his/her mind off certain thoughts; obsessions (describe): _____	0 1 2	40.	Hears things that aren't there (describe): _____ 55		
0 1 2	10.	Can't sit still, restless, or hyperactive 25	0 1 2	41.	Impulsive or acts without thinking		
0 1 2	11.	Clings to adults or too dependent	0 1 2	42.	Likes to be alone		
0 1 2	12.	Complains of loneliness	0 1 2	43.	Lying or cheating		
0 1 2	13.	Confused or seems to be in a fog	0 1 2	44.	Bites fingernails		
0 1 2	14.	Cries a lot	0 1 2	45.	Nervous, highstrung, or tense 60		
0 1 2	15.	Cruel to animals 30	0 1 2	46.	Nervous movements or twitching (describe): _____		
0 1 2	16.	Cruelty, bullying, or meanness to others					
0 1 2	17.	Day-dreams or gets lost in his/her thoughts					
0 1 2	18.	Deliberately harms self or attempts suicide	0 1 2	47.	Nightmares		
0 1 2	19.	Demands a lot of attention	0 1 2	48.	Not liked by other children		
0 1 2	20.	Destroys his/her own things 35	0 1 2	49.	Constipated, doesn't move bowels		
0 1 2	21.	Destroys things belonging to his/her family or other children	0 1 2	50.	Too fearful or anxious 65		
0 1 2	22.	Disobedient at home	0 1 2	51.	Feels dizzy		
			0 1 2	52.	Feels too guilty		
0 1 2	23.	Disobedient at school	0 1 2	53.	Overeating		
0 1 2	24.	Doesn't eat well					
			0 1 2	54.	Overtired		
0 1 2	25.	Doesn't get along with other children 40	0 1 2	55.	Overweight 70		
0 1 2	26.	Doesn't seem to feel guilty after misbehaving		56.	Physical problems without known medical cause:		
0 1 2	27.	Easily jealous	0 1 2	a.	Aches or pains		
0 1 2	28.	Eats or drinks things that are not food (describe): _____	0 1 2	b.	Headaches		
			0 1 2	c.	Nausea, feels sick		
			0 1 2	d.	Problems with eyes (describe):		
0 1 2	29.	Fears certain animals, situations, or places, other than school (describe): _____	0 1 2	e.	Rashes or other skin problems 75		
			0 1 2	f.	Stomachaches or cramps		
			0 1 2	g.	Vomiting, throwing up		
0 1 2	30.	Fears going to school 45	0 1 2	h.	Other (describe): _____		

PAGE 3   **Please see other side**

Figure 5.2 (continued)

additional problems. Many of these children have secondary developmental and conduct problems in addition to their attention-related difficulty. Barkley (1981a) collected data on the Child Behavior Checklist from parents of 60 boys identified as hyperactive. The group profile on the Child Behavior Checklist obtained by Barkley appears in Figure 5.4. Kirby and Grimley (1986) also obtained a typical

0 = Not True (as far as you know)	1 = Somewhat or Sometimes True	2 = Very True or Often True

0 1 2	57.	Physically attacks people	0 1 2	84. Strange behavior (describe): _____
0 1 2	58.	Picks nose, skin, or other parts of body (describe):		
		80	0 1 2	85. Strange ideas (describe):
0 1 2	59.	Plays with own sex parts in public 16		
0 1 2	60.	Plays with own sex parts too much	0 1 2	86. Stubborn, sullen, or irritable
0 1 2	61.	Poor school work	0 1 2	87. Sudden changes in mood or feelings
0 1 2	62.	Poorly coordinated or clumsy	0 1 2	88. Sulks a lot 45
0 1 2	63.	Prefers playing with older children 20	0 1 2	89. Suspicious
0 1 2	64.	Prefers playing with younger children	0 1 2	90. Swearing or obscene language
0 1 2	65.	Refuses to talk	0 1 2	91. Talks about killing self
0 1 2	66.	Repeats certain acts over and over; compulsions (describe):	0 1 2	92. Talks or walks in sleep (describe):
			0 1 2	93. Talks too much 50
0 1 2	67.	Runs away from home	0 1 2	94. Teases a lot
0 1 2	68.	Screams a lot 25	0 1 2	95. Temper tantrums or hot temper
0 1 2	69.	Secretive, keeps things to self	0 1 2	96. Thinks about sex too much
0 1 2	70.	Sees things that aren't there (describe):	0 1 2	97. Threatens people
			0 1 2	98. Thumb-sucking 55
			0 1 2	99. Too concerned with neatness or cleanliness
			0 1 2	100. Trouble sleeping (describe):
0 1 2	71.	Self-conscious or easily embarrassed		
0 1 2	72.	Sets fires		
0 1 2	73.	Sexual problems (describe):	0 1 2	101. Truancy, skips school
			0 1 2	102. Underactive, slow moving, or lacks energy
		30	0 1 2	103. Unhappy, sad, or depressed 60
0 1 2	74.	Showing off or clowning	0 1 2	104. Unusually loud
0 1 2	75.	Shy or timid	0 1 2	105. Uses alcohol or drugs (describe):
0 1 2	76.	Sleeps less than most children		
0 1 2	77.	Sleeps more than most children during day and/or night (describe):	0 1 2	106. Vandalism
			0 1 2	107. Wets self during the day
0 1 2	78.	Smears or plays with bowel movements 35	0 1 2	108. Wets the bed 65
0 1 2	79.	Speech problem (describe):	0 1 2	109. Whining
			0 1 2	110. Wishes to be of opposite sex
0 1 2	80.	Stares blankly	0 1 2	111. Withdrawn, doesn't get involved with others
			0 1 2	112. Worrying
0 1 2	81.	Steals at home		113. Please write in any problems your child has that were not listed above:
0 1 2	82.	Steals outside the home		
0 1 2	83.	Stores up things he/she doesn't need (describe):	0 1 2	70
		40	0 1 2	
			0 1 2	

PLEASE BE SURE YOU HAVE ANSWERED ALL ITEMS. PAGE 4 UNDERLINE ANY YOU ARE CONCERNED ABOUT.

Figure 5.2 (continued)

profile for children in their ADD sample. Both studies concurred with Achenbach and Edelbrock's results in finding that this population of children scored extremely high on externalizing scales.

ADD Children also presented difficulty on the social withdrawal and obsessive/-compulsive scales. This, too, makes sense. For example, items on the obsessive/

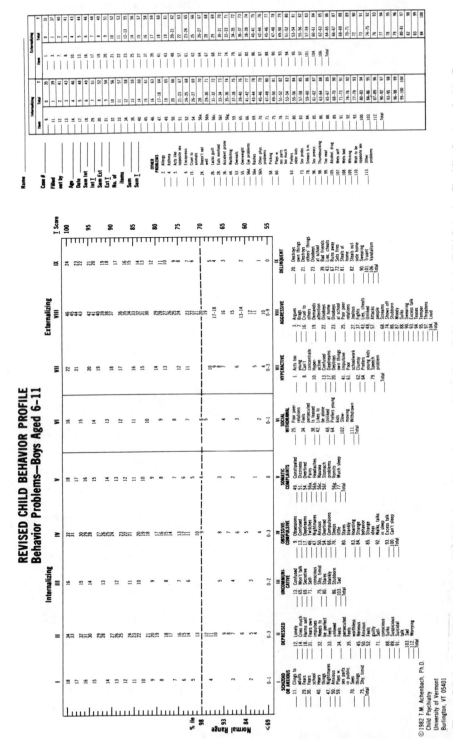

Figure 5.3 Revised child behavior profile: Behavior problems, boys ages 6–11. From T. M. Achenbach, Child Behavior Checklist for Ages 6–11—Parent Form. Copyright 1982. Used by permission of the author and the publisher.

108

REVISED CHILD BEHAVIOR PROFILE
Social Competence—Boys Aged 4-5, 6-11, 12-16

ACTIVITIES
I. A. # of sports
   B. Mean of participation and skill in sports
II. A. # of nonsports activities
    B. Mean of participation and skill in activities
IV. A. # of jobs
    B. Mean job quality
Total

SOCIAL
III. A. # of organizations
     B. Mean of participation in organizations
V. 1. # of friends
   2. Frequency of contacts with friends
VI. A. Behavior with others
    B. Behavior alone
Total

SCHOOL
VII. 1. Mean performance
     2. Special class
     3. Repeated grade
     4. School problems
Total
*Not scored for 4-5-year-olds

Name ___
Case # ___
Age ___
Date CBCL filled out ___
CBCL filled out by ___
Sum of social competence scores ___
Sum I ___

T Score

Figure 5.3 (continued)

© 1982 T.M. Achenbach. Ph.D.
Child Psychiatry
University of Vermont
Burlington, VT 05401

109

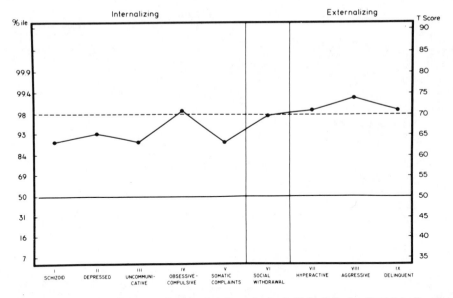

Figure 5.4 Profile for 60 hyperactive boys on the Achenbach Child Behavior Checklist—Parent Form. From R. Barkley, *Hyperactive Children* (p. 26). Copyright 1981 by Guilford Press. Used with permission of the author and publisher.

compulsive scale include difficulty with daydreaming, talking excessively, perseverating on thoughts or ideas, having difficulty with sleep and, at times, odd or different behavior. All of these behaviors are frequently characteristic of attention-disordered children as are problems with peer relations. Scores on the hyperactive scale have also been found to correlate significantly with high symptom scores for ADD based upon a child assessment interview (Hodges, Kline, Stern, Cytryn & McKnew, 1982).

Home Situations Questionnaire

This questionnaire (Figure 5.5) was developed by Russell Barkley (1981a) as a means of assessing the impact of the child's attention and related deficits upon home and community-based situations. As with the School Situations Questionnaire, this form allows the practitioner to make the important connection between the child's difficulties and the specific situations in which those difficulties cause problems. This form is invaluable during the history session as the practitioner attempts to understand the approaches that parents use to manage the child's behavior in various situations and settings. Barkley developed this questionnaire to provide the practitioner with qualitative as opposed to quantitative data. Barkley noted that attention-disordered children present with problems in at least 50% of most home situations. Breen (1986) has developed normative data for the Home Situations Questionnaire for children ranging in age from 4 to 11 years. The data is presented in Table 5.1. Breen's data suggests that of the 16 situations, the average non-ADHD child experiences, at most, mild problems in only a few situations.

HOME SITUATIONS QUESTIONNAIRE

Name of Child _____

Person Completing This Form _____
/ / Mother   / / Father   / / Foster Parent

Does the child or adolescent present problems in any of these situations? If so, indicate the severity of the problem and a brief description if possible.

Situation	Yes/No (Circle One)	If yes, how severe? (Circle One) Mild								Severe
When playing alone	Yes No	1	2	3	4	5	6	7	8	9
When playing with other children	Yes No	1	2	3	4	5	6	7	8	9
When at meals	Yes No	1	2	3	4	5	6	7	8	9
When getting dressed	Yes No	1	2	3	4	5	6	7	8	9
When washing/bathing	Yes No	1	2	3	4	5	6	7	8	9
When you are on the telephone	Yes No	1	2	3	4	5	6	7	8	9
When watching TV	Yes No	1	2	3	4	5	6	7	8	9
When visitors are in your home	Yes No	1	2	3	4	5	6	7	8	9
When you are visiting someone else	Yes No	1	2	3	4	5	6	7	8	9
When in supermarkets, stores, church, restaurants, or other public places	Yes No	1	2	3	4	5	6	7	8	9
When asked to do chores at home	Yes No	1	2	3	4	5	6	7	8	9
When going to bed	Yes No	1	2	3	4	5	6	7	8	9
When in the car	Yes No	1	2	3	4	5	6	7	8	9
When with a babysitter	Yes No	1	2	3	4	5	6	7	8	9
When at school	Yes No	1	2	3	4	5	6	7	8	9
When asked to do school homework	Yes No	1	2	3	4	5	6	7	8	9

Figure 5.5 Home Situations Questionnaire. From R. Barkley, *Hyperactive Children*. Copyright 1981 by Guilford Press. Used with permission of the author and publisher.

A significant percentage of attention-disordered children experience difficulty when playing with others, at meals, when parents are on the telephone, when visitors are in the home, when visiting someone else, when accompanying parents in public places, when asked to do chores at home and when going to bed (Barkley, 1981a). Attention-disordered children are least likely to experience problems when playing alone. This makes sense since they have no one to disagree with, and

TABLE 5.1.   Normative Data for the Home Situations Questionnaire

Age	n	Number of Problem Settings	Mean Severity
Boys:			
4–5	162	3.1 (2.8)*	1.7 (1.4)
6–8	205	4.1 (3.3)	2.0 (1.4)
9–11	138	3.6 (3.3)	1.9 (1.5)
Girls:			
4–5	146	2.2 (2.6)	1.3 (1.4)
6–8	202	3.4 (3.5)	1.6 (1.5)
9–11	142	2.7 (3.2)	1.4 (1.4)

*Note: These entries are means with standard deviations in parentheses.
Breen, M. J. "Norms for the Home Situations Questionnaire" Copyright 1986 by *ADD/Hyperactivity Newsletter*. Used by permission of the publisher.

so long as they can find something to interest them or multiple tasks to engage in that do not threaten their own safety, they can frequently occupy themselves. Barkley (1981a) suggests that if problems occur in specific home situations, the examiner should question parents concerning what it is about the child's behavior that disturbs them, how they respond, what the child does next, how often the problem occurs and how the problem is finally dealt with.

Social Skills Assessment

The Social Skills Assessment (Goldstein, 1988a) was developed to assist the practitioner in gaining descriptive data about the child's social behavior. (See Figure 5.6.) As with the Teacher Social Skills Assessment, this form is used qualitatively and no normative data has been collected by the author. Discussing their responses on this questionnaire with parents during the history session is helpful. This questionnaire also helps the practitioner make specific treatment recommendations for the development of deficient social skills.

Additional Parent Report Questionnaires

There are additional questionnaires that practitioners may find helpful. The Werry-Weiss-Peters Activity Scale (Werry, 1968) presents seven behavioral categories, five of which relate to situations in the home (i.e., doing homework, playing, sleeping) and two for areas of activity in situations outside of the home (i.e., behavior at school and in the community). Ross and Ross (1982) suggest that this scale is a measure of inappropriate activity rather than of total activity. It is therefore useful in the assessment of the hyperactive component of attention-deficit disorder. The scale was shortened by Routh, Schroeder and O'Tauma (1974). Normative data has been collected for children ranging in age from three to nine years.

SOCIAL SKILLS ASSESSMENT
(Parent Form)

Name _____   Date _____

Individual Completing this Form _____
                         / / Mother   / / Father   / / Foster Parent

Description: Please check any statements which you feel describe your child or
             adolescent. Please make note if there are differences in your child's
             behavior with siblings or peers.

Not True	Sometimes True	Frequently True	My child:
___	___	___	appears socially isolated. For example, he or she spends a large proportion of time engaged in solitary activities, and may be judged independent and capable of taking care of himself/herself.
___	___	___	interacts less with friends, appearing shy and timid. My child can be described as somewhat overanxious with others.
___	___	___	spends less time involved in activities with other children due to a lack of social skills and/or appropriate social judgment.
___	___	___	appears to have fewer friends than other children due to negative, bossy or annoying behaviors which "turn off" others.
___	___	___	spends less time with friends than most due to awkward or bizarre behaviors.
___	___	___	disturbs others: teases, provokes, fights, interrupts others.
___	___	___	openly strikes back with angry behavior to the teasing of other children.
___	___	___	can be argumentative and must have the last word in verbal exchanges.
___	___	___	displays physical aggression towards objects or persons.
___	___	___	will manipulate or threaten peers.
___	___	___	speaks to others in an inpatient or cranky tone of voice.
___	___	___	says uncomplimentary or unpleasant things to others. For example, may engage in name calling or ridicule.

-over-

Figure 5.6 Social Skills Assessment—Parent Form. From S. Goldstein, Social Skills Assessment
Questionnaire. Printed with permission of the author. Copyright applied for.

The Personality Inventory for Children (Wirt et al., 1977), contains a reasonably
good hyperactivity scale. This questionnaire is considered to be the childhood
equivalent of the Minnesota Multiphasic Personality Inventory. The inventory is
completed by parents based on observations of their children. The 600 true/false
items on the inventory yield 14 clinical subscale scores and 2 validity subscale
scores. Normative data has been collected for children ranging in age from 3 to 16

Social Skills Assessment
Page two

Not True	Sometimes True	Frequently True	My child:
___	___	___	will respond when other children initiate conversation.
___	___	___	will engage in long conversations.
___	___	___	will share laughter with friends.
___	___	___	will spontaneously contribute to a family discussion.
___	___	___	can take a leadership role at home.
___	___	___	will work with family members on projects
___	___	___	can verbally initiate with family members.

Additional Comments: _____

_____

_____

_____

_____

_____

_____

_____

_____

_____

_____

_____

_____

Figure 5.6 (continued)

years. The hyperactivity subscale is comprised of 36 of the 600 items. Because the length of the questionnaire was seen as a disadvantage by many practitioners, the authors recently published normative data for a shortened form. The Personality Inventory for Children has proven to be a difficult questionnaire for parents with literacy problems. However, when a child is presenting a complex or confusing pattern of behavioral problems, it may be helpful in assisting with differential diagnosis. Additionally, Voelker, Lachar and Gadowski (1983) collected data suggesting that the Personality Inventory for Children may be useful in predicting response to stimulant treatment.

The SNAP Checklist (Pelham et al., 1981b) has been structured primarily from the diagnostic criteria for attention-deficit disorder contained in the DSM-III (APA,

1980). The authors suggest that either these items can be read to parents or parents can complete the questionnaire on their own. The questionnaire can also be used with teachers. The authors collected brief normative teacher data for elementary school children. A similar 15-item questionnaire also using DSM-III criteria was developed by Ozawa and Michael (1983).

With preschoolers, attempts at assessing temperament, as distinct from behavior that has been primarily shaped and influenced by the environment, are also helpful for gaining insight into the child's behavior. Temperament questionnaires developed by Thomas and Chess (1977) and Carey (1970) have been norm-referenced and are useful as part of a clinical assessment. The practitioner is cautioned, however, not to arbitrarily assume that patterns of behavior generated on the basis of these questionnaires are primarily or solely a function of temperament versus environmental experience. The practitioner is also cautioned that the older the child, the more likely it is that the environment has played a role in shaping the child's behavior.

Suggested Combination of Questionnaires

In addition to the completed history form, a combination of the Child Behavior Checklist, Conners Parent's Questionnaire, Home Situations Questionnaire and Social Skills Assessment provides quantitative and qualitative behavioral descriptions of the child in the home and community. The history form and questionnaires should be completed by parents before the parent interview/history session so that the information is available at that time for review and clarification. In addition, the history form and completed questionnaires provide an essential organizing framework for conducting the parent interview/history session.

PARENT LOG

During the parent interview/history session it is often readily apparent to the practitioner when an ADHD child's parents are contributing significantly to their child's behavioral problems. In some situations, however, despite the history and questionnaires, that determination is not easily made. In those situations it may be beneficial for the practitioner to request parents to maintain a log or diary covering two or three of the most problematic behaviors and situations in which they occur. A parent data sheet can be constructed fairly simply. It is suggested that the behavior to be observed be operationally defined at the top of the sheet. The sheet can then be divided into four columns containing the date, time, parent's action and child's response. It is important for the practitioner to assist parents in operationally defining the problems and to help them understand that the time spent collecting this data is useful not only for the diagnostic process but also for developing a treatment plan. Data-gathering can help parents accurately track their responses to problematic behaviors. Parents can be encouraged to attempt a number of different interventions and to evaluate their impact by monitoring the child's responses. It is suggested that initially parents track only one of the more significant behavior problems. As they become more proficient in data collection, two or three behavioral problems can be tracked at the same time.

PARENTING-STYLE INTERVIEW

If the practitioner suspects that parental expectations, interactional style or general behavior play a significant role in the development and maintenance of the ADHD child's problems, it may be beneficial to conduct a separate interview concerning parenting style. Data gathered during such an interview can prove invaluable in helping parents understand the role they may play in their child's behavioral difficulty and in making them more effective facilitators of behavioral change in their child. The purpose of the interview is not only to gain practical data concerning parent problem solving skills but also to develop an understanding of the parents' philosophy and perception of parenting.

It may be beneficial to begin the interview by asking the parents whether or not they have some particular philosophy about how children should be raised. Parents often find that a challenging question, but after a few moments of thought, their answers may be quite revealing about the manner in which they interact with their children. The extreme responses may range from the view that children should be seen and not heard to the view that children should be allowed to do whatever they want because these are the formative years and discipline may stifle their future creativity.

Frequently, parents are not aware of the impact their behavior has on their children's personality development and future behavior. In many cases, parents inadequately describe their own behavior and, more importantly, the reasons that motivated their behavior. The goal of this type of interview is to gather information about parenting style. Determining whether parental style is good or bad is not the issue. Instead, the practitioner attempts to understand parental style and the way it shapes the child's behavior.

Through experience, the authors have identified ten parenting variables that appear to underlie and affect the manner in which parents interact with their children. The best way to obtain information concerning these underlying parent variables is to provide parents with examples of hypothetical problem situations and interpret their responses. Each variable will be defined and an illustrative problem situation that the practitioner can use to gain data about the variable will be provided. For each sample situation, a number of multiple-choice responses are offered, but it is suggested that hypothetical situations be presented without these responses. If parents have difficulty generating a response, multiple-choice alternatives can be helpful in providing them with a structure for responding.

Variable One: Consistency

Consistency is a critical parenting behavior. Research has found that children can tolerate a variety of adult behavior so long as that behavior is predictable.

Children have greater difficulty tolerating inconsistency. If children are dealt with inconsistently by their parents, they will have a difficult time dealing effectively with people in other areas of their lives, including adults and children at school and personal friends. Because of the unpredictability of their behavior ADHD children are at significant risk to be dealt with inconsistently by even the most competent parents. The combination of an ADHD child and an inconsistent parent frequently leads to significant behavioral problems. It is important for the practitioner to develop some understanding of the parent's behavior as it relates to consistency. A sample situation for a young child follows.

> Assume the rule in your house is that toys must be put away when young children are finished playing with them. Your child is slow to put away his toys and you must leave the house with your child. You would:

a. quickly help the child clean up;

b. allow the child to clean up later when you return;

c. wait until the child is done, no matter how long the child takes;

d. punish the child by taking the toys away and then leave;

e. put all the toys away yourself.

The rigidly consistent parent will wait until the child is completed, no matter how long it takes. The inconsistent parent will put the toys away herself. The flexibly consistent parent will assist the child but insist that the toys be put away before leaving.

Variable Two: Passivity/Democracy/Autocracy

Parents usually deal with their children in one of three manners. They may be democratic, making decisions with the child's input; autocratic, making decisions without the child's input; or passive, allowing the child to make decisions alone. Both autocratic and passive parents often encounter great difficulty with their children's adjustment. Autocratic parents often end up in significant power struggles with their ADHD children. The ADHD child is frequently unable to meet the autocratic parent's demands. Over time, a significant pattern of oppositional, resistant behavior develops as the child repeatedly fails and is punished. Alternatively, some parents of ADHD children become passive over time and set minimal limits rather than engage in repeated conflicts with the child. Although the passive parent avoids conflict, in the long run passivity does not help the child develop an internal sense of responsibility and maturity. Autocratic parents make decisions for the child; passive parents play little or no role; democratic parents provide input and work cooperatively with the child to reach decisions. A sample question for an adolescent follows.

> Your teenager has the opportunity to choose between two summer jobs with very different responsibilities but similar salary. You are aware of the choices she faces. You:

a. say nothing, allowing her to choose;
b. insist on discussing it with her, citing pros and cons, but allowing her to choose;
c. make the decision for her based upon your greater experience;
d. strongly recommend one choice, allowing her to have the final say;
e. offer to discuss it with her but allow her to choose regardless.

Variable Three: Conformity

From infancy, parents subtly or directly teach their children to think for themselves or to routinely behave in the manner expected by others. In the extreme, completely conforming children have difficulty thinking for themselves. Many parents, especially those stressing conformity, may pressure the ADHD child to "fit in" and meet the expectations of others. These children, who are temperamentally nonconforming, often experience difficulty following rules and limits. Additionally, because of their inability to meet the expectations of others and their repeated failures, ADHD children may become excessively nonconforming as a means of coping with their environment. The combination of a rigidly conforming parent and an ADHD child may lead to an exponential increase of problems. A sample question for a preschool child follows.

At snack time in kindergarten, milk is routinely served with cookies. Your child complains that he doesn't like milk and he doesn't want to drink it at school. You then:

a. insist that he must drink milk at school like everyone else;
b. discuss it with him in an attempt to reach a compromise for him to drink at least some of the milk;
c. restrict cookies at school unless milk is drunk;
d. discuss alternatives with the child and then present them to the teacher, attempting to reach a compromise;
e. tell the child he doesn't have to drink the milk, should have his cookie and send a note stating so to his teacher.

Insisting the child must drink milk at school like everyone else fosters blind conformity to society's rules and limits. At the other extreme, allowing the child to avoid the milk issue altogether may foster too much nonconformity.

Variable Four: Self-Esteem

Many factors influence the way a child feels about herself. These include the manner in which she is parented and the success she has with friends and teachers. Since a child does not often think about or evaluate herself, she usually responds in a manner that reflects how she has been dealt with by others. Without realizing it, many parents of ADHD children subtly undermine and sabotage the child's self-esteem. Inability to meet parental demands causes the ADHD child to receive a significant amount of negative feedback related to competence and worth, typically characterized by comments such as, "Quit it, stop it, cut it out, don't do that, can't you do anything right?" A sample question for an elementary age child follows.

> Your child experiences the loss of a close friend. She expresses concern to you that she won't be able to make another close friend ever again. You:
>
> a. discuss what she may have done to lose that friend;
> b. reassure her that friends are easy to make;
> c. discuss with her how she made and kept that friendship, emphasizing her worth as a person;
> d. point out that she has other friends;
> e. do nothing, she will get over it.

Allowing the child to understand the role she may play in friendships and realistically praising her past successes while building her self-confidence and motivation for future social contacts is an important self-esteem builder.

Variable Five: Responsibility

ADHD children have great difficulty developing an internal sense of responsibility because of their skill deficits and repeated failures. They frequently remain externally controlled. As children grow, we hope that they will internalize control and learn to deal appropriately with society, not because they have to, but because they want to. The development of responsibility is often a sore point for many parents of ADHD children. A sample question for an adolescent follows.

> Your son agrees to fill in for a friend at work on a Saturday. At the last minute your son is invited to go water skiing. Water skiing is a very special event. He is uncertain what he should do and wants your recommendation. You:
>
> a. tell him he must work;
> b. tell him to go skiing;
> c. encourage him to find someone else to fill in at work;
> d. tell him to go skiing if he can get a friend to work;
> e. review all of the alternatives and allow him to make the decision.

Fostering responsibility requires parents to help their ADHD children develop a sense of obligation to themselves and to others. Telling the child what to do does not foster responsibility. Providing alternatives for children and being supportive of their choices but allowing them to experience the natural consequences of these choices certainly fosters responsible behavior. The practitioner must be aware however that ADHD children may require specific educational training to ameliorate their incompetencies in addition to experiencing natural consequence for their actions. More information will be provided concerning this point in the intervention chapters.

Variable Six: Sexual Stereotypes

The emphasis on sexual stereotypes in our society is not surprising. Research has indicated that even as young as two years of age, children are bombarded with messages to behave in ways consistent with and expected for their sex. ADHD males are often excused for their behavior problems with the saying, "He is just a boy." However, sexual stereotypes and stereotypic behavior often impede children in many situations. A sample question for an elementary age child follows.

> Your daughter comes home and wants to join the local little league baseball team. She is a fairly athletic child. You:
>
> a. tell her baseball is only for boys and end the discussion;
> b. offer her an alternative activity such as volleyball;
> c. discuss the pros and cons with her and let her make the decision;
> d. take her right down and sign her up;
> e. seek out an all-girl baseball team.

It has been suggested that children with fewer sexual stereotypes have better potential to succeed socially and academically. The ability to combine what have been typically defined as male and female characteristics has been found to be a positive personality trait. It is beneficial to avoid teaching children sexually stereotypic behavior.

Variable Seven: Emotions

Many adults have difficulty dealing with and expressing their feelings. It is not surprising, therefore, that many children have the same problem. Researchers suggest that individuals unable to express their feelings and emotions appropriately are at increased risk for psychological stress and physical responses such as ulcers. ADHD children, who typically express their emotions quickly and intensely, may constantly receive messages to repress rather than control their feelings and emotional reactions. A sample question for a preschool child follows.

> Your child's grandparent passes away. You:
>
> a. show no emotion in front of the child;
> b. discuss your feelings with the child;
> c. openly display grief and anguish in front of the child;

d. act as if nothing happened in front of the child;

e. display your emotions and discuss them with the child.

Variable Eight: Problem Solving

To deal effectively with the world it is important for children to recognize a problem, define it effectively, review alternatives and make appropriate decisions. Effective problem solving is important in all areas of our lives. Their impulsive, inattentive nature makes ADHD children typically poor problem solvers. Often, parents do not realize that the manner in which they deal with their own problems can have a positive or negative effect on the development of the child's problem-solving behavior. A parent modeling effective problem solving increases the chances of even an ADHD child becoming a more effective problem solver. A sample question for an elementary age child follows.

Your child comes home with a social studies project. You:

a. tell her to work on it whenever she wants to, as long as it gets done by the deadline;

b. sit down and plan out a work schedule for the child to complete the project in small parts;

c. assist the child in determining a work schedule;

d. threaten restrictions if the work isn't completed by the deadline;

e. tell the child to get started and check on her progress periodically.

Variable Nine: Reward

Most parents have at least a superficial awareness that behavior that is reinforced or rewarded is strengthened and will be exhibited at a later time. Parents are often unaware of the subtle reinforcement and rewards they provide for many behaviors their children exhibit. With ADHD children it is fairly common for a pattern of negative reinforcement to develop between the parents and child. Parents do not recognize the complexity of this type of behavior. Sample questions dealing with positive reinforcement for an adolescent and negative reinforcement for a latency age child are provided.

Your teenage daughter, generally a good student, comes home with an A− average on her final report card. You are pleased and you:

a. send her on a trip for the summer;

b. take her on a limited clothing/shopping trip;

c. do nothing except tell her what a good job she has done and to keep up the good work;

  d. give her a few choices for rewards to choose from;

  e. extend her curfew by one hour.

You send your eight-year-old son into his room to get dressed. Ten minutes later you check on him, and although he had begun to prepare his clothes, he did not begin dressing and had begun looking at a favorite book. You:

  a. tell him to get started again, watch to see that he does and then leave;

  b. tell him to get started again and walk out;

  c. threaten to restrict television that evening if he does not finish dressing immediately and walk out;

  d. tell him to start dressing again and stay there until he completes the task;

  e. say nothing to him but just walk out.

A discussion of rewards must focus on the parent's ability to choose appropriate rewards and use them effectively. Some parents fail to acknowledge significant achievement; others over-reward for minor accomplishments. With ADHD children, it is especially important to review the issue of negative reinforcement with parents, helping them understand that pattern of behavior and the role they may play in reinforcing their child for beginning but not completing tasks. Guidelines for dealing with negative reinforcement problems will be reviewed in the intervention chapters.

Variable Ten: Punishment

Parents usually attempt to develop good behavior in their children by first offering rewards. When this fails, they resort in a reactionary manner to their second choice, punishment. Punishment requires the occurrence of an aversive consequence following a particular behavior. Punishment can be an effective intervention, but it must be appropriate and followed by giving the child the opportunity first to learn and then to exhibit the appropriate alternative behavior. ADHD children frequently may be punished for nonpurposeful behavior that results from incompetence. Punishing the child without affording the opportunity to learn more appropriate behavior often leads to an increasing spiral of failed punishments in an attempt to change the child's behavior. A sample question for a preschool child follows.

Your child continues to hit his sister after a positively stated direction to stop. You:

  a. warn him again;

  b. send him to his room, telling him he can come out when he can behave himself;

  c. spank him;

  d. time him out for one minute and allow him to continue playing with his sibling;

e. immediately restrict a privilege such as watching television later in the evening.

The final part of the parenting style interview may consist of providing the parents with typical child behavior problems and assessing their general strategy and capacity to respond. Gardner (1982b) provides a set of 16 typical child behavior problems as part of a maternal discipline interview. The Maternal Discipline Techniques—Self-Report Instrument appears in Appendix 2.

NECESSARY DATA FOR CONFIRMING ADHD

In making the diagnosis of ADHD within the home setting, it is recommended that a child be approximately two standard deviations higher than the same sex-and-age normative group for the hyperkinesis index on the Conners Parent's Rating Questionnaire. It is additionally recommended that problems with attention and overarousal should cause the child difficulty in at least 50% of home and community situations. The majority of ADHD children also experience chronic problems with attention and arousal from infancy. These problems are recognized before the child enters an organized school setting. A careful collection of behavioral data referenced to a variety of specific situations and an analysis of parenting style assist the practitioner in beginning to make a differential diagnosis between temperamental problems and environmentally reinforced difficulty.

SUMMARY

This chapter provided a model for the collection of home data, including the child's behavior, functioning within the community and relationship with parents and peers. Assessment of ADHD within the home must involve the collection of a careful parental history to determine whether the etiological sequence of behavioral events is characteristic for ADHD children. Parent questionnaires, including the Conners Parent's Rating Scale and Achenbach Child Behavior Checklist, are invaluable in providing a norm-referenced measure of the child's home behavior. Assessment is even more complex for preschoolers and adolescents. The former group usually has not had sufficient interaction with the community for the examiner to obtain useful data from adults other than parents. The latter group typically has had a very long history of problems, making it difficult to separate a temperamental disorder from the development of an inappropriate behavioral repertoire primarily as a result of negative interactions with the environment. With complex behavioral problems, an indepth parenting-style interview and a parent log are often helpful in providing insight into parent-child interaction. Direct observation of the interaction between parents and child is usually obtained in an unstructured manner during the history session or as part of the evaluative process.

CHAPTER 6

Clinical Evaluation of Attention Problems

The development of a norm-referenced psychometric assessment battery for attention problems has been an elusive goal for researchers and practitioners. Some believe that an attention-related battery is an attainable goal (Gardner, 1982a). Others argue that psychometric tests for children experiencing attention problems without concomitant learning disability are unnecessary (Barkley, 1981a). This text's definition of attention disorder incorporates the proposition that the child's attention and reflection disabilities must be observed on standardized, norm-referenced assessment instruments. Structured psychometric testing also affords the practitioner the opportunity to interact with the child in a well-defined situation, which adds additional qualitative data. A clinical or school psychologist is best qualified to administer psychometric instruments. The majority of instruments presented in this chapter are fairly simple, and other professionals with appropriate training, including physicians, nurses, speech pathologists and neuropsychology technicians, can administer them efficiently and effectively. Interpretation of the test scores is a more complex process, especially in the area of attention deficit. The practitioner must be able to integrate quantitative performance, qualitative observations of the child's style and motivation and other sources of assessment data.

This chapter will provide a brief overview of research in this area, presenting specific tests and batteries of tests that have been developed to measure attentional skills. Suggestions for observing the child's behavior during the evaluation and making inferences about motivation, attention and emotional status will be described. Clinical instruments, listed according to the specific type of attentional skill they appear to measure, will be reviewed. The chapter will conclude with suggestions for a clinical interview and assessment of the child's personality and emotional adjustment. The practitioner must always be sensitive to the fact that chronic problems with attention span, impulsivity, frustration and overarousal will have a pervasive impact on personality style and overall test performance.

ASSESSMENT OF ATTENTIONAL SKILLS

It is well recognized by the experienced practitioner that there is a marked degree of heterogeneity in problems with attentional skills for the population of children diagnosed as ADHD. Mesulam (1985) notes that there is an advantage and practical value in assessing the various components of attention separately. The assessment of attentional skills provides a backdrop against which other skills are measured. For example, hypothesized cognitive impairments resulting from assessment of an inattentive, impulsive child are certainly suspect. The development of an appropriate treatment plan designed specifically for each child necessitates the objective assessment of various attentional skills.

The clinical evaluation of the potential ADHD child includes a number of components. The most common psychometric tests used for the attention-deficient child include tasks measuring reflection, vigilance and sustained attention. There are a number of tasks that also measure selective, divided and focused attentional skills. None of these tests are a pure measure of attentional ability, and critics have argued that many tests designed to measure attentional skills focus on reliability, often at the expense of validity (Werry, 1978). The majority of psychometric tests presented in this chapter were not designed as primary measures of attention and reflection capability, but do appear to have face validity. A wide sample of psychometric tests is presented in this chapter to acquaint the practitioner with their attentional components and to allow the practitioner to experiment and eventually determine which instruments he or she finds to be sensitive indicators during clinical assessment. For example, research has demonstrated that maze tasks are sensitive measures of reflective capability and can be of assistance in making the ADHD diagnosis. Some practitioners find maze tasks helpful and use them; others do not. At the close of the chapter, the authors will present the assessment instruments that they typically use during psychometric testing.

It is a valid point that qualitative inferences of a child's attention and reflection capabilities can be made based on that child's interaction with any psychometric measure, structured task or interview. The clinical evaluation, therefore, must also include a qualitative assessment by the examiner of the child's attentional, problem-solving and reflection skills. In some situations it is helpful to obtain information concerning the child's or adolescent's insight into his or her problems. A structured self-report questionnaire or incomplete-sentences task in addition to the clinical interview can prove helpful in obtaining this type of information.

It is not the intent of this chapter to provide a broad outline of psychological or psychometric testing. The psychometric tests presented are offered specifically to assist in the measurement and observation of attention and reflection skills. During an in-depth assessment of a child experiencing attention, learning and/or behavior problems, these tasks must be integrated into the overall evaluation. A complete psychometric or psychological battery for such a child might additionally include the full administration of the Wechsler Intelligence Scale for Children—Revised; measures of motor, perceptual and academic skills; and an in-depth assessment of the child's personality.

AN OVERVIEW OF ASSESSMENT TASKS

A brief overview will acquaint the practitioner with the breadth and scope of research efforts in the area of assessment of attention. Over the past 30 years, researchers have attempted to develop laboratory tasks that could measure a specific component of attention or reflectional skill (Rosenthal & Allen, 1978). For example, reaction tasks involving either immediate or prolonged attention by the child to visual stimuli presented on a screen yield data suggesting that inattentive children make more errors that go uncorrected (Douglas, 1972). The most sensitive of these measures is the Continuous Performance Test, which was developed by Rosvold, Mirsky, Sarason, Bransome and Beck (1956). The test was originally designed to be a measure of brain injury, but both the auditory and visual components of this test appear sensitive as measures of vigilance and reflective capability (Douglas, 1972).

The concept of the original Continuous Performance Test has been revised and expanded a number of times. Gordon (1983) developed a portable apparatus, the Gordon Diagnostic System, using a continuous performance task. Garfinkel and Klee (1983) developed a continuous performance test as part of an attentional battery. This battery also includes a computerized progressive maze task and a task of sequential organization. Shapiro and Garfinkel (1986) found this attentional battery to discriminate between a nonreferred normal population and children experiencing attentional problems. The battery, however, was not able to discriminate between a group of children with attention problems and a second group experiencing specific conduct problems.

Goldberg and Konstantareas (1981) developed the Operant Vigilance Task. The task requires the child to push a button that initially presents a stimulus picture of a clown. The child must then push another button if the clown is missing a nose. Children with attention problems were slower to respond and made more errors of commission when the stimulus was intact.

A large body of research data (Douglas, 1972; 1974; Cohen, Weiss & Minde, 1972) eventually demonstrated that it is the inattentive child's lack of persistence, not necessarily distractions in the environment, that draws the child off task. Despite this research, tests of distractibility continue to be of interest. A number of these tasks are also sensitive measures of divided attention. Color distraction tasks (Stroop, 1935; Santostefano & Paley, 1964) assess the child's ability to name items or colors when the stimuli being presented are interfered with by distracting cues. Douglas (1972) found that children with attentional problems make more errors of commission that go uncorrected. When the inattentive group was receiving stimulant medication, the difference between the normal and inattentive groups did not measure as statistically significant.

Complex visual tasks that require a degree of reflective strategy for successful performance and that are designed to produce frustration have been found to be sensitive discriminators between inattentive and normal children. Mazes are an example of this type of task. The most widely researched and clinically used of these reflective tasks is the Matching Familiar Figures Test (Kagan, Rosman, Day, Albert & Phillips, 1964). Although the Matching Familiar Figures Test has its critics (Egeland & Weinberg, 1976; Berry & Cook, 1980), there is extensive data that attention-deficient children are more disorganized, respond quicker and make more matching errors on this task than normal children. Kuehne (1985) found that both the Matching Familiar Figures Test and the Porteus Mazes Test significantly discriminated between attention-disordered and normal children.

The Children's Embedded Figures Test (Karp & Konsteadt, 1971) represents another class of tests that appear to be sensitive to sustained attention and organizational skill. The Visual Closure Subtest of the Illinois Test of Psycholinguistic Abilities is a similar measure. These tests require the child to locate stimulus items that are hidden in a larger visual field. These tasks also require adequate visual/perceptive skills. Kirby and Grimley (1986) found the Children's Embedded Figures Test to be a sensitive discriminator between inattentive and normal children.

The majority of research based assessment instruments in this area have been designed for, and used with, children (6 to 12 years of age). Assessment of preschool children with attentional problems more often focuses on observation of the child in the laboratory or preschool setting. Campbell et al. (1982) observed inattentive two-and three-year-olds shifting activity more readily in a free play setting and exhibiting more problems with restlessness, out-of-seat and off-task behavior in structured situations where reflection and sustained attention are required. In adolescents, a careful history is often the most valuable component of assessment for attentional problems.

Kaufman (1979), based upon factor analytic research, suggests that three of the Wechsler Intelligence Scale for Children-Revised subtests (Arithmetic, Coding and Digit Span) may cluster, demonstrating deviation in a negative direction from the overall Verbal, Performance or Full-Scale intellectual scores. Kaufman arbitrarily applied the label Freedom From Distractibility to this factor. Even though the deviations on these subtests may not be significant, if all three subtests present in a similar manner, deficient performance may result from an inability by the child to focus attention on the task at hand. Kaufman, however, does not make a clear distinction between the various components of attentional difficulty that could account for a poor performance on these three subtests. He notes that low scores on this factor could also be caused by sequencing difficulty, anxiety problems or an inability to manipulate numerical symbols. The practitioner is cautioned to use behavioral observation and the quality of the child's responses in attempting to explain poor performance on these three subtests. The practitioner is also cautioned not to blindly assume that if these subtests are low the child must be experiencing attention deficit.

In an interesting study, Massman, Nussbaum and Bigler (1988) found that for children between ages 6 to 8 years, there was no significant association between hyperactivity and attentional problems and poor performance on these subtests. For children 9 to 12 years of age, there was a significant correlation for these problems and poor test performance. The data suggests that ADHD problems may have an increasing negative effect on the child's performance on these tests with increasing age. It is also of interest to note that these authors found similar results for performance on the Arithmetic subtest of the Wide-Range Achievement Test. Performance on this task has been found to be positively correlated with Kaufman's Freedom From Distractibility factor (Stedman, Lawlis, Cortner & Achterberg, 1978). These findings would suggest that the practitioner use caution when interpreting results from the Wide Range-Achievement Arithmetic subtest with ADHD children.

Many test tasks have proven to be effective discriminators of ADHD on a group basis, but they have not made the transition into clinical utility, in part because it has been difficult to establish normative data. Other measures, such as the Continuous Performance Test, have not lent themselves to clinical use because of machinery or computerized requirements necessary to administer the tasks. Still other measures have not been researched sufficiently enough that the majority of practitioners are aware of their existence.

BEHAVIORAL OBSERVATION DURING ASSESSMENT

The psychometric assessment may last anywhere from one to three hours and may be completed in one or two sessions. It is important for the practitioner to qualitatively evaluate the child's or adolescent's behavior from the moment of meeting until the close of the evaluation. A number of published forms designed to organize the practitioner's observations during assessment are available. Goldstein and Goldstein (1985) have developed a simple one-page form to meet this need. It appears as Figure 6.1.

It is important for the practitioner to observe the child's initial response to meeting the practitioner in a waiting room or classroom, as well as the child's ability to separate and accompany the practitioner to the testing room. Observation of the child's physical size and appearance should be made. The majority of ADHD children without additional psychiatric problems have no difficulty separating from their parents or classroom and accompanying the practitioner into the testing room. As noted in Chapter 5, in some situations parents are invited to directly observe the evaluation. It is important for the practitioner to clearly note the parent's presence as this may have an impact on the child's performance.

The practitioner should observe the child's ability to make appropriate eye contact, as well as initiate and maintain conversation. Even in a one-to-one setting, many ADHD children have difficulty focusing on the practitioner and may frequently look around the room even as they respond to the practitioner's questions. General observation of the child's receptive language skills, voice quality, expressive syntax and articulation is also suggested.

The practitioner must note if the child presents as excessively anxious or unhappy. At times it is difficult to distinguish excessive mobility and restless behavior, which is characteristic of the ADHD child, from signs of anxiety. When questioned, anxious children will usually openly acknowledge that they are feeling uncomfortable. The ADHD child denies these feelings. This subjective data is important in making the distinction between anxiety or inattention. Further, anxious children often engage in behaviors characteristic of anxiety such as hand wringing, while attention-disordered children engage in behaviors such as wiping the desk with their arms, kicking the desk, and fidgeting excessively in their seats. Some children are overly concerned about their performance. Others lack emotion and appear quite constricted. Some children are extremely labile, jumping from one

GOLDSTEIN BEHAVIORAL OBSERVATION CHECKLIST

Name _____ Age _____ Date _____
Size _____ Appearance _____
Apprehension accompanying E _____ Entering Room _____
Alert _____ Attention _____ Concentration_____
Cooperation _____ Attempt _____
    Eye Contact _____ Tearfulness _____
Startle Response _____ Tremulousness _____
Expression: Anxious _____ Sad _____ Miserable _____
    Unhappy _____ Calm _____ Concerned about performance _____
    Lack of Affect _____ Labile _____ Other _____
Preoccupation with topics of: Anxiety _____
    Depressive _____ Aggressive _____
Muscular tension: Clinching jaw _____
    Sitting stiffly in chair _____
    Gripping Table of Chair _____
    Gripping hands together _____ Other _____
Habitual mannerisms: Tics_____ Rocking _____
    Twisting hair _____ Facial mannerisms _____
    Sucking _____ Flapping arms _____
Activity: Underactive, little spontaneous movement _____
    Normal _____ Tendency to increased activity _____
    Markedly overactive relative to situation _____
    Extremely overactive, tempo of activity increases _____
Fidgetiness: Normal _____ Occasional squirming or wriggling _____
    Marked fidgetiness _____
Persistence: Normal _____ Needs occasional prompting _____
    Needs continuous examiner praise and encouragement _____
    Inconsistent effort _____
Motivation _____ Maturity _____
Emotional Stability _____
Distractibility: not distracted _____ occasionally distracted _____
    easily distracted _____ seeks distraction _____
Orientation to purpose of testing: _____
Self-Confidence: Extremely confident _____ Overly confident _____
    Moderately confident _____ Inclined to distrust abilities _____
    Very Insecure _____
Speech and Language: Receptive _____ Expressive Syntax _____
    Expressive Articulation _____ Maintains Conversation _____
    Initiates Conversation _____
Comprehension _____
Relationship with Examiner _____
Emotional Responsiveness to Examiner _____
Smiling: Smiles appropriately _____ Smiles only occasionally _____
    No, or very little smiling _____
Orientation to Testing: _____
Final Adjustment: _____
Thought Processes: Logical _____ Focused _____ Relevant _____
NOTES: _____
_____
_____
_____

Figure 6.1 Goldstein Behavioral Observation Checklist. From S. Goldstein and M. Goldstein, *The Multi-Disciplinary Evaluation and Treatment of Attention Disorders in Children: Symposium Handbook.* Copyright 1985 by Neurology, Learning and Behavior Center. Used with permission of the publisher.

extreme of emotion to another. Typically, ADHD children do not have significant problems with these emotional characteristics. Problems in these areas are often signs of additional emotional disturbance.

The practitioner must note if the child is alert. Based on the mental-status assessment (Strub & Black, 1977), being alert directly refers to the ability to remain awake. The practitioner must also note if the child is able to pay attention for short periods sufficient to follow task instructions. Observations of sustained attention, also referred to as concentration or vigilance by some, must also be made. Frequently, during a psychometric assessment the majority of the assessment instruments administered take only a few minutes to complete, and many ADHD children can remain on task for a sufficient amount of time to complete them.

The practitioner must also note if the child is cooperative. Some children are passively resistant, agreeing with the examiner but dawdling and not completing tasks. Others are openly defiant, refusing to complete tasks. These behaviors are not characteristic for most ADHD children. The majority of ADHD children cooperate but simply lack persistence. They are willing to attempt most tasks and are motivated. They frequently lack persistence and may need prompting from the examiner in the form of praise or encouragement. In a well-controlled, structured examination room, these children may be occasionally distracted. It is also important for the practitioner to observe if the child is actively seeking distraction as a means of avoiding the tasks being presented.

The practitioner must observe the child's degree of muscular tension, habitual mannerisms and activity level. A distinction may be made between restless fidgeting while remaining seated and excessive activity that results in the child being frequently out of his seat and moving about the room excessively.

It is also beneficial for the practitioner to attempt to observe the child's level of self-confidence. Some ADHD children are overly confident and do not have an understanding of their skills or abilities. At times, it is difficult for the practitioner to determine whether the child's tendency to give up quickly as task complexity increases results from impulsive frustration or feelings of helplessness. Frequently, direct questioning of the child will help make this distinction. The Child Behavior Profile—Parent and Teacher Forms can also be of assistance in interpreting observable behavior as stemming from anxiety, helplessness or attention disorder.

It is frequently helpful to attempt to determine how well oriented the child is to the purpose of evaluation. Some children will present with very poor orientation but will accept your explanation of the need for assessment. Others will deny a need for assessment, even in the face of problematic home and school data. The child's ability to relate to the practitioner is observed by whether the child smiles and how well the child progresses emotionally through the evaluation. Assessment of the child's thought processes, determining whether they are logical, focused on the tasks at hand and relevant to the examiner's questions, is also useful. An overall observation of the child's final adjustment and orientation during the close of the evaluation should also be made.

CLINICAL MEASURES OF ATTENTIONAL SKILLS

Each of the tasks reviewed in this section measures a component of attentional skill. None of these tasks are considered pure tests of attention. No such tasks exist. In fact, attentional skills are a necessary precondition for successful performance on any type of evaluative measure. Therefore, attention can be inferred based on observing the child's approach to the entire testing procedure. These measures are presented not only because they have a high loading of attentional skill required for successful performance, but because they have proven clinically useful by allowing the practitioner to draw normative-based conclusions. For quick reference purposes, Table 6.1 contains a list of these tests organized by the primary attentional skill they appear sensitive in measuring. Some tests are sensitive in measuring more than one type of attentional skill and are listed repeatedly.

Measures of Vigilance

Vigilance is a measure of the child's capacity to be ready to respond and to sustain that readiness over time. Successful performance on all types of tests requires efficient vigilance (Lezak, 1983). Some measures of vigilance tap the child's readiness to respond by requiring the child to consistently attend to a sequential presentation of auditory or visual stimuli and respond when a target stimulus is observed; others require the child to be ready to attend to increasingly longer sequences of stimuli with breaks between stimulus presentations.

Detroit Test of Auditory Attention Span for Unrelated Words

This task, from the original Detroit Tests of Learning Aptitude (Baker & Leland, 1967), is a measure of auditory vigilance and immediate auditory sequential memory. Increasingly longer sequences of single-syllable words are read at a rate of one word per second. Immediately following the examiner's presentation, the child must repeat the series of stimulus words. Scores of the total number of correct stimuli repeated and the number of stimuli repeated in proper sequence can be tabulated. The former score appears to be the more sensitive measure of vigilance. Children with specific language problems, auditory discrimination or other processing dysfunction may also experience problems performing this task successfully. Normative data, though somewhat outdated, is available for this test for individuals 3 through 18 years of age. The Detroit Tests were recently revised (Hammill, 1985). The Auditory Attention Span for Unrelated Words Test was altered and retitled as Word Sequences. Credit for the total correct number of stimuli recalled was eliminated, and only those stimulus items repeated in correct sequence are counted. It appears that the restructuring and scoring of this task has resulted in it becoming a better measure of sequential memory but possibly not as good a measure of vigilance.

Detroit Test of Visual Attention Span for Objects

In addition to measuring visual vigilance and persistence, this is a task of visual sequential memory. The child is exposed to increasingly longer sequences of simple, visual objects at an exposure rate of one second per object. The child must immediately respond with verbal labels for what has been seen. As with the Auditory Attention Span for Unrelated Words Test, scores of total recall and sequential recall can be obtained, with norms available for ages 3 through 18 years.

TABLE 6.1. Assessment Measures Sensitive to Attentional Skills

Vigilance

Detroit Test of Auditory Attention for Unrelated Words
Detroit Test of Visual Attention for Objects
Wechsler Intelligence Scale for Children—Revised,
   Digit Span Subtest
Seashore Rhythm Test
Speech-Sounds Perception Test
Gordon Diagnostic System-Vigilance Task

Sustained Attention

Rapidly Recurring Target Figures Test
Wechsler Intelligence Scale—Revised, Coding Subtest
Seashore Rhythm Test
Speech-Sounds Perception Test
Symbol Digit Modalities Test
Halstead Trail-Making Test
Visual Closure Subtest of the Illinois Test of Psycholinguistic
   Abilities (ITPA)
Gardner Motor Steadiness Test

Focused Attention

Stroop Color Distraction Test
Visual Closure Subtest of the Illinois Test of Psycholinguistic
   Abilities
Halstead Trail-Making Test
Rapidly Recurring Target Figures Test

Selective Attention

Rapidly Recurring Target Figures Test

Divided Attention

Wechsler Intelligence Scale for Children—Revised,
   Arithmetic Subtest
Wechsler Intelligence Scale for Children—Revised,
   Digit Span Subtest
Halstead Trail-Making Test

Impulsivity

Matching Familiar Figures Test
Wechsler Intelligence Scale for Children—Revised,
   Mazes Subtest
Gordon Diagnostic System-Delay Task
Halstead Trail-Making Test

Children with perceptual difficulty or dysnomia, as well as ADHD children, may also perform poorly on this task.

It is frequently useful to compare the child's performance on the visual and auditory tasks. The child's visual and auditory performances typically reflect the relationship between the child's Verbal and Performance I.Q.s on the Wechsler Intelligence Scale for Children—Revised. It would be expected that a child will perform at approximately the same level on these two tasks as on the Wechsler. The Wechsler can therefore be used as a standard measure for comparison. The practitioner must be careful, however, in making comparisons, as the normative data for the Detroit tests is quite old, yielding only chronological age scores. The data has not been converted to standard scores, which would allow a better comparison with Wechsler scores.

Clinical observations have suggested that ADHD children typically have equal difficulty on both the auditory and visual tasks (Goldstein,"personal communication," 1988). Their approach to these tasks is often disorganized and inconsistent. Children with visual perception problems or dysnomia perform better on the verbal task, while children with auditory processing or language disability perform better on the visual task. The revised Detroit has retitled the Visual Attention Span for Object Test as Object Sequences. Although the stimulus items are the same, instead of the child verbally recalling the sequence of items, a second stimulus card is shown and the child must correctly point to the sequence of items as they appeared on the original card. Hammill (1985) notes that the original intent of this subtest was to measure visual memory. The restructuring of this subtest seems to make it a better measure of visual memory, but as with the auditory attention span test, not as good a measure of vigilance. A sample set of stimulus items for the Object Sequences Test appears in Figure 6.2.

WISC-R Digit Span Subtest

The Digit Span subtest requires the child to recall increasingly longer sequences of digits. It is a measure of both vigilance and immediate auditory sequential memory. The Wechsler Digit Span task is complicated by the fact that both the child's score in recalling digits forward and the score in recalling digits in reversed sequences are combined to obtain one summary score. The efficient recall of digits in reverse is considered by some practitioners to be an even better measure of vigilance and concentration than digits forward (Gardner, 1979) and a measure of efficient mental tracking by others (Lezak, 1983). Gardner (1979) provides separate normative data for digits forward and digits reversed.

Seashore Rhythm Test

The Seashore Rhythm Test is part of the Halstead-Reitan Neuropsychological Battery (Reitan & Wolfson, 1985). The test was adapted from the Seashore Test of Musical Ability (Seashore, Lewis & Saetveit 1960). The child listens to a tape recording presenting 30 pairs of rhythmic beats. The child has to record on the answer sheet whether the second group of beats in each pair was the same or different from the first group. While it is obvious that successful performance

PRACTICE B

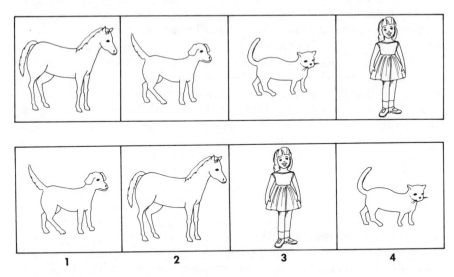

Figure 6.2 Object Sequences Test. From D. Hammill, *Detroit Tests of Learning Aptitude—2*. Copyright 1985 by Pro-Ed. Used with permission of the publisher.

involves the child's auditory memory and ability to discriminate between different patterns of nonverbal sounds, the test also clearly requires components of vigilance and coordination between the ear, eye and hand. Normative data is available for ages nine years through adulthood.

Speech-Sounds Perception Test

This task is also a component of the Halstead-Reitan Neuropsychological Battery. It, too, is administered with a tape recorder. The child has a response sheet with 60 groups of four nonsense words, all of which contain the **ee** sound. The child must listen and underline the correct nonsense word. The stimuli in this task are verbal, and the pace is somewhat slower than the Seashore Rhythm Test. The childhood version of this task requires completion of the first 30 items. This is a simpler task than the Seashore Rhythm Test. There is a component of auditory vigilance and coordination between the ear, eye and hand required for successful performance. Children with auditory processing or auditory discrimination dysfunction may also experience difficulty on this task. Normative data is available for ages nine years through adulthood.

Gordon Diagnostic System-Vigilance Task

The Gordon Diagnostic System (Gordon, 1983; Gordon & Mettelman, 1987) is a portable electronic device designed to assess deficits in vigilance and impulse control in children. Normative data is available from 4 through 16 years of age, with increasing data available for older adolescents and adults. The vigilance task is a measure of readiness to respond and of persistence. The child views a series of digits flashing one at a time on an electronic display and is required to press a button every time the number one is followed by the number nine. Younger children are instructed to respond every time they see the number one. A related distractibility task, which provides a more complex measure of vigilance, was recently added in an attempt to obtain better discriminative data for adolescents and adults. On the distractibility task, subjects are instructed to respond to the one/nine combination only when it appears in the center of the screen. The Gordon Diagnostic System has been reported to differentiate accurately between children experiencing ADHD and those classified in the school setting as reading disabled, overanxious or normal (Gordon & McClure, 1983). Although its use by practitioners is increasing, the expense of the Gordon device has limited its widespread use at this time.

Measures of Sustained Attention

Sustained attention requires the child to persist at a task until it is successfully completed. Many ADHD children, either because of a low frustration threshold or an impulsive style of responding, lack task persistence. The lack of persistence frequently results in underestimates by practitioners of the child's skills and abilities. Regardless of the title of a test, many tests administered to ADHD children are better measures of the child's persistence and reflection than of the skills the tests are supposed to be measuring.

Cancellation of Rapidly Recurring Target Figures Test

Originally developed by Rudel, Denckla and Broman (1978) as part of a research project to differentiate reading and learning disorders in children, the Diamond and 592 tasks of the Cancellation of Rapidly Recurring Target Figures Test are simple tasks that are good measures of visual persistence. Successful performance on these tasks also requires a certain degree of reflection and visual discrimination. The Diamond subtest (Figure 6.3) requires the child to locate and mark all of the diamond figures placed randomly among an array of 140 geometric forms. The total amount of time the child takes to complete the task and the number of errors, including omissions and commissions (marking a nondiamond) are recorded. The 592 subtest (Figure 6.4) requires the child to scan an array of 140 three-digit numbers, all beginning with the number five and having second digits of six or nine. The child is instructed to place a line through only the 592 sequence. Completion time, as well as combined omission and commission errors, are obtained. Table 6.2 contains normative data for both the Diamond and 592 subtests.

It is also helpful for the practitioner to make qualitative observations of the child's approach to these tasks. By the age of six, most children are fairly well organized, beginning in the upper-left corner and proceeding either vertically or horizontally on this task. Most children will also check their answers, since the instructions are to find all of the target stimuli as quickly as possible but to make certain that all of the stimulus items are found before stopping. Poorly motivated children will casually scan the stimuli, mark one or two, and announce that they are

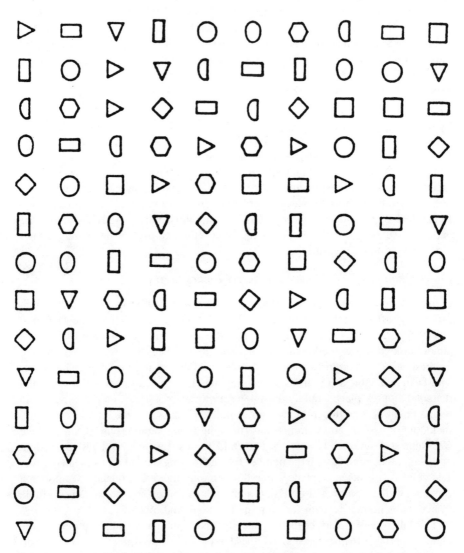

Figure 6.3 Cancellation of Rapidly Recurring Target Figures Test—Diamond Form. From R. Rudel, M. Denckla and M. Broman, Rapid Silent Response to Repeated Target Symbols by Dyslexic and Non-Dyslexic Children. Copyright 1978, *Brain and Language*. Used by permission of the publisher.

569	562	598	561	591	564	563	591	569	561
564	561	592	599	562	594	591	562	598	592
599	593	563	564	591	598	562	564	569	599
563	599	594	569	561	591	592	599	592	564
561	564	591	562	599	599	561	569	598	594
594	592	563	569	594	564	594	599	561	563
569	562	569	599	598	563	591	564	599	592
563	592	561	563	591	561	569	598	562	569
562	591	594	564	592	563	599	592	599	591
598	561	592	599	562	594	564	562	563	598
564	563	599	598	594	569	592	561	599	562
598	592	569	591	564	562	594	598	594	591
561	563	564	562	592	598	563	592	564	562
569	591	598	594	561	569	591	594	561	563

Figure 6.4 Cancellation of Rapidly Recurring Target Figures Test—592 Form. From R. Rudel, M. Denckla and M. Broman. Rapid Silent Response to Repeated Target Symbols by Dyslexic and Non-Dyslexic Children. Copyright 1978. *Brain and Language*. Used by permission of the publisher.

TABLE 6.2. Cancellation of Rapidly Recurring Target Figures—Normative Data

| | DIAMOND | | | | |
| | Total Errors | | | Time (Seconds) | |
Age	Mean	S.D.		Mean	S.D.
4–5	12	(4)		—	—
6–7	5	(3)		103.43	(46,30)
8–9	4	(3)		66.26	(21.63)
10–11	3	(3)		70.10	(24.55)
12–13	2	(3)		40.90	(8.88)
			592		
	Total Errors			Time (Seconds)	
Age	Mean	S.D.		Mean	S.D.
4–5	13	(4)		—	—
6–7	6	(3)		200.76	(81.51)
8–9	2	(2)		116.00	(33.71)
10–11	2	(2)		90.70	(24.66)
12–13	2	(2)		67.13	(15.76)

From R. Rudel, M. Denckla and M. Broman. Rapid Silent Response to Repeated Target Symbols by Dyslexic and Non-Dyslexic Children. Copyright 1978. *Brain and Language*. Used by permission of the publisher.

finished. Some children who have difficulty accurately assessing task demands may perceive the Diamond subtest as very simple and not carefully scan the stimulus items. This results in more errors of omission. On the 592 subtest, however, these children recognize the task's complexity, exert more effort and perform competently. It is frequently characteristic for ADHD children to use a random search strategy and not check their performance. The inattentive, disorganized, but not significantly impulsive ADHD child may remain on this task a significantly long period of time but because of an ineffective approach to the task may make many errors of omission.

WISC-R Coding Subtest

Both the simpler form for children under age 8 and the more complex form for children age 8 through 16 require matching one's own performance to sample stimuli for success. This task is considered a good measure of persistence, new learning capacity and visual discrimination. Children with learning problems stemming from perceptual difficulty or difficulty efficiently manipulating a pencil may also perform deficiently on this task. Poorly motivated children will dawdle on this task. The Coding subtest is one of the three subtests that, based on Kaufman's factor analysis, loaded on the Freedom From Distractibility factor. This task is also sensitive to visual memory since efficient performance requires the child to quickly learn the code and write it from memory rather than having to continuously check back with the sample. The usefulness of Wechsler subtests as attentional measures is increased by the excellent normative data available. Figure 6.5 contains a sample of both coding tasks.

Symbol Digit Modalities Test

The Symbol Digit Modalities Test (Smith, 1973) is similar to the coding subtest of the WISC-R but reverses the presentation of material so that the symbols are presented as stimulus items and numbers must be written by the child. This enables the child to respond with more common elements, numbers. The design of this task also provides for the parallel measurement of oral performance by having the child point to each stimulus item and say the corresponding number as quickly as possible. The oral trial follows the administration of the written trial. Symbol Digit Modalities is a sensitive measure of persistence, visual discrimination, new learning capacity and efficient pencil control. Comparing the child's written and oral performance is frequently helpful in making comparisons between visual/motor and verbal skills. Normative data is available from age 8 through adulthood for males and females.

ITPA Visual Closure Subtest

The Visual Closure subtest of the Illinois Test of Psycholinguistic Abilities (Kirk, McCarthy, & Kirk, 1968), which involves identifying partially visible objects embedded in a complex background, was designed as a measure of visual perception and short-term visual memory. Because of the complexity of the task it is obvious that this is also a measure of reflection and persistence capability.

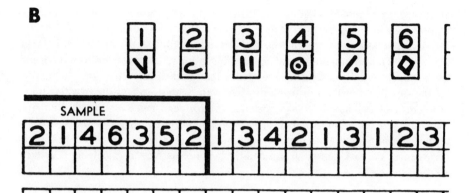

Figure 6.5 Wechsler Intelligence Scale for Children—Coding subtest. From D. Wechsler, *Wechsler Intelligence Scale for Children—Revised.* Copyright 1974 by The Psychological Corporation. Used with permission of the publisher.

(See Figure 6.6.) The test allows the child a 30-second exposure to each of the five stimulus displays. Observing the child's approach to the task as well as her ability to make use of additional time often provides qualitative insight into the child's persistence and reflection capabilities. Children with complex perceptual problems may also have difficulty performing this task successfully. Normative data is available for children ages 2½ through 10 years.

Gardner Steadiness Test

Gardner, Gardner, Caemmerer, and Broman (1979) developed a measure of motor steadiness by modifying an instrument originally designed by Knights (1966). The child is required to insert a stylus in a somewhat larger hole and hold it there as steady as possible. Contact duration of the stylus with the hole's perimeter is

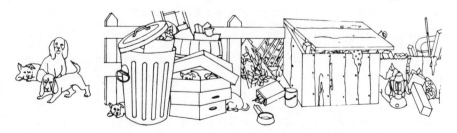

Figure 6.6 Visual Closure subtest of the Illinois Test of Psycholinguistic Abilities. By S. Kirk, J. McCarthy and W. Kirk, *The Illinois Test of Psycholinguistic Abilities (Revised Edition).* Copyright 1968 by University of Illinois Press. Used by permission of the publisher.

electronically recorded. Gardner (1979) suggests that while the steadiness tester is a good measure of motor persistence, resting tremors and choreiform movements, it is also a measure of hyperactivity and difficulty with task persistence. It is Gardner's belief that motor impersistence, resting tremors and choreiform movements are relatively uncommon in children with attention disorder. Therefore, he considers the steadiness tester a measure of drive from within, suggesting that steadiness problems reflect a lack of task persistence. Motor persistence has not been a major focus in the evaluation of attention problems in children; therefore the steadiness tester has not gained widespread acceptance. For practitioners interested in motor persistence, the task can be useful and there is normative data available (Gardner, 1979).

Measures of Focused Attention

The ability to focus attention and free oneself from distractibility is a skill that is usually inferred by the practitioner through observation of the child in a natural setting, feedback from parents or teachers, and behavioral observation of the child during clinical assessment.

Trail-Making Test

The Trail-Making Test is a timed paper-and-pencil test that has been found to be a sensitive measure of brain injury (Reitan, 1958). The test consists of two parts, A and B. There is normative data and a simpler version designed for children 9 through 15 years of age, as well as the parallel version for older adolescents and adults. On Part A, the child is required to sequentially connect dots in numerical order. On Part B, the child must not only connect dots in numerical order but also track the alphabet in order, creating an alternating sequence of numbers and letters. Both parts of this test require persistence. Part B is also a good measure of focused and divided attention. Mesulam (1985) considers the Trail-Making Test a good measure of response inhibition and vulnerability to interference. Normative data for the Trail-Making Test has been extensively collected (Fromm-Auch & Yeudall, 1983). Reitan (1987) has developed a parallel form of this test utilizing geometric shapes for children five through eight years of age. Both the Progressive Figures Test and the Trail-Making Test are also sensitive measures of flexibility of thinking, new learning capacity and visual/motor speed.

Stroop Color Distraction Test

This novel task measures distractibility. The child is first asked to read as quickly as possible 100 color words (red, blue, green), printed in black and white and arranged in random sequence. This establishes a response tendency. Then a second response tendency to name colors is developed by having the child read 100 colored dots (red, blue, green). In the third, or distraction, condition the child is presented with 100 color words, each of which is printed in a color other than the one spelled by the letters. So, for example, the word green is printed in red ink. The time to complete this third task is recorded. Comalli, Wapner, and Werner (1962) obtained normative data for both children and adults. Trenerry, Crosson, DeBoe and Leber (1989) recently published a new two-part version of this test.

Measures of Divided Attention

To perform competently on this skill, the child must be able to simultaneously track two different sources of information. The child's ability to follow numbers and letters sequentially and simultaneously on Part B of the Trail-Making Test is a good example of divided attention. Recent data (Van Zomeren, 1981) suggests that difficulty with divided attention is also frequently characteristic of the head-injured individual. It may also be a consistent, often undetected problem for the ADHD child.

WISC-R Arithmetic

The Arithmetic subtest of the WISC-R also loads on Kaufman's Freedom From Distractibility factor. All but the first four and last three questions on this task are presented verbally by the examiner. The first four questions are accompanied by a visual stimulus. The last three questions must be read aloud by the child. All of the child's responses are verbal. The use of paper and pencil is not allowed. As problem complexity increases, the child must listen carefully and integrate and organize various key aspects of the problem questions while computing an answer. This task is also a measure of simple arithmetic reasoning, vigilance, persistence and reflection. ADHD children frequently respond impulsively as task complexity increases on this subtest. Limit testing frequently reveals that they possess the arithmetic skill to respond correctly when they are forced to slow down and think each problem through.

Measures of Impulsivity

Impulsivity results in increased errors caused by a lack of effective time spent before responding. Reflection is just the opposite skill, and involves increased preresponse time and cognition resulting in a greater likelihood of correct responses and reduced errors.

Matching Familiar Figures Test

This was designed specifically as a measure of reflection and impulsivity (Kagan, 1964). A number of alternate forms have been developed. Normative data has been collected for children and adults. Kagan's original task consisted of 12 items. Each item contains a stimulus picture of an object and six similar pictures, only one of which matches the stimulus picture exactly. (See Figure 6.7.) The child selects a response and is allowed to continue responding until a correct choice has been made. The child's time from stimulus exposure to the initial response is recorded along with the number of errors per item. Messer (1976) has collected extensive normative data on the Matching Familiar Figures Test. Messer notes that impulsive children present short reaction times and make many errors. Reflective

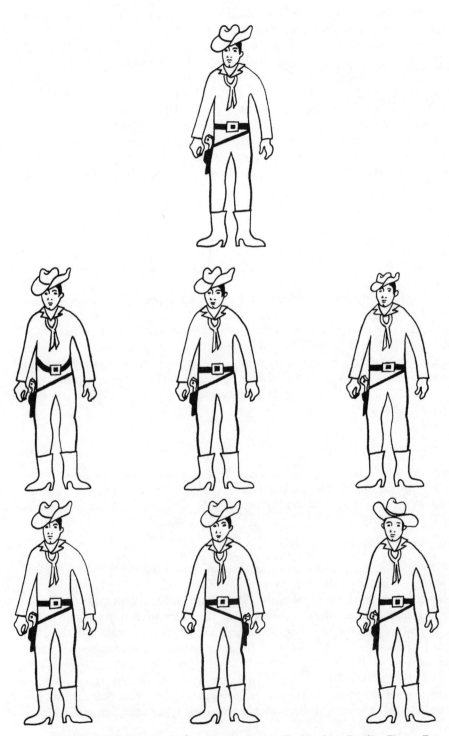

Figure 6.7 Matching Familiar Figures Test. From J. Kagan, *The Matching Familiar Figures Test.* Copyright 1964. Used by permission of the author.

children have longer reaction times and make few errors. Some children respond very quickly and are accurate; others take a very long time to respond but are most inaccurate. Children with this latter response style characteristically have difficulty with attention, organization and an efficient approach to tasks, but are not necessarily impulsive.

WISC-R Mazes Subtest

Maze performance is considered a measure of reflection as well as visual/motor speed and coordination. Kaufman's research also suggests that maze performance is a measure of perceptual organization. A child's score results from the number of blind alleys entered and the crossing of barriers. Poor planning is readily observed in the impulsive child's approach to this task. A sample of the Mazes subtest appears in Figure 6.8.

Gordon Diagnostic System-Delay Task

This is the initial task of the Gordon Diagnostic System. The task requires the child to inhibit responding in order to earn points. The child's delay from the time an instruction is given until the button may be pushed must be at least six seconds. The number of responses, the number of correct responses and the percentage of correct responses is recorded.

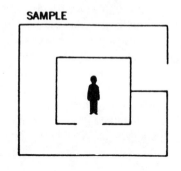

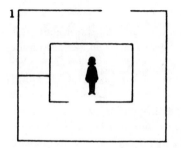
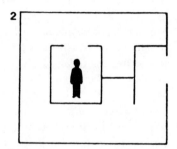

Figure 6.8 Wechsler Intelligence Scale for Children—Mazes subtest. From D. Wechsler, *Wechsler Intelligence Scale for Children—Revised.* Copyright 1974 by The Psychological Corporation. Used with permission of the publisher.

IMPACT OF ATTENTIONAL PROBLEMS ON OVERALL TEST PERFORMANCE

The practitioner inexperienced in evaluating attention-deficient children may be led to draw inaccurate or erroneous conclusions about the child's skills and abilities based on test performance. For example, the Motor Free Visual Perception Test is a commonly used assessment instrument designed to assess the elementary school child's visual/perceptual skills. It is a visual, multiple-choice task. ADHD children may parallel the performance of perceptually impaired children as they respond correctly on the first few simple items in each category but then proceed to get many of the remaining items wrong. Actually, what is occurring is that the child is capable of performing the task, but as task complexity increases, the child's low frustration threshold and impulsive tendency take over. Rather than carefully viewing the four stimulus choices to select among them, the ADHD child responds impulsively to one aspect of the stimulus item. In a situation such as this, misinterpretation may be further compounded by the administration of a visual/motor task, such as the Bender Visual Motor Gestalt Test. ADHD children frequently plan poorly on this test, and their productions may be impulsively drawn, yielding additional errors, and appear to support hypotheses of perceptual/motor impairment.

To avoid such problems, it is strongly recommended that the practitioner test the child's limits routinely throughout psychometric testing. This is especially important if the child has demonstrated consistent problems on tasks of attentional skill. It is not uncommon during limit testing on the WISC-R subtests to determine that the ADHD child knows more information, can locate more missing items, can sequence cards or puzzle pieces more efficiently and has better social judgment than is revealed during standardized assessment. While the improved performance cannot be counted or considered when tests are scored, the data is certainly important in helping the practitioner understand that the assessment obtained is an underestimate of the child's potential. In such situations, an accurate assessment of the ADHD child's capabilities may be impossible because of her deficient attentional system.

MEASUREMENT OF ACADEMIC SKILLS

Frequently, academic and achievement information can be obtained through group or individual assessment within the school setting. Since there is an increasing likelihood that the older ADHD child will experience some degree of academic deficiency, it is beneficial for the practitioner to obtain some measure of the child's academic skills. If in-depth data is not available and deficiencies are suspected, the child's word reading, spelling and arithmetic capability can be quickly screened using the Wide Range Achievement Test (Jastak & Wilkinson 1984). As noted earlier, however, the practitioner is cautioned in using any academic screening instrument that requires the child to work independently for more than a few minutes at a time.

If specific areas of weakness are observed, the academic section from the Wood-cock-Johnson Psycho-Educational Assessment Battery (Woodcock and Johnson, 1977; Woodcock, 1989), Peabody Individual Achievement Test (Dunn & Mark-wardt, 1970), Woodcock Reading Mastery Tests (Woodcock, 1973), Gray Oral Reading Test (Gray, 1967) or Key Math Diagnostic Inventory (Connoloy et al., 1976) can be helpful in providing a definition of the child's academic achievement and reasons for possible academic delays.

ASSESSMENT OF PERSONALITY AND EMOTIONAL ADJUSTMENT

In response to their increased problems dealing successfully with the environment, ADHD children present an increased risk for the development of helplessness, depression, poor self-esteem and oppositional problems. As part of the evaluation for attention disorder, it is recommended that the practitioner obtain at least a general overview of the ADHD child's self-awareness, emotional adjustment and coping and problem-solving skills. A number of self-report and interview measures are beneficial for this part of the evaluation.

Self-Report Measures

Achenbach and Edelbrock (1983) have developed a parallel form of the Revised Child Behavior profile designed to be filled out by children 11 through 18 years of age. The Youth Self-Report at this time is primarily a research instrument, and normative data is not available. The report requires at least a fifth-grade reading level to be completed. Qualitative assessment of the adolescent's responses is often helpful since questions on the profile deal with peer relations, community activities, fears, emotional problems and attention difficulty.

The Children's Depression Inventory (Kovacs, 1983) is a 26-item, self-report measure requiring the child to check one of three descriptors in each item that best characterizes that child over the past two weeks. For example, the child may be asked to respond whether he was less happy, as happy or more happy than others. Normative data has been collected by Finch, Saylor and Edwards (1985) for males and females from grades two through eight (Table 6.3). Based on their responses to the Children's Depression Inventory, attention-disordered children, in comparison to a normal control group, acknowledged significantly more depressive symptoms (Borden, Brown, Jenkins & Clingerman, 1987). These authors also found that in comparison to normal children, ADD children demonstrated more external attribution for both positive and negative experiences. With 13 to 18 year old adolescents, the Reynolds Adolescent Depression Scale (Reynolds, 1987) is an equally effective depression survey.

The Children's Depression Inventory is a sensitive instrument for identifying the quality and severity of depressive ideation. With a child not excessively using denial as a psychological defense, it may also prove helpful in allowing the practitioner to develop an understanding of the child's awareness of the severity of her problems and the level of contact with her feelings. Based on a recent

TABLE 6.3.   Children's Depression Inventory Means and Standard Deviations by Sex and Grade

Grade	Males			Females			Combined		
	n	M	SD	n	M	SD	n	M	SD
2	49	11.18	5.93	45	6.84	4.70	94	9.11	5.77
3	38	8.03	6.65	52	8.07	7.81	90	8.06	7.30
4	136	11.26	7.41	150	8.94	6.85	286	10.04	7.20
5	159	10.46	8.44	153	9.61	7.66	312	10.05	8.06
6	131	9.28	6.85	134	8.36	6.65	265	8.81	6.75
7	123	10.27	7.32	118	8.81	6.64	241	9.56	7.02
8	69	10.99	8.91	106	10.64	6.96	175	10.78	7.63
Total	705	10.33	7.59	758	9.01	6.97	1,463	9.65	7.30

Finch, A., Saylor, C. and Edwards, G., "Children's Depression Inventory: Sex and Grade Norms for Normal Children." Copyright 1985 by *Journal of Consulting and Clinical Psychology*. Used with permission of the publisher.

study, the practitioner is cautioned that the Children's Depression Inventory may not accurately discriminate between children with major depression and those with conduct disorders. Woodside, Brownstone and Fisman (1987) found that both of these clinical groups demonstrated elevated scores on this inventory. It may be that both of these clinical groups share many of the problems covered on this inventory.

Conners and Wells (1985) have developed a 100-item Adolescent Self-Report Scale. The scale contains items dealing with concentration difficulty, restlessness, self-control, anger, confidence, friends, learning and emotions. Uniquely, the scale also has a number of items asking the adolescent to note his assets and strong points, as well as specific family problems. There is no normative data available, but as with the Youth Self-Report, qualitative observations of the adolescent's responses are often of diagnostic significance. Gittelman (1985) has also developed a self-evaluation report for teenagers. The report has 27 items and uses a four-point Likert response scale similar to the Conners Questionnaires.

Piers and Harris (1984) have recently revised the Piers-Harris Self-Concept Scale. The scale is subtitled "The Way I Feel about Myself." It was developed as a brief self-report measure to evaluate self-concept in children and adolescents. Many consider it a measure of self-esteem. The 80-item true-false questionnaire is designed to evaluate children's conscious feelings about themselves. Item content includes questions about behavior, school status, physical appearance, anxiety, popularity and happiness. This instrument can be used with children as young as eight years of age. The practitioner must be cautious, however, since children using psychological defenses of projection, denial and intellectualization may provide overly positive profiles.

Millon, Green and Meagher (1982) developed the Millon Adolescent Personality Inventory to evaluate adolescent personality, behavior and concerns. This inventory consists of 150 items and is designed for adolescents 13 through 18 years of age. The inventory generates 22 scales dealing with personality styles; concerns such as self-concept and peer and family relations; and behavioral issues such as poor social conformity and impulse control.

Clinical Interview

Barkley (1981a) notes that it is important for the practitioner to pay close attention to the child's style and the quality of the child's responses during an interview. ADHD children frequently respond impulsively, thus revealing their immediate feelings but not necessarily their ability to respond accurately to the practitioner's questions. Nonetheless, observation of the child's or adolescent's ability to interact in a semi-structured clinical interview is an essential component of the evaluation.

Some children enjoy a verbal presentation by the practitioner of a series of incomplete sentences in which the practitioner begins the sentence and the child must complete the sentence with the first thing that comes to mind. This activity can be a useful ice breaker. Other children may respond more openly and personally if a sentence-completion task is administered toward the end of the assessment. The practitioner needs to be aware that children with limited intellectual skills or language problems may find an open-ended task such as this extremely difficult. Adolescents are usually provided with the incomplete sentences form and asked to write their responses. Figure 6.9 contains a sample set of incomplete sentences. Rotter (1950) developed an incomplete sentence form specifically for adolescents. Information concerning self-image, family relations, motivation, outlook concerning school and adult relations can be obtained. Although there is not a profile of responses characteristic of ADHD children, the practitioner can make inferences concerning the child's or adolescent's view of the world based upon her responses.

In lieu of incomplete sentences, some practitioners may find presentation of storytelling cards a useful ice breaker. Some practitioners find the presentation of photographs or line drawings depicting children engaged in various home, social and school activities helpful in eliciting information concerning the child's social perception and problem-solving skills. Children are asked to either tell stories about the pictures or place themselves in the situation and explain how they would respond. With young children, the Plenk Storytelling Test (Plenk, 1975) or the Children's Apperception Test (Bellak & Bellak, 1968) can be used to elicit a wide variety of information. The Thematic Apperception Test (Morgan & Murray, 1935) can be a useful projective instrument with older adolescents. The stimulus cards on the Thematic Apperception Test are extremely ambiguous, but there are certain themes considered to be normally elicited by each. The 20 stimulus cards can be used in a variety of combinations and may be somewhat difficult for a younger adolescent. For both male and female children, the Robert's Apperception Test (Roberts, 1982) provides a wide variety of stimulus pictures. Although lacking in ambiguity, which is the basis for some of the projective picture tests, the Robert's Apperception Test is often quite revealing concerning the ADHD child's limited social perception and poor problem or conflict resolution skills.

It is suggested that the clinical interview begin with fairly general, novel questions designed to increase the child's interest in the interview process. The child can be asked if she had three wishes what she would wish for. ADHD children's responses are typically impulsive and not well thought out. This is true for most of their answers during the clinical interview. The child can then be asked if she were going to a deserted island, who she would like to take and what single object

INCOMPLETE SENTENCES

NAME _____ **AGE** _____ **DATE** _____

I like _____

I dislike _____

When I go to bed _____

My mother _____

Working is _____

School _____

Most boys _____

When I am mad _____

Fighting _____

I want to know _____

My father _____

Most girls _____

I would like to forget _____

I wish my mother _____

My friends _____

When I grow up _____

My parents _____

I can not _____

At home _____

My teacher _____

I need _____

I am afraid _____

My family _____

I wish my father _____

My looks _____

Grown-ups _____

I worry _____

I like people who _____

When I cannot have my way _____

Babies are lucky because _____

Nobody likes children who _____

If I had a gun _____

Sometimes I make believe _____

Even the best parents may forget _____

Children are usually certain that _____

If only people knew how much _____

There would be fewer divorces if _____

The worst thing that could happen to a family is _____

The best kinds of homes are the ones that _____

Figure 6.9 Incomplete Sentences. From S. Goldstein, *Incomplete Sentences*. Copyright 1987. Used with permission of the author.

she would take. Older children will typically choose a friend. At times a child's response to this question is quite revealing. It is not uncharacteristic for a child experiencing significant family and social problems to choose a pet, despite the fact that the question asks for a person. One child experiencing significant social and family problems responded that he would not take anyone since no one would want to go with him and people would be better off without him. This is an extremely revealing response concerning the child's feelings about himself and others.

The interview can then continue by asking the child what kind of an animal she would like to be; what one thing she would like to change about herself; what person she might like to be for a day; and what she likes to do best. Novel questions include asking the child what a fly might say if it followed the child around all day and if the walls of the child's house could talk what they would say about the child and her family. These two questions come from the Talking, Feeling and Doing Game (Gardner, 1978).

It is often useful to try to elicit data concerning the child's self-image by asking the child what she feels she is best at or does better than other children. Children experiencing self-image problems may have difficulty suggesting something they do better than others. A brief discussion of emotions might include asking the child whether she feels she is as happy as others and what kinds of things make her feel happy. The child can then be asked if she is ever sad and what makes her sad, as well as whether or not she becomes angry and why. It may also be helpful to ask the child to name specific things she likes about herself, as well as attempt to identify something she doesn't like about herself. Answers to this latter question for some ADHD children are often quite revealing. Many children may suggest their "hyperness" or their "problems doing what people tell them to do."

A discussion of friends is an integral part of the clinical interview. It is suggested the child be initially asked if she has a best friend and then the relationship between the child and best friend explored in terms of what they like about each other and their favorite activities. It is helpful to ask whether or not the child feels she has as many friends as others and if not, why not. The child can be asked if she is satisfied with her friends and if she feels her friends at home or school are different and why. Because of their lack of insight, it is not uncommon for ADHD children to recognize their difficulty with friends but lack an understanding of the impact their behavior has upon others, which results in socialization problems.

A discussion of school can follow, initially asking the child to identify her favorite and least favorite parts. Characteristic answers concerning favorite parts of school for children experiencing learning and attention problems include recess, lunch, final bell of the day, physical education or vacations. When asked about his least favorite part of school, one ADHD child impulsively but insightfully noted "sitting still." A child can also be asked if she perceives that she is as smart as the other children and if not why not; as well as whether or not she learns as well as other children. Questions specific to attention-related problems might include asking the child if she perceives that she has difficulty finishing work at school, whether or not the teacher frequently tells her she isn't listening; whether she has difficulty playing with one friend or one thing for a long period of time; whether she has problems waiting her turn; whether she has difficulty staying seated; and whether she perceives that she has more energy than other children. One child, when asked if he had difficulty waiting his turn said, "Oh no! I just run right to the front of the line so I am always first."

For the practitioner desiring a more in-depth interview specifically focusing on attentional issues, Kirby and Grimley (1986) developed a 16-item child interview form based on the DSM-III Attention-Deficit Disorder diagnostic criteria. Miller and Bigi (1979) developed an even longer structured interview designed to assess a child's understanding of the concept of paying attention.

The interview can then proceed with a discussion of the child's home and family relations, asking the child what she likes and doesn't like about each parent; the best and worst thing that has happened to her in the family; and relationships with specific siblings. Given recent trends in child suicide, it is also recommended that the practitioner broach the question of death, asking the child if she has thought about death and specifically if she has thought about killing herself. If the practitioner questions the adequacy of the child's reality testing, further assessment concerning the child's experiencing auditory or visual hallucinations may also prove fruitful. Initially, the child can be asked if she ever hears or sees things that other people cannot. Clarification and further explanation can proceed if the child responds affirmatively.

CLINICAL CRITERIA FOR CONFIRMING ADHD

In making the diagnosis of ADHD based on the clinical evaluation, it is suggested that problems with vigilance and sustained attention should be observed during the assessment. Impairment with these two skills has been hypothesized as the primary attentional deficits hyperactive children experience (Douglas & Peters, 1979). Problems with divided attention and impulsivity and observations of restlessness during the assessment are supporting but not essential data. A clinical interview can assist the practitioner in developing an understanding of the child's insight and awareness of his attention and arousal-related problems.

During the clinical assessment for attention problems, the authors routinely use Matching Familiar Figures, Detroit Auditory and Visual Attention Span, Rapidly Recurring Target Figures Test, Trail-Making, and the Wechsler subtests of Arithmetic, Digit Span, Coding and Mazes. It is rare that a child with significant attention and arousal-related problems performs successfully on the majority of these tasks. In many cases, successful performance on these tasks coupled with inefficient attention in the environment leads to discovery of an emotional basis for the child's problems. Psychometric tests assist the skilled practitioner in making the distinction between the child who may have skills but chooses not to use them and the ADHD, skill-deficient child. Chapter 7 will provide a structured model to facilitate this and other diagnostic distinctions. Appendix 2 contains a list of the tests reviewed in this section and sources where they may be obtained.

SUMMARY

This chapter outlined procedures to assist the practitioner in structuring the clinical evaluation. Assessment instruments sensitive to different types of attentional skills were reviewed, and a model for behavioral observation and for the clinical interview was presented. These procedures assist the practitioner to draw conclusions concerning the child's attentional skills and to determine the degree to which attentional factors influence psychometric test performance and personality style. Given the combination of psychometric instruments and interview techniques recommended, a psychologist is the ideal practitioner to obtain this type of data for the attention evaluation.

CHAPTER 7

Making the Diagnosis of ADHD

The previous three chapters presented a model and specific methods for collecting data essential for making a diagnosis of ADHD. This chapter will provide a framework to organize and interpret that data. The practitioner must be aware that it is not one specific score or observation that confirms or rules out the presence of ADHD. Additionally, collection of in-depth data facilitates the practitioner's ability to deal with the issue of false positives. Many of the attention and arousal-related problems attributed to ADHD are also commonly associated with other emotional and adjustment problems in children. Careful review and integration of all collected data, using the five components of the working definition, provides the framework for a logical etiology and helps to avoid the occurrence of false positives. Conversely, concerns about a false negative diagnosis constitute a less significant issue. It would be rare for the presentation of multiple attention and overarousal problems to be overlooked, and almost automatically they would be considered to reflect ADHD.

Figure 7.1 contains an overview of the working definition integrated into a checklist format (Goldstein, 1989). Components of the definition include the DSM-III-R diagnostic criteria for ADHD, home and school rating scales, objective data, situational problems and alternative etiological factors that must be considered in the differential diagnosis of attention and overarousal problems. The checklist is designed as a tool to be used by the practitioner to integrate the data. It is not a statistical tool and there is no absolute minimum or maximum number of variables that must be present for the diagnosis of ADHD to be made. In the majority of situations in which the diagnosis of ADHD is made, all five of the criteria are met to the practitioner's satisfaction. Each section of the ADHD Diagnostic Checklist will be reviewed with an extended presentation concerning the issue of differential diagnosis. At the close of the chapter, case studies will illustrate the manner in which data is collected and integrated. A number of cases will be presented that include some various types of compounding problems to assist the practitioner in gaining an understanding of the complexity of this disorder and its interaction with other disorders of childhood.

DSM-III-R DIAGNOSTIC CRITERIA FOR ADHD

The DSM-III-R diagnostic criteria for ADHD has been extensively reviewed and critiqued in Chapter 1. In order to use the criteria effectively, the practitioner must possess an understanding of behavioral differences at various developmental levels. For example, restless fidgeting is generally a common phenomenon in

ADHD DIAGNOSTIC CHECKLIST

Ia. DSM III-R Diagnostic Criteria for ADHD

    A. Eight of the following fourteen must be present:

       _____ 1. Restless fidgeting

       _____ 2. Problems remaining seated

       _____ 3. Easily distracted by extraneous stimuli

       _____ 4. Problems taking turns

       _____ 5. Impulsive responding

       _____ 6. Problems completing things

       _____ 7. Difficulty with sustained attention

       _____ 8. Shifts from one uncompleted activity to another

       _____ 9. Difficulty playing quietly

       _____ 10. Talks excessively

       _____ 11. Interrupts frequently

       _____ 12. Doesn't seem to listen

       _____ 13. Is disorganized

       _____ 14. Takes high risks

  ____ B. Onset before age seven

  ____ C. Not part of a pervasive developmental disorder

  ____ D. Duration over six months

    E. Severity:

       _____ Mild

       _____ Moderate

       _____ Severe

or

Figure 7.1 ADHD Diagnostic Checklist. From S. Goldstein. *ADHD Diagnostic Checklist*. Copyright 1989. Used with the author's permission.

young children but is not often observed in adolescents. Much of the data used by the practitioner to substantiate that the child exhibits at least 8 of the 14 behavioral descriptions in Part A is obtained through the observations and comments of others, including parents and teachers. The practitioner is also cautioned that on Part A, the inattentive, but not necessarily significantly impulsive or hyperactive child may

ADHD Diagnostic Checklist (continued)

Ib. DSM III-R Diagnostic Criteria for Undifferentiated **ADHD**

_____ Persistent Inappropriate Inattention

_____ Not Result of Other Disorder (e.g., Mental Retardation)

II. Rating Scales

A. Home:

_____ 1. Conners Hyperkinesis Index (at or above
2 standard deviations)

_____ 2. Achenbach Hyperactivity Factor for males ages
6-16 years and females ages 4-16 years or
Immaturity and Aggression Scale for males
ages 4-5 years (at or above 98th percentile)

B. School:

_____ 1. Conners Hyperkinesis Index (at or above
2 standard deviations)

_____ 2. (or) ACTeRS (Attention score below 20th percentile)

_____ 3. Achenbach Inattentive Factor (at or above
the 98th percentile)

III. Objective Data. Problems with:

_____ A. Vigilance

_____ B. Sustained attention (persistence)

_____ C. Divided attention

_____ D. Focused attention

_____ E. Selective attention

_____ F. Impulsivity

IV. Situational Problems (difficulty observed in over 50% of
common situations).

_____ A. Home

_____ B. School

_____ C. Community

Figure 7.1 (continued)

ADHD Diagnostic Checklist (continued)

V.   Differential Diagnosis. Rule out or consider contribution of:

_____   A.   Emotional/Adjustment problems

_____   1.   Oppositional problems

_____   2.   Conduct problems

_____   3.   Depression

_____   4. · Anxiety

_____   5.   Adjustment problems

_____   6.   Inadequate or abusive parenting

_____   B.   Learning/Developmental problems

_____   1.   Language difficulty

_____   2.   Auditory processing dysfunction

_____   3.   Memory problems

_____   4.   Other specific learning disabilities

_____   5.   Achievement deficits

_____   6.   General intellectual deficits

_____   C.   Specific cognitive deficits

_____   1.   Problems with speed of information processing

_____   2.   Difficulty with flexible thinking

_____   3.   Problems with concept formation

_____   D.   Medical Factors

_____   1.   History of head trauma

_____   2.   Physical illness or disease

Figure 7.1 (continued)

meet a number of the criteria. Such a child will meet the DSM-III-R diagnostic criteria for undifferentiated attention-deficit disorder.

Sufficient data must be collected to convince the practitioner that the onset of these behavioral problems began before age seven. For children in whom symptoms appear to initially arise in kindergarten and increase in severity as the child progresses through school, a careful review of differential diagnostic etiology, including learning problems, must be considered. A majority of children with histories of attention and arousal-level problems exhibit significant symptoms before entering the school system. The practitioner must be aware that attention related problems are also frequently characteristic of children with significant or pervasive developmental impairments. Children with language, socialization, cognitive and behavioral difficulties that are the result of atypical development often exhibit attention-related problems. They may develop attention and overarousal problems as the result of frustration generated by difficulty interacting with and meeting the demands of the environment (Goldstein & Hinerman, 1988).

Finally, symptoms must be observed for a duration of over six months. If the child appears to meet the diagnostic criteria but symptoms have arisen suddenly, the practitioner must consider the possibility that an emotional or adjustment problem may be the source of symptomatic attention and overarousal difficulty.

The DSM-III-R is extremely general in providing guidelines for rating severity of problems. In determining severity, the practitioner may wish to consider variables such as the number of situations in which the child experiences problems, multiple types of attention difficulty observed, the length of time the child has been experiencing difficulty (i.e., onset very early in life) and the possibility that a number of factors are contributing to symptomatic problems with attention and overarousal.

RATING SCALES

The recommended rating scales were reviewed in Chapters 4 and 5. The practitioner may find general scales, such as the Achenbach Child Behavior Checklist and Personality Inventory for Children, extremely useful in providing a general description of the child's functioning in relation to others. In settings or situations in which time is limited, it is recommended that at the very least parents complete the Conners Parent's Questionnaire and Achenbach Child Behavior Checklist. School data should include the Conners Teacher's Questionnaire or the ADD-H: Comprehensive Teacher Rating Scale. The practitioner must keep in mind that noncompliant, oppositional or conduct-disordered children will frequently present with elevated attention and overarousal problems on all of these questionnaires.

OBJECTIVE DATA

Chapter 6 extensively reviewed assessment instruments that are sensitive to various types of attention problems. It is uncharacteristic for attention-disordered children to perform well normatively or in comparison to their other skills across a sample of these types of tasks. In making the diagnosis of ADHD, it is essential that the attention-disordered child demonstrate difficulty on tasks of this nature. Attempting to assess each type of attention skill separately may provide the practitioner with a better description or operational definition of the child's attentional deficits and assist with specific treatment recommendations.

SITUATIONAL PROBLEMS

It is uncharacteristic for children with ADHD to exhibit severe problems in one situation but be relatively free of problems in other situations. The practitioner must keep in mind that the number and severity of problems the child exhibits is frequently determined by the demands placed upon the child by the environment. It is not uncommon for an attention-disordered child to experience more problems in one situation than in another. Frequently, attention-disordered children have more difficulty in school than at home. School is more demanding and restrictive. On the other hand there are children who demonstrate minor prolems at school but have difficulty at home because of their inability to meet parental expectations. The working definition requires consistent observation of problems in at least 50% or more of common situations in the home, school and community. The practitioner may also wish to use Breen's data (see Chapters 4 and 5) to make statistical comparisons to a normative sample concerning the severity of stituational problems.

Interpretation of the actual number and severity of situational problems within the home must be based on the practitioner's assessment of the parents' expectations and disciplinary style. At the extremes, the overly rigid, unrealistic parent may report a significant number of situational problems for a child with fairly mild attention and overarousal difficulty. The extremely unstructured, possibly attention-disordered parent may report very little difficulty with a severe ADHD child, because the parent makes no effort to structure or set limits. Finally, there are parents that naturally or intuitively are able to understand the ADHD child's incompetencies and adapt their expectations and parenting style to meet the child's abilities. Frequently, these parents will acknowledge the severity of their child's problems but report few situational difficulties given the manner in which they manage the child. Often, asking parents to compare the child to siblings or same-age peers will result in an explanation that the parents understand the degree of their child's disabilities but have restructured their expectations to reduce problematic behavior.

DIFFERENTIAL DIAGNOSIS

In order to make the differential diagnosis of ADHD, the practitioner needs to evaluate a variety of situational and medical factors.

Emotional/Adjustment Problems

Oppositional Problems

It is not surprising that a large percentage of ADHD children develop a pattern of oppositional behavior. Their behavior frequently does not meet the expectations of others; thus, they receive a very high percentage of negative feedback concerning the inadequacy or inappropriateness of their behavior. Eventually this pattern of feedback leads to frustration and an attitude on the part of the child to oppose or push back. Often, parents may initially perceive a large percentage of their child's behavior as stemming from purposeful opposition. Closer scrutiny frequently reveals that this behavior for most ADHD children results from inability to conform rather than planned opposition. It would be rare that a child placed in such a position would not develop some pattern of oppositional attitude or behavior. Over time, bad fit between the child's competencies and parental expectations leads to inappropriate parental demands and escalating punishment. The result is an angry, frustrated child who may become negative, provocative and oppositional with parents and other authority figures.

Temperamentally, some children may be more difficult to manage. Children with a strong need to control would be more likely to engage in power struggles with authority figures and to develop a repertoire of oppositional behaviors. It is not uncharacteristic for children with expressive language problems to develop strong controlling needs because of their inability to use language to effectively manipulate their environment. For the majority of ADHD children, a pattern of oppositional behavior is not a pre-existing condition but develops over time as a result of the unique aspects of the ADHD child's interactions with the environment.

The DSM-III-R cites the essential feature of an oppositional defiant disorder as a "pattern of negativistic, hostile and defiant behavior without the more serious violations of the basic rights of others that are seen in conduct disorder" (p. 56). Oppositional children are argumentative with adults, frequently lose their temper and seem angry, resentful, and easily annoyed by others. They tend to project the blame for their mistakes onto others. Characteristic of this disorder is the fact that these patterns of behavior are exhibited more commonly towards adults and other children whom the oppositional child interacts with on a regular basis. This pattern of behavior is rarely seen in a clinical setting with an unfamiliar practitioner. The DSM-III-R notes that this disorder is often associated with ADHD. Recent research (Shapiro & Garfinkel, 1986) suggests that there may be a significant overlap in children presenting with inattentive-overactive symptoms and those presenting with more serious oppositional and conduct problems. This will be discussed further in the following section on conduct problems.

According to the DSM-III-R definition oppositional defiant disorder typically begins by eight years of age. It frequently may evolve into a conduct or mood disorder. The child experiencing an oppositional defiant disorder presents at least five of the following nine behaviors with considerably greater frequency than would be common for children of the same mental age. These include:

1. Often loses temper
2. Often argues with adults
3. Often actively defies or refuses adult's requests or rules, e.g., refuses to do chores at home
4. Often deliberately does things that annoy other people, e.g., grabs other children's hats
5. Often blames others for his mistakes

6. Is often touchy or easily annoyed by others
7. Is often angry and resentful
8. Is often spiteful or vindictive
9. Often swears or uses obscene language (APA, 1987, p. 57)

A number of these criteria are frequently characteristic of ADHD children. Additionally, since many adults misinterpret the ADHD child's problems as resulting from purposeful misbehavior, they may report that a number of these other criteria have been met. A careful review of the child's history will often yield an etiology strongly suggesting that attention and arousal-related problems occurred first and were a major contributing force in the development of the child's pattern of oppositional behavior. It is rare that a child with only an oppositional defiant disorder will present sufficient behavioral, situational, and objective data to meet the criteria for an attention-deficit hyperactivity disorder.

Conduct Problems

The DSM-III-R defines the essential feature of conduct disorder as a "persistent pattern of conduct in which the basic rights of others and major age-appropriate societal norms or rules are violated" (p. 53). These problems are considered more serious than those seen in oppositional defiant disorder. Physical aggression, cruelty, destruction of property, confrontation with the victim and even physical violence may be present. Truancy and other school problems are observed. Drug, alcohol and sexual problems may also develop. The DSM-III-R also notes that "attentional difficulties, impulsiveness and hyperactivity are very common, especially in childhood, and may justify the additional diagnosis of attention-deficit hyperactivity disorder" (p. 54). Although DSM-III-R states that attention-deficit hyperactivity disorder is a commonly associated diagnosis, no prevalence and overlap occurrence data is provided in the manual. The DSM-III-R does observe that "antecedent attention-deficit hyperactivity disorder" may often be a predisposing factor (p. 54). Onset of conduct disorder for males is usually prior to puberty. Postpubertal onset is considered more common among females.

It is not surprising that there is a significant overlap in the presentation of attention-deficit and conduct disorder symptoms. In a nonreferred elementary school population, Shapiro and Garfinkel (1986) determined a prevalence of inattentive-overactive symptoms at 2.3% of the population. Children with aggressive and oppositional symptoms suggesting conduct disorder presented at a prevalence of 3.6%. An additional 3% demonstrated symptoms of both attention deficit and conduct disorder. Although symptomatic problems for these three groups were different, most assessment measures did not reflect group differences. A standardized questionnaire such as the Conners could differentiate the three groups, but a computerized attention battery was unsuccessful in doing so. It is for this reason that practitioners must be cautious in data interpretation. For example, when using the Conners, children with high hyperkinesis indices may also be presenting with a high degree of noncompliant behavior, which elevates their score.

The DSM-III-R describes both a group type of conduct disorder in which the essential feature is conduct problems that occur among members of a group and a solitary, aggressive type in which the essential feature is the predominance of physically aggressive behavior initiated by the child individually. There is a third undifferentiated type for children whose problems are a mixture. To meet the DSM-III-R diagnostic criteria for conduct disorder, the child or adolescent must present conduct problems lasting at least six months in which at least three of the following are present:

1. Has stolen without confrontation of a victim on more than one occasion (including forgery)
2. Has run away from home overnight at least twice while living in parental or surrogate home (or once without returning)
3. Often lies (other than to avoid physical or sexual abuse)
4. Has deliberately engaged in fire setting
5. Is often truant from school (for older person, absent from work)
6. Has broken into someone else's house, building or car
7. Has deliberately destroyed other's property (other than by fire setting)
8. Has been physically cruel to animals
9. Has forced someone into sexual activity with him or her
10. Has used a weapon in more than one fight
11. Often initiates physical fights
12. Has stolen with confrontation of a victim (e.g., mugging, purse-snatching, extortion, armed robbery)
13. Has been physically cruel to people (APA, 1987, p. 55)

Again, as noted for children with oppositional disorders, some of these diagnostic criteria are frequently met by ADHD children. Their impulsivity may lead ADHD children to steal, lie or engage in other impulsive behaviors such as initiating physical fights. Although the DSM-III-R provides criteria for severity of conduct disorder ranging from mild to severe, there is a very great difference in a child who meets the conduct disorder criteria because of minor theft, lying or fighting and a child meeting these criteria because of rape or extortion. Again, because the nonthinking, impulsive and nonpurposeful behavior of many ADHD children is often interpreted by many adults as planned, it would be easy for a number of these behaviors to be misinterpreted. The seriously conduct-disordered child is destructive and aggressive and with malicious forethought consistently engages in activities designed to hurt others for his own gain.

As with oppositional defiant disorder, the majority of children and adolescents presenting with conduct disorder did not present an early and significant history of attention-related problems. There is, however, a significant group of conduct-disordered children and adolescents who began with a progression of problems including inattention, impulsivity and overarousal. Problems may have been exacerbated as the result of a bad fit between child and parent temperament; a misinterpretation by parents, teachers and other authority figures concerning the cause of the child's problems; and a subsequent lack of effective, multidisciplinary intervention. The majority of children or adolescents presenting with conduct disorder and ADHD in all likelihood displayed ADHD and oppositional problems preceding the onset of serious conduct disorder.

The diagnosis of conduct disorder should be reserved for children and adolescents committing serious and persistent violations of the rights of others. When a question of ADHD etiology is unclear, the child or adolescent with conduct disorder will present a pattern of inattention, impulsivity and overarousal inconsistently across situations, and attention deficits will not be easily documented through objective data. The practitioner must use caution in determining direction of etiology since the majority of conduct-disordered individuals, especially angry, openly defiant, school-age adolescents, would appear to easily meet the DSM III-R diagnostic criteria for ADHD.

Although researchers have agreed that it may be difficult to generate test scores to differentiate conduct disorder and ADHD, behaviorally these disorders are very different (Hinshaw, 1987). Milich, Whidiger and Landau (1987) suggested that certain behaviors are more valuable as inclusionary, others as exclusionary, diagnostic criteria. Some behaviors can be used both ways. For example, the presence of stealing strongly suggests conduct problems, while its absence strongly suggests that a conduct disorder is not present. Lying and suspension from school, however, are not distinguishing factors and occur as frequently in conduct disorder and ADHD children. Lying, however, appears to be an efficient symptom for ruling out conduct disorder. If the child did not lie, it was highly unlikely in this study that he was having serious conduct problems. Similar observation was made for setting fires. The authors pointed out that the absence of symptoms such as "doesn't listen," "acts without thinking" and "easily distracted" was useful in excluding the conduct disorder diagnosis. If these behaviors did not occur, it was unlikely the child was experiencing a conduct disorder.

Depression

It has been reported that symptoms of attention deficit occur in up to 60% of depressed children (Stanton & Brumback, 1981). Weiss et al. (1971) found a high incidence of sadness, helpless feelings and poor self-image in children identified as hyperactive. It is important to note, however, that it has recently been reported that few attention-deficit symptoms are observed in boys experiencing major depressive disorder; however, depression symptoms are commonly noted in ADHD children (Jensen, Burke, & Garfinkel, 1988). These authors also suggest that children diagnosed with ADHD on the basis of impulsive symptoms rather than inattention symptoms may actually be depressed. Based on this data, it is strongly suggested that the practitioner carefully consider the contribution of depression in the etiology of attention-disordered symptoms. The administration of depression rating scales should be routinely considered when questions of depression arise.

Sometimes the practitioner is faced with the need to determine whether the child is presenting with depression or ADHD. When depression is a factor, there is frequently a positive family history for depressive episodes. The DSM-III-R criteria note that in order to make a diagnosis of major depressive episode the child must present a change in previous functioning over a two-week period in which at least one of the symptoms is either depressed mood or loss of interest or pleasure. These are important differentiating criteria for the practitioner to consider. The majority of problems the ADHD child is experiencing are chronic and persistent. On this basis alone, the majority of ADHD children would not be considered to experience single-episode major depression, unless there is an acute change in their presentation. Also using this criteria, it would be rare for the majority of ADHD children to present with recurrent major depression since the primary criterion for this disorder involves two or more major depressive episodes, each separated by at least two months or more of usual functioning. Again, the majority of ADHD children present chronic problems. Characteristic ADHD symptoms that overlap with depression include sleep problems, irritability, hyperactivity, impulsivity and difficulty with concentration.

The DSM-III-R also provides diagnostic criteria for a related mood disorder, dysthymia. Dysthymic children during periods of depression present with at least two of the following symptoms:

1. Poor appetite or overeating
2. Insomnia or hypersomnia
3. Low energy or fatigue
4. Low self-esteem
5. Poor concentration or difficulty making decisions
6. Feelings of hopelessness (APA, 1987, p. 232)

While many ADHD children may present with at least two of these behaviors, diagnostic criteria for dysthymia also include irritability or depressed mood "for most of the day, more days than not" (APA, 1987, p. 232). For children, this pattern of depressed mood must be consistently present during a one-year period, and the child must not be without these symptoms for more than a two-month period at a time. Again, it is rare for the majority of ADHD children to meet all of the criteria necessary for a diagnosis of dysthymia.

In considering the diagnosis of dysthymia, the practitioner must be cautioned that the key diagnostic issue may be determining whether irritable mood stems from symptoms of helplessness and depression or is simply a characteristic of the ADHD child's overarousal and impulsivity. The majority of depressed or dysthymic children will not present with significantly elevated attention rating scales or objective data clearly indicative of attention deficit. ADHD children with significant overarousal and hyperactivity problems and long histories of environmental failure appear at greatest risk to develop symptoms of dysthymia. The DSM-III-R notes that in children and adolescents ADHD is a predisposing factor for dysthymia.

Dysthymia is also often observed to begin with a clear onset and a chronic course. Differential diagnosis is further complicated by the fact that depressed children may exhibit confrontive negative behavior towards others and be poorly motivated and inattentive at school.

Anxiety

The DSM-III-R provides diagnostic descriptions for three specific anxiety-related disorders of childhood or adolescence. These involve problems with separation anxiety, avoidance or overanxious response. DSM-III-R also provides additional diagnostic categories for adults, some of which may be used with children, including phobias and post traumatic stress disorder. The DSM-III-R notes that children with ADHD "may appear nervous and jittery, but are not unduly concerned about the future" (p. 64).

Again we have the issue of differential diagnosis. For the ADHD child, apparent nervousness is related to a physiological state that occurs steadily and is often independent of environmental events. Children experiencing an overanxious disorder typically have excessive somatic complaints, marked self-consciousness, an excessive need for reassurance and feelings of tension or inability to relax. Practitioners insensitive to the restless, seemingly anxious behavior of the ADHD child are at risk to interpret behaviors, including pulling of clothing, wiping back and forth with an arm across a desk or fidgeting in a chair, as signs of excessive anxiety, when in fact they represent symptoms of ADHD. The reverse may also be true. As noted in Chapter 6, standardized questionnaires such as the Achenbach Child Behavior Checklist, as well as direct inquiry about the child's fears, anxieties and current emotional status, is the best way of providing a differential diagnosis. It is rare for an ADHD child to develop serious anxiety-related symptoms. It is also rare for the child experiencing specific anxiety problems to present the range of attention and overarousal problems that characterize most ADHD children.

Adjustment Problems

The DSM-III-R provides descriptions for nine adjustment disorders. The primary feature of adjustment problems "is a maladaptive reaction to an identifiable psycho-social stressor or stressors that occurs within three months after the onset of the stressor and has persisted for no longer than six months" (APA, 1987, p. 329). The diagnostic criteria include impairment in school functioning, social activities and relationships with others. Symptoms can vary but are in excess of what is normal and expected. The disturbance must also not be one instance of a pattern of over reaction to stress. The diagnostic criteria for adjustment disorder also indicate that "the disturbance does not meet the criteria for any specific mental disorder" (APA, 1987, p. 330). This has resulted in this diagnostic category being used as a catch-all for children experiencing symptomatic problems not severe enough to warrant other psychiatric diagnoses. Adjustment disorders include several subtypes with differing manifestations: problems with anxious or depressed mood, disturbance of conduct, mixed disturbance of emotions and conduct, mixed emotional features, physical complaints, withdrawal, work or academic inhibition and a ninth category for other adjustment problems that do not fit any of those specific descriptions.

Many ADHD children, in response to the stress of school, develop a repertoire of mixed emotional problems. Frequently, these problems are not strong enough in severity to warrant diagnoses of depression, anxiety, opposition or conduct problem but do appear to meet the diagnosis of adjustment disorder. In this case the specific stress is school. The ADHD child's adjustment problems are frequently cyclical but do not actually represent single instances in a pattern of overreaction to stress. More accurately, these problems represent the number of forces acting upon the ADHD child and the child's ability to meet the demands of the environment. Summer brings fewer demands, and many ADHD children function better. They begin school and after a number of months of failure begin demonstrating increased emotional difficulty. Once school ends they again have a period of relative freedom and decreased demands. In response, their emotional difficulties diminish.

Many practitioners use the adjustment disorder diagnoses as a means of providing additional diagnostic labels for some of the emotional and behavioral problems ADHD children experience. Although the diagnostic criteria indicate that the maladaptive reaction should persist for no longer than six months, the DSM-III-R notes "that if the stressor persists . . . , as in a chronic physical illness, it may take much longer to achieve a new level of adaptation" (p. 330). With this qualifier in mind, the diagnosis of adjustment disorder can be used to define and set apart emotional or behavioral problems an ADHD child may experience.

By definition, adjustment disorders do not represent a pattern of chronic disability. It is therefore rare for a child experiencing only adjustment problems to present as if he had a history of attention and arousal difficulty on a long-term basis. As with many other disorders of childhood, ADHD children experiencing adjustment disorders stemming from a specific stressor such as death in the family or a move to a new home usually present with a pre-existing pattern of attention and arousal problems. The adjustment difficulties arise from the new demands placed upon the ADHD child and the child's inability to meet those demands.

Learning/Developmental Problems

Language Difficulty

Research by Baker and Cantwell (1987) suggests that as children with significant speech and language problems mature, a significant percentage, as high as one-third, appear at risk to develop patterns of inattention and overarousal. Many of these children develop this pattern of behavior in response to the stress and frustration that arises as a result of their difficulty communicating.

The emergence of complex language skills coincides with a child's improvement in self-control. As verbal abilities improve, children are able to more effectively process information and express their needs. Language becomes a substitute for action. When language development is abnormal, the development of behavioral control is potentially disrupted. Many parents and clinicians do not understand the connection between language development and a child's behavioral self-control. Children with language impairments are frequently placed in situations where their ability to respond appropriately is compromised, not because of a lack of motivation or an attention deficit but because of specific language disability. When parents and teachers inadvertently continue to place pressure upon the language-disordered child to conform behaviorally, a chronic pattern of behavioral, attention and arousal-level problems may develop. Parental frustration over the child's inability to follow directions may lead to anger and exaggerate the language-impaired child's level of frustration, which leads to characteristic temper tantrums.

In the preschool years, more subtle and complex language impairments frequently go unrecognized by parents and many professionals. Frequently, the child's misbehavior may end up being the focus of treatment, resulting in interventions directed at symptomatic behavior rather than the underlying cause of that behavior. As the public's awareness of overarousal and attention problems in children increases, it is also increasingly likely that the practitioner will be asked to evaluate a young child by a parent who believes that the source of the child's overarousal and attention problems stems from an attention-deficit hyperactivity disorder. Even behaviorally disordered children with clear-cut histories of speech and language problems are frequently thought to be "hyperactive" without any consideration that their behavioral problems might arise from language disability. The errant focus on the source of the child's problems precipitates a frustrating cycle of interventions that may be misdirected. It is important for practitioners to recognize that delayed or deviant language development can lead to a wide range of behavioral problems, including symptoms mimicking attention-deficit hyperactivity disorder.

Differential diagnosis for both younger and older language-impaired children is difficult. When preschool children experience both language and attention difficulty, the practitioner may be unable to clearly determine which disability came first. With these preschoolers, it is judicious to initially assume, unless the history strongly suggests otherwise, that a significant component of the child's attention and overarousal difficulty stems from specific language impairments. For such children, the focus and intervention must initially be language-based, providing both professional remediation and parent training. Such children must be monitored closely as they enter school. Many two- and three-year-olds with significant language problems accompanied by serious temper outbursts improve significantly in behavior when an appropriate course of language intervention is provided.

With school-age children, language processing impairments are significantly more subtle. They may be difficult for the practitioner to detect. The frustrated, language-impaired child presenting symptoms of attention deficit is frequently not significantly hyperactive. Although based on parent or teacher ratings the child may receive elevated attention-deficit scores, he usually performs well on objective measures of attention. Characteristically, he presents as significantly weaker on tasks of auditory and verbal attention, as opposed to tasks of visual or perceptual attention. His verbal subtest scores on the Wechsler are frequently lower than his performance scores.

Auditory Processing Dysfunction

Efficient operation of the auditory system involves not only adequate acuity and the collection of auditory information but the efficient capacity to transmit, decode and integrate signals received along the aural pathway. Impairment in the auditory processing system can result in poor auditory attending skills, deficits in discrimination, limitations in auditory memory and retrieval, and delays in receptive and expressive language development. In a home or classroom setting, children with specific auditory processing dysfunctions related to attention and memory may appear to present many of the same symptoms as the attention-disordered child without hyperactivity. These children rarely become overemotional and are not terribly impulsive. Other family members may experience similar disorders. These children usually have normal hearing acuity, but poor auditory association, retention, closure, discrimination and recall. They may or may not have more observable speech and language disorders such as articulation difficulty.

Recent research has suggested that auditory processing disorders in children reflect nothing more than specific attention deficits (Burd & Fisher, 1986; Gascon, Johnson & Burd, 1986). This is a heated topic of debate among audiologists, with lines of opinion clearly drawn. Clinical opinion supports the hypothesis that auditory processing dysfunction is a separate disorder that may or may not occur in conjunction with ADHD (Harward, "personal communication," 1987). Children with auditory processing disorders typically do not have significantly elevated behavioral scales for attention and overarousal problems, do perform well on tasks of visual attention and are not usually described as experiencing numerous situational problems of strong severity.

Memory Problems

Norman (1969), in his excellent text on memory and attention, notes that all paths of human processing lead to memory. Attention is considered the initial step in the process. Children with attentional problems will not process as much information and therefore will not have the opportunity to store and recall that information. Attention-disordered children may then appear to have memory deficits. Conversely, children with memory disorders but intact capacity to pay attention may, based on their poor recall, be accused of faulty attentional skills. Differential diagnosis for the practitioner is a complex and difficult process.

Memory, much like attention, is an extremely complex process that is used in all of our interactions with the environment. Psychology has not yet developed a widely accepted, comprehensive model of memory processes and specific types of memory skills. We make a rough distinction between auditory and visual memory, as well as between immediate, short-term and long-term memory. The complexity of memory processes is reflected in the fact that there are no comprehensive memory assessment batteries for children. Memory is frequently inferred by a child's performance on a variety of auditory, visual and motor tasks. Children with memory difficulty, but not attention problems, will present with lower scores on attention-related behavior checklists and minimal situational problems. They usually perform well on tasks of persistence, sustained attention and divided attention. For example, on tasks such as the Detroit Auditory and Visual Attention Span Tests, the child with impaired memory will consistently recall just so many stimulus items and consistently demonstrate the ability to recall the first few and last few items in each presentation. This reflects a serial position learning effect. Conversely, the ADHD child will be very inconsistent in his performance; for example, demonstrating the ability to recall a sequence of five stimulus items one moment but only two or three the next moment. In objectively making the differential diagnosis for memory problems, the revised Stanford Binet (Thorndike, Hagen & Satler, 1986) may be of assistance with younger children, and the Denman Neuropsychology Memory Scale (Denman, 1984) can be very helpful with older children and adolescents.

Achievement Problems

Children with attention and overarousal problems resulting from the frustration of academic failure will rarely present histories of this type of problem before entering an organized school program. For the practitioner, this is often essential differential data. Learning-disabled children with attention and overarousal problems resulting from frustration may have elevated attention-deficit behavior checklist scores, but on direct assessment will often perform well on measures of attention span. Tarnowski, Prinz and Ney (1986) in a comparative study found that ADD children with and without learning disabilities experience problems with sustained attention. However, learning disabled children without ADD did not experience problems with sustained attention but appeared to have difficulty with selective attention and short-term memory. The group of children experiencing both ADD and learning disability presented with the largest range of attentional problems.

Behavioral observation will also yield data suggesting that the child's lack of persistence and attention results from feelings of helplessness and incompetence rather than an inability to stay on task. Cunningham and Barkley (1978a) presented a theory to explain the presence of attention and overarousal problems in children experiencing persistent academic difficulty and failure. Hyperactivity, difficulty with attention and emotionality are considered symptoms of academic failure in Cunningham and Barkley's model. Aggression and impulsivity, which frequently occur in ADHD children, are regarded as responses to the frustration of classroom failure. This model is probably accurate in describing the development of attention and overarousal problems in children with other forms of developmental impairment that may impede academic achievement or language development. Baker and Cantwell's (1987) research suggested a marked increase in difficulty with attention and overarousal problems over a five-year period in children continuing to experience significant language problems and learning difficulty. This longitudinal data suggests that a percentage of this population developed symptomatic problems with attention and overarousal in response to environmental stress.

General Intellectual Deficits

It is not surprising, since attention is a complex process in the brain, that children with intellectual deficits experience attention-related problems. The more intellectually impaired a child is the more likely it is that the entire brain is dysfunctional and the greater difficulty there will be with related skills such as attention span. For this population, difficulty with attention is a symptom of faulty intelligence. Such a population of children will present with elevated scores on attention-sensitive behavior checklists, multiple situational problems and difficulty on objective measures of attention and reflection, and may, on a superficial level, meet the DSM-III-R diagnostic criteria for ADHD. The majority of these children, however, do not experience primary attention deficit. When their behavior and test performance is compared to their mental age, they do not present with significantly different problems from other intellectually handicapped children. However, there are some intellectually handicapped children who, even when this comparative adjustment is made, continue to appear to have attention and overarousal problems that are significantly greater than other children of their chronological age and cognitive skills. This small population of intellectually handicapped children may be experiencing significant attention problems relative to their overall cognitive abilities. Although treatment for the attention difficulty must be approached with caution, this population of children may be benefited by stimulant medications and training to improve on task behavior.

For the practitioner, differential diagnosis of intellectual deficit versus ADHD is based on a careful history. The history may demonstrate a long standing pattern of developmental delays that were present before the observation or onset of attention and arousal-related problems. Considering the child's mental age also assists in making the differential diagnosis.

Specific Cognitive Deficits

Problems with Speed of Information Processing

The speed at which a child can process incoming stimulation is not an attentional skill. However, children who are slow information processors may appear not to be paying attention in classroom situations. Efficient information processing is an essential cognitive skill (Ben-Yishay, Rattok & Diller, 1979). The speed with which a child can assimilate and integrate information from his environment is directly, but not completely, related to his intellectual capacity. There is a population of learning-impaired children with adequate intellect but impairment in the speed with which they can assimilate information from the environment. Such children often have difficulty on tasks such as the Wechsler Coding subtest, the Symbol Digit Modalities Test and the Trail-Making Test. In classroom settings these children are described by their teachers as slow to grasp or understand instructions, and they experience difficulty completing tasks in the assigned amount of time. For the practitioner, the differential determination that must be made is between this type of problem and the ADHD child's lack of persistence. Both problems may yield performance results that look similar. Differentially, if additional instruction is provided and sufficient response time is allowed, the slow processors will remain on task and persist. However, unlike that of the persistent ADHD child, whose persistence does not pay off because of disorganization, the quality of the slow information processing child's work will be adequate, but the work will be slow-in-coming. Lifting time limits will often reveal the difference since the ADHD child, even if he remains on task, will be disorganized and the quality of his work may not reflect the extra time taken.

Difficulty with Flexible Thinking

In discussing cognitive skills, flexibility implies the child's ability to deal with new or novel stimulation in an efficient manner. Children with problems in this area often struggle when faced with even simple novel tasks. Such children have difficulty on the Trail-Making Test and the Progressive Figures Test. They may also experience problems on tasks of concept formation such as the Categories Test from the Halstead-Reitan Battery, the Visual-Verbal Test (Feldman & Drasgow, 1981) or the Test of Non-Verbal Intelligence (Brown, Sherbenou and Dollar, 1983). It is not uncommon for ADHD children to have problems with flexibility in thinking. This problem, however, is insufficient to explain the severity and extent of the ADHD child's problems. When this problem is present in an ADHD child, that child frequently has increased difficulty. Even when she is paying attention it may be difficult for her to handle and approach novel tasks, which results in increasing frustration and an exacerbation of overarousal and inattentive problems.

Problems Forming Concepts

The ability to develop rules and relationships about the world is an essential component for efficient learning and appropriate behavior. Often, ADHD children appear to have difficulty with concept formation because of the fact that their impulsivity results in repetitive mistakes. Differentially, these children understand the concept required for successful performance, but when the time comes to make a decision, they are influenced by their impulsive need for gratification rather than an internal sense of responsibility to plan and follow task rules. When the practitioner makes an extended effort to ensure that the child is paying attention, ADHD children and adolescents usually do not have problems performing tasks of reasoning, judgment and concept formation such as the Category Test, Visual-Verbal Test (Feldman & Drasgow, 1981), or the Test of Non-Verbal Intelligence (Brown, Sherbenou & Dollar, 1983). When care is not taken to control for impulsivity, ADHD children may make increased errors of commission that result from an impulsive response style. Such a pattern can be easily observed and differentiated by the practitioner during assessment.

Medical Factors

As explained in Chapter 3, the practitioner must make certain that the child's attention and arousal-related problems are not primarily caused by a specific physical or neurological abnormality. It is rare for such problems to be the cause of ADHD. Nonetheless, a thorough medical evaluation is important to allow the physician to rule out these potential causes.

The most common of these rarely occurring contributing medical factors appears to be head trauma. As such, there is a strong likelihood that practitioners will be faced with children presenting attention and arousal-level problems as a consequence of a head injury. It has also been observed that children with mild attention and arousal problems appear at risk to develop a full-blown pattern of difficulty with these behaviors following head trauma. It is important for the practitioner to rule out the contribution of a specific neurological trauma in the development of the ADHD child's problems. If trauma appears to be the source of attention and arousal problems, the practitioner must make additional effort to provide a well-documented overview of specific attentional skills. Frequently, children with attention-related problems stemming from head trauma present a checkerboard pattern of attention difficulty in which certain attention skills have not been affected, while others are significantly impaired. For many head-trauma children, problems with speed of information processing and concept formation may contribute to observations of attention deficit. Often this population of traumatically induced ADHD exhibits significantly high levels of overarousal and behavioral problems. Such children often are an enigma for their parents and teachers. For such children, a careful evaluation is essential to define problems and facilitate treatment planning.

INTEGRATING THE DATA

The most helpful approach for understanding the complexity of attentional problems, integrating the data, making the diagnosis and understanding commonly associated problems is through case studies. The remainder of this chapter will be devoted to specific cases describing children with attention difficulty and other specific cognitive or behavioral problems. The greatest risk the practitioner faces is making the diagnosis of ADHD based on a narrow scope of evaluation, limited review of the data presented or an inappropriate emphasis on specific elements of historical, behavioral or testing data to the exclusion of other relevant data. The risk of false diagnosis is minimized when a systematic approach such as the Diagnostic Checklist is used. In such a situation, children meeting the DSM-III-R diagnostic criteria but not presenting with elevated rating scales, extensive situational problems or objective data suggesting attention difficulty will not be diagnosed as ADHD, and other sources for their problems will be sought. Similarly, children presenting with elevated rating scales and situational problems but not objective data problems or behavior meeting the DSM-III-R diagnostic criteria will also not be diagnosed as ADHD. The two biggest problems facing the practitioner in making the diagnosis occur when it is difficult to clearly rule out alternative etiologies and when the objective data does not consistently suggest attention problems. Because ADHD is a common disorder of childhood, it is more likely than not that the majority of children experiencing emotional, learning or cognitive problems with concomitant symptoms of ADHD have presented with foundational attention and arousal problems prior to or in conjunction with these other difficulties.

As previously discussed, it is not uncommon for ADHD children over time to develop a pattern of oppositional behavior in response to their frustration. The diagnosis of oppositional defiant disorder may often be made to describe the behavioral problems many ADHD children develop. Many ADHD children may also experience specific developmental disorders. These are the two most commonly associated diagnoses. The cases presented will describe not only these coexisting problems but other less frequently encountered problems that may occur concomitantly with ADHD.

It is not unusual for an ADHD child to present strengths in some attentional skills but weaknesses in others. As noted earlier, the majority of ADHD children have problems with vigilance and sustained attention. As the case studies will demonstrate, some ADHD children are not particularly impulsive and can sustain attention. However, they have difficulty with vigilance, divided attention and disorganization while they are persisting with a task. The practitioner must keep in mind that the Diagnostic Checklist is meant as an organizational tool, not as a normative or score-based checklist upon which to make the diagnosis of ADHD. It is essential for a child to present problems in the first four areas and for the practitioner to rule out causative problems in the fifth area. The severity of problems and the specificity of those problems is left to the practitioner's decision in terms of how different this child is from children of the same chronological age or developmental level. Use of the ADHD Diagnostic Checklist provides the practitioner with a solid framework to consider the diagnosis of ADHD in childhood and adolescence.

DEALING WITH THE DATA: CASE STUDIES

APPARENT ADHD AND LANGUAGE DISORDER: THE CASE OF T. H.

T. H., a 3-year-old child, was referred by her speech pathologist. At three years of age, T. H.'s receptive language skills appeared approximately six to eight months delayed, with expressive language skills appearing approximately fourteen to sixteen months delayed. After a normal infancy, T. H., at two years of age, began demonstrating a pattern of inattention, impulsivity and overarousal. Parents reported problems with eye contact and a dislike for cuddling. Multiple daily temper outbursts, sleep problems and oppositional behavior primarily directed at her mother were also reported. Further assessment of parenting strategies reflected an inconsistent, confrontive approach by the mother, which appeared to be reinforcing increasing oppositional problems.

Parent responses to the questionnaires indicated significant attention and arousal-related problems. Preschool observations did not suggest significant difficulties in these areas. Temperament assessment suggested a somewhat overactive child with increased negative mood, difficulty fitting routines and a strong intensity of reaction. Parent and preschool observations of social skills noted social isolation,

NAME ___T.H._____ D.O.B. _____ AGE 3 yr 0 mo DATE _____

HISTORY

Age of Onset _____2_____
Average Independent Attention Span
  (Minutes) _____3_____
Easily Overaroused ___Yes___
Impulsive ___Yes___
S̶ Not Effective ___Yes___
Other 1. Normal Infancy
  2. Problems with eye contact
  3. Disliked cuddling
  4. Late milestones
  5. Speech and language problems
  6. Multiple daily temper outbursts
  7. Sleep problems 8. Oppositional

QUESTIONNAIRES   w/mother

Parent Conners   Above 98th %ile
Teacher Conners   50th   %ile
ACTeRS: Attention   %ile
       Hyperactivity   %ile
       Social Skills   %ile
       Oppositional   %ile
Parent Achenbach: Scales Above 98th %ile
Social withdrawal
Aggression
_____   _____
_____   _____
_____   _____

Teacher Achenbach: Scales Above 98th %ile
_____   _____
_____   _____
_____   _____
_____   _____

Home Situations Problems:
Number of Situations   11
Average Severity Moderate
School Situations Problems:
Number of Situations
Average Severity
Parent Social Skills: Type of Problems
1. Argumentative
2. Socially isolated
3. Lacks social and communication
   skills

Teacher Social Skills: Type of Problems
1. Prefers to play alone
2. Withdrawal from group
3. Limited vocabulary
_____

Observation During Assessment
1. Delayed receptive & expressive skills
2. Good attention span
3. Emotionally responsive
4. Cooperative
5. Tested mother's limits at close
   of assessment

PERSONALITY OR EMOTIONAL FACTORS
1. Normal range of emotional response
   observed
_____
_____
_____

WECHSLER

Verbal	S.S.	Performance	S.S.
Information	____	Picture Completion	____
Similarities	____	Picture Arrangement	____
Arithmetic	____	Block Design	____
Vocabulary	____	Object Assembly	____
Comprehension	____	Coding	____
Digit Span	____	Mazes	____
Verbal I.Q.	____	Performance I.Q.	____
	Full Scale I.Q.	____	

MOTOR SKILLS

Purdue Pegboard: Preferred Hand   %ile
           Non-preferred hand   %ile
           Both hands   %ile
           Assembly   %ile
Developmental Test of Visual Motor
  Integration   50th %ile
Bender Visual Motor Gestalt Test   %ile
Benton Visual Retention Test   %ile
Detroit Test:
  Auditory Attention Span
  Visual Attention Span   _____
  Notes on Performance   _____
_____

Matching Familiar Figures Test:
  Errors   %ile
  Completion Time   %ile
Peabody Picture Vocabulary Test   19th %ile
Trail Making Test: Completion Time   %ile
          Errors   %ile
Progressive Figures Test   %ile
Rapidly Recurring Target Figures:
  592: Completion Time   %ile
     Errors   %ile
  Diamond: Completion Time   %ile
     Errors   %ile
Motor Free Visual Perception Test   %ile
Hand Preference ____ Left   X Right

ACADEMICS

Test	Grade	%ile
_____	_____	_____
_____	_____	_____
_____	_____	_____
_____	_____	_____

OTHER TESTS OR QUESTIONNAIRES

Test	Score or %ile
1. Parent Temperament: Overactive, strong	
intensity of reflection, doesn't fit	
routines well, negative mood.	
2. Stanford-Binet - I.Q. = 100	
Strength in visual skills	
Weakness in verbal skills	

ADHD Diagnostic Checklist Criteria

I	Situationally	III	No
II	Situationally	IV	Home
	V Language & Parenting		

Figure 7.2 Apparent ADHD and language disorder: The case of T. H. ADHD Worksheet by S. Goldstein. Copyright 1989. Used in this and all subsequent figures with permission of the author.

a delay in basic social communication and argumentative behavior, primarily with her mother.

Observation during assessment reflected significant receptive and expressive language problems. T. H. was very cooperative and remained seated for a one hour period during the assessment. She demonstrated a good attention span and was cooperative and emotionally responsive to the examiner. At the close of the evaluation she was somewhat oppositional with her mother, but when a limit was clearly set by the examiner, T. H. responded appropriately. A normal range of emotional response and interaction was observed with the examiner.

Assessment revealed a child with average intellectual skill. Despite significant language impairments, the development of average intellect suggested that T. H.'s intellectual potential was probably somewhat better than the average. Her receptive vocabulary, as measured by the Peabody Picture Vocabulary Test, was delayed. Fine motor speed and coordination tested in the average range. Despite impaired language, the quality of T. H.'s play with the examiner during the assessment was appropriate.

T. H. appeared to exhibit attention problems within the home. Objective data did not suggest significant attention problems. Medical evaluation was unremarkable. The DSM-III-R criteria were met if the home situation was viewed independently from this child's behavior during the assessment or from behavior in the preschool. The complication of a child with a difficult temperament, receptive and expressive language problems and ineffective parent intervention appeared to be the source of the majority of T. H.'s attention and arousal-related problems. Based on the history, behavioral observation and test data, a diagnosis of receptive and expressive language disorder was made with a recommendation that T. H.'s development be closely monitored and parenting intervention be initiated.

APPARENT ADHD, OPPOSITIONAL DISORDER, AUDITORY PROCESSING DYSFUNCTION AND MILD LANGUAGE-BASED LEARNING DISABILITIES: THE CASE OF J. S.

J. S., a 7-year, 4-month old first grader, was referred by a family friend. J. S.'s mother was concerned that her ex-husband was causing J.S. to become emotionally disturbed. J. S.'s parents had been divorced 3 1/2 years previously. During the last few years of their marriage, J. S. was exposed to considerable family discord. Since the divorce, he had seen his father infrequently; however, he had continued to observe bickering and arguing between his parents. J. S.'s mother blamed his father for not coming to visit him, while making it very difficult for J. S.'s father to arrange weekly visits. J. S.'s father withheld child support money as a means of retaliation. Both parents described J. S. as caught in the middle.

J. S. had a normal infancy. He experienced problems as soon as he entered school and repeated kindergarten because of immaturity. J. S.'s mother provided the developmental and behavioral history. She reported having no problems with J. S. in the home. J. S.'s father, however, reported that during visits with him, J. S. was extremely manipulative and controlling. If he could not have his way he would immediately have a tantrum. Upon further questioning, J. S.'s mother

NAME ___J.S._____ D.O.B. _____ AGE _7 yr 4 mo_ DATE _____

HISTORY

Age of Onset ____5____
Average Independent Attention Span
 (Minutes) ___15___
Easily Overaroused ___Yes___
Impulsive ___Yes___
S Not Effective ___Yes___
Other 1. Parents divorced 3. years
2. Continued stress between parents
3. J.S. in the middle
4. Normal infancy
5. Repeated kindergarten
6. Reportedly not causing mother
 significant problems

QUESTIONNAIRES

Parent Conners	85th	%ile
Teacher Conners	95th	%ile
ACTeRS: Attention		%ile
Hyperactivity		%ile
Social Skills		%ile
Oppositional		%ile

Parent Achenbach: Scales Above 98th %ile
Aggression _____ _____
_____ _____
_____ _____
_____ _____

Teacher Achenbach: Scales Above 98th %ile
Unpopular _____ _____
Inattentive _____ _____
Aggressive _____ _____
_____ _____

Home Situations Problems:
 Number of Situations ___3___
 Average Severity ___Mild___
School Situations Problems:
 Number of Situations ___9___
 Average Severity ___Moderate___
Parent Social Skills: Type of Problems
1. Argumentative
2. Negative
3. Bossy

Teacher Social Skills: Type of Problems
1. Manipulative and coercive
2. Controlling
3. Aggressive
4. Poor judgment

Observation During Assessment
1. Calm
2. Related well to examiner
3. Attempted to control evaluation
 session

PERSONALITY OR EMOTIONAL FACTORS
1. Immature
2. Egocentric
3. Lacks conscience
4. Aggressive view of problem solution
5. Poor social perception
6. Unresolved divorce issues

WECHSLER

Verbal	S.S.	Performance	S.S.
Information	9	Picture Completion	13
Similarities	15	Picture Arrangement	13
Arithmetic	9	Block Design	15
Vocabulary	14	Object Assembly	17
Comprehension	9	Coding	12
Digit Span		Mazes	
Verbal I.Q.	107	Performance I.Q.	129
	Full Scale I.Q.	119	

MOTOR SKILLS

Purdue Pegboard: Preferred Hand ___60th %ile___
 Non-preferred hand ___10th %ile___
 Both hands ___50th %ile___
 Assembly ___60th %ile___
Developmental Test of Visual Motor
 Integration _____ %ile
Bender Visual Motor Gestalt Test ___85th %ile___
Benton Visual Retention Test _____ %ile
Detroit Test:
 Auditory Attention Span _____
 Visual Attention Span _____
 Notes on Performance _____
_____

Matching Familiar Figures Test:
 Errors ___50th %ile___
 Completion Time ___37th %ile___
Peabody Picture Vocabulary Test _____ %ile
Trail Making Test: Completion Time _____ %ile
 Errors _____ %ile
Progressive Figures Test _____ %ile
Rapidly Recurring Target Figures:
 592: Completion Time ___50th %ile___
 Errors ___50th %ile___
 Diamond: Completion Time ___50th %ile___
 Errors ___50th %ile___
Motor Free Visual Perception Test _____ %ile
Hand Preference ___X___ Left _____ Right

ACADEMICS

Test	Grade	%ile
WRAT-Reading		25th
WRAT-Arithmetic		32nd
Letter & Numberwriting		2 mirror image reversals

OTHER TESTS OR QUESTIONNAIRES

Test	Score or %ile
Wepman Auditory Discrimination	4 errors
Visual Aural Digit Span Test	35th %ile

ADHD Diagnostic Checklist Criteria

I	Yes	III	No
II	Yes (Situational)	IV	No
	V	No	

Figure 7.3 Apparent ADHD, oppositional disorder, auditory processing dysfunction and mild language-based learning disabilities: The case of J. S.

acknowledged that the easiest way of managing J. S. in the home was to let him do whatever he wanted. She described J. S. as having on the average an attention span of 15 minutes for independent activities. She acknowledged that he was easily overaroused and impulsive. She indicated that rewards were effective in changing his behavior.

School data suggested more significant problems than J. S.'s mother was reporting. Questionnaires suggested significant problems with attention and arousal level. More difficulty with aggression and manipulative behavior was noted at school. J. S.'s mother acknowledged that with peers he could be argumentative, negative and bossy. Schoolteachers reported that he was manipulative and often acted in a way designed to hurt others. Only mild situational problems were noted in the home, but moderate problems were noted in almost all school situations. J. S. was not completing his school work.

During the evaluation, J. S. superficially related to the examiner. He was generally calm and not labile. He frequently tried to control the course of the evaluation by attempting to engage the examiner in conversation or to change tasks. He was willing to respond to limits set by the examiner.

Assessment data revealed an extremely intelligent child with a significant weakness in verbal skills. Lateralizing measures supported a relative left-brain weakness. For example, J. S.'s nonpreferred hand performance on the Purdue Pegboard was significantly lower than his ability to work with his preferred hand or his ability to use both hands together. Objective assessment did not suggest significant problems with reflection or attentional skills. Brief academic screening yielded low-average academic achievement scores, well below expectation based on J. S.'s intellectual capacity.

It was clear from all the data collected that J. S. was a pawn in his parents' ongoing problems. His passive mother was reinforcing his controlling, oppositional behavior. He then unsuccessfully attempted to exert this control in other areas of his life. School data was of concern, suggesting the early onset of more serious conduct problems. Assessment data did not indicate significant problems with attention or reflection skills but suggested a relative weakness with verbal/linguistic skills. Further assessment by the audiologist documented significant auditory processing dysfunction. Medical evaluation did not identify a specific physical problem.

Additionally, J. S.'s exceptionally good intellect combined with his low academic skills appeared to be creating additional stress at school. Often J. S. was unable and, at times, unwilling to begin or to persist with academic tasks. Although historical and questionnaire data suggested that J. S. met the DSM-III-R diagnostic criteria for ADHD, objective assessment did not yield attention-related problems, and J. S.'s family history appeared to be the primary cause of attention and arousal-level difficulties. Diagnoses of oppositional disorder and developmental learning problems were made.

ADHD IN A CHILD WITH HIGH INTELLECTUAL SKILLS: THE CASE OF D. W.

D. W., an 11½-year-old fifth grader, was referred by his pediatrician, following an unremarkable medical evaluation, for a history of attention problems, over-

NAME _____ D.W. _____ D.O.B. _____ AGE 11 yr 6 mo DATE _____

HISTORY

Age of Onset _____ 2 _____
Average Independent Attention Span
  (Minutes) _____ 10 _____
Easily Overaroused _____ Yes _____
Impulsive _____ Yes _____
S Not Effective _____ Yes _____
Other 1. Family history of ADHD _____
2. Problems not purposeful _____
3. Increasing school problems _____
_____
_____

QUESTIONNAIRES

Parent Conners _____ above 99th %ile
Teacher Conners _____ above 99th %ile
ACTeRS: Attention _____ %ile
        Hyperactivity _____ %ile
        Social Skills _____ %ile
        Oppositional _____ %ile
Parent Achenbach: Scales Above 98th %ile
Hyperactivity _____ _____
Aggression _____ _____
_____
_____
_____

Teacher Achenbach: Scales Above 98th %ile
_____
_____
_____
_____

Home Situations Problems:
  Number of Situations _____ 14 _____
  Average Severity _____ Moderate _____
School Situations Problems:
  Number of Situations _____ 5 _____
  Average Severity _____ Moderate _____
Parent Social Skills: Type of Problems

1. Lacks social skill
2. Tries to be center of attention
_____
_____

Teacher Social Skills: Type of Problems
1. Overwhelms peers
2. Incompetent
_____
_____

Observation During Assessment
1. Related well to examiner
2. No significant problems during
   evaluation
3. Tried
4. Adequate motivation
_____

PERSONALITY OR EMOTIONAL FACTORS
1. Aware of attention problems
2. Desires more friends
3. Immature
4. Poor problem solving skills
5. Adequate emotional development

WECHSLER

Verbal	S.S.	Performance	S.S.
Information	14	Picture Completion	13
Similarities	13	Picture Arrangement	8
Arithmetic	11	Block Design	18
Vocabulary	11	Object Assembly	16
Comprehension	10	Coding	8
Digit Span		Mazes	8
Verbal I.Q.	111	Performance I.Q.	118

Full Scale I.Q. _____ 116 _____

MOTOR SKILLS

Purdue Pegboard: Preferred Hand _____ 60th %ile
                 Non-preferred hand _____ 65th %ile
                 Both hands _____ 20th %ile
                 Assembly _____ 80th %ile
Developmental Test of Visual Motor
  Integration _____ %ile
Bender Visual Motor Gestalt Test _____ %ile
Benton Visual Retention Test _____ %ile
Detroit Test:
  Auditory Attention Span _____ 11 yr 0 mo
  Visual Attention Span _____ 11 yr 0 mo
  Notes on Performance _____
_____

Matching Familiar Figures Test:
  Errors _____ 81st %ile
  Completion Time _____ 12th %ile
Peabody Picture Vocabulary Test _____ %ile
Trail Making Test: Completion Time _____ 50th %ile
                   Errors _____ 50th %ile
Progressive Figures Test _____ %ile
Rapidly Recurring Target Figures:
  592: Completion Time _____ 50th %ile
       Errors _____ 50th %ile
  Diamond: Completion Time _____ 50th %ile
           Errors _____ 50th %ile
Motor Free Visual Perception Test _____ %ile
Hand Preference _____ Left _____ XX _____ Right

ACADEMICS

	Test	Grade	%ile
SAT -	Reading		80th
	Arithmetic		85th
	Language		78th
	Listening		90th
	Overall		82nd

OTHER TESTS OR QUESTIONNAIRES

Test	Score or %ile
Symbol Digit Modalities Test:	
Oral	50th
Written	50th

ADHD Diagnostic Checklist Criteria

I	Yes	III	Yes
II	Yes	IV	Yes
		V	Yes

Figure 7.4 ADHD in a child with high intellectual skills: The case of D. W.

arousal and poor social skills. The family history was positive for attention diffi-culty in siblings and parents. Parents observed problems in D. W. at two years of age. His independent attention span presently was estimated to be ten minutes. He became overaroused easily and was impulsive, and rewards did not change his behavior. D. W.'s parents felt that his problems were not purposeful. They were concerned, however, that as he was progressing through the elementary grades, he was experiencing increasing difficulty functioning effectively at school. His parents noted that they were concerned about D. W. before he entered kindergarten. In a preschool setting, he was aggressive as well as inattentive. Aggressive problems were not noted in kindergarten or first grade. D. W. had frequent temper outbursts at home that resulted from frustration. He did not appear to learn well from his experiences and was more active than his siblings.

Parent and teacher questionnaires reported significant attention and arousal-level problems. Within the home, problems of moderate severity were noted in almost all situations. Within the school, problems of moderate severity were primarily noted during work times. Parents noted that D. W. lacked social skills and attempted to be the center of attention. Teachers observed that he tended to overwhelm his peers and seemed incompetent in social situations.

During the evaluation, D. W. related well to the examiner. He was motivated to perform and was persistent. No significant behavioral problems were observed. Assessment data suggested that D. W. was a child of, at the very least, high-average intellectual skills. Because of his age and intellect, he was able to perform in the average range on many of the tasks designed to assess attention span and reflection. For D. W., however, average performance was well below expectation given his exceptionally good intellect. D. W. appeared aware of his attention difficulty and the impact it was having on his home behavior, school performance and social relations. Although he exhibited a pattern of inattention and impulsivity, D. W. appeared to have relatively adequate emotional development. He was somewhat immature for his chronological age and intellect and had poor problem-solving skills.

D. W.'s history and current functioning met the DSM-III-R diagnostic criteria for ADHD. Situational problems were consistent in both the home and the school. Objective assessment pointed to relative weaknesses in attention and reflection skills. The test data and history did not suggest that D. W. was experiencing other cognitive or psychiatric problems. D. W.'s social problems appeared to result from his inattentive, impulsive style. Given his exceptionally good intellect, D. W. was able to enter school and function adequately in the first few grades. When the demands of school began to overwhelm D. W., he was unable to remain on task long enough to keep up and make effective use of his intellect. A diagnosis of ADHD was made.

ADHD AND LEARNING PROBLEMS: THE CASE OF J. T.

J. T., a 7½-year-old second grader, was referred by his pediatrician because of a history of inattention, overarousal and learning difficulty. The pediatrician

NAME _____ J.T. _____ D.O.B. _____ AGE 7 yr 6 mo DATE _____

HISTORY

Age of Onset ____ Infancy _____
Average Independent Attention Span
  (Minutes) _____ 5 _____
Easily Overaroused ___ Yes _____
Impulsive _____ Yes _____
S`Not Effective _____ Yes _____
Other 1. Parents divorced, father
  remarried
2. Mother rejected as infant
3. Problems in nursery school
4. Active
5. No form of discipline works well
6. Family history of ADHD

QUESTIONNAIRES

Parent Conners _____ 98th %ile
Teacher Conners ___ Above 98th %ile
ACTeRS: Attention _____ 8th %ile
    Hyperactivity Below 5th %ile
    Social Skills _____ 18th %ile
    Oppositional _____ 21st %ile
Parent Achenbach: Scales Above 98th %ile
Hyperactive _____
Aggressive _____
Delinquent _____
Obsessive-Compulsive _____

Teacher Achenbach: Scales Above 98th %ile
Unpopular _____ Aggressive _____
Self-Destructive _____
Obsessive/Compulsive _____
Inattentive _____
Nervous-Overactive _____
Home Situations Problems:
  Number of Situations __ 16 ____
  Average Severity ___ Moderate __
School Situations Problems:
  Number of Situations __ 7 _____
  Average Severity ____ Severe ___
Parent Social Skills: Type of Problems
1. Teases siblings
2. Mildly aggressive
_____
_____

Teacher Social Skills: Type of Problems
1. Significant problems
2. Teases, provokes, fights, argues
3. Aggressive
_____

Observation During Assessment
1. Poor attention
2. Overactive
3. Easily distracted
4. Impulsive
5. Disorganized

PERSONALITY OR EMOTIONAL FACTORS
1. Immature
2. Dependent
3. Easily frustrated
4. Poor social perception

WECHSLER

Verbal	S.S.	Performance	S.S.
Information	12	Picture Completion	10
Similarities	13	Picture Arrangement	13
Arithmetic	12	Block Design	15
Vocabulary	11	Object Assembly	10
Comprehension	9	Coding	6
Digit Span		Mazes	7
Verbal I.Q.	108	Performance I.Q.	105

Full Scale I.Q. _____ 107

MOTOR SKILLS

Purdue Pegboard: Preferred Hand _____ %ile
             Non-preferred hand _____ %ile
             Both hands _____ %ile
             Assembly _____ %ile
Developmental Test of Visual Motor
  Integration _____ 25th %ile
Bender Visual Motor Gestalt Test __ 40th %ile
Benton Visual Retention Test _____ %ile
Detroit Test:
  Auditory Attention Span ___ 4 yr 0 mo
  Visual Attention Span _____ 6 yr 3 mo
  Notes on Performance ___ inconsistent
_____

Matching Familiar Figures Test:
  Errors _____ 88th %ile
  Completion Time _____ 30th %ile
Peabody Picture Vocabulary Test ____ %ile
Trail Making Test: Completion Time ___ %ile
             Errors _____ %ile
Progressive Figures Test _____ %ile
Rapidly Recurring Target Figures:
  592: Completion Time _____ 10th %ile
      Errors _____ 86th %ile
  Diamond: Completion Time _ 10th %ile
      Errors _____ 98th %ile
Motor Free Visual Perception Test __ %ile
Hand Preference _____ Left _____ Right

ACADEMICS

Test	Grade	%ile
WRAT-Reading		below 1st %ile
WRAT-Spelling		1st %ile
		55th %ile

OTHER TESTS OR QUESTIONNAIRES

Test	Score or %ile
Reversals Frequency Test	all 3 parts
	below 10th %ile

ADHD Diagnostic Checklist Criteria

I	Yes	III	Yes
II	Yes	IV	Yes
		V	Yes

Figure 7.5 ADHD and learning problems: The case of J. T.

did not identify a specific remediable medical problem. Parents reported problems in infancy, including difficulty fitting routines, overactivity and irritability. J. T. was described as a difficult infant. For a period of a year he was emotionally neglected by his mother. J. T.'s parents subsequently divorced, and he now lived with his father and stepmother. J. T.'s average attention span for an independent activity was five minutes. He was active, impulsive and easily overstimulated. Additionally, rewards had not been effective in changing his behavior. Parents noted that frequently J. T.'s behavior appeared nonpurposeful. No particular form of discipline had worked well in changing his behavior. He began experiencing problems in nursery school. He entered kindergarten and was immediately referred for special education services because of attention problems and academic delay. Attentional difficulties increased despite special education services. Parents noted a history on mother's side of the family of attention and arousal-level problems. J. T.'s ten-year-old brother, Donald, had previously been diagnosed as experiencing ADHD.

Parent and teacher questionnaires were consistent for attention and activity-level problems. Greater problems with aggression and poor social interaction were noted at school than at home. Consistent moderate problems were noted in all home situations, and severe problems were noted in all classroom work-related situations. Teachers also reported significant problems with aggression, teasing, provoking and arguing.

During assessment, J. T. presented as a child with normal physical development. He was, however, inattentive, impulsive, disorganized, overactive and easily distracted. He seemed immature and displayed a low frustration tolerance.

Assessment data revealed a child of above-average intellectual skill who exhibited significant problems with reflection, vigilance and persistence. A mild to moderate degree of perceptual difficulty was observed, with the greatest perceptual problems occurring in relation to the auditory recognition and recall of linguistic material. Academic assessment reflected significant reading and spelling difficulty but average arithmetic achievement. J. T. presented as a child with generally adequate emotional development; however, at the same time, his immaturity was clearly revealed by his impulsivity and inability to effectively modulate his emotions and deal with frustration.

J. T.'s history, current functioning and assessment data met the DSM-III-R diagnostic criteria for ADHD. Consistent situational and objective skill problems were observed. Although J. T.'s history was compounded by possible rejection during infancy, the early onset of attention and arousal-level problems strongly suggested a physiological basis for J. T.'s current problems. A diagnosis of ADHD and learning disorder was made. J. T.'s increasing behavioral problems at school appeared to result from his inability, both behaviorally and academically, to meet the demands of school.

ADHD AND MILD PERCEPTUAL LEARNING DISABILITY: THE CASE OF D. B.

D. B., an 8-year-old first grader, was referred by a pediatric neurologist for continued problems with inattention and overarousal. Medical evaluation was

NAME _____ D.B. _____   D.O.B. _____   AGE 8 yr 2 mo DATE _____

HISTORY

Age of Onset _____ Birth _____
Average Independent Attention Span
  (Minutes) _____ 10 _____
Easily Overaroused _____ Yes _____
Impulsive _____ Yes _____
S̃ Not Effective _____ Yes _____
Other 1. Difficult infant
  2. Poor fine and large motor skills
  3. Problems began in kindergarten
  4. High activity level
  5. Family history of attention problems
  6. Discipline not effective

QUESTIONNAIRES
  *With Ritalin
Parent Conners _____ 99th %ile
Teacher Conners _____ %ile
*ACTeRS: Attention _____ 10th %ile
         Hyperactivity _____ 30th %ile
         Social Skills _____ 50th %ile
         Oppositional _____ 60th %ile
Parent Achenbach: Scales Above 98th %ile
Hyperactivity _____
Obsessive-Compulsive _____
Depression _____
_____
_____

*Teacher Achenbach: Scales Above 98th %ile
Teacher well organized. Effective
at managing in the classroom.
He requires significant teacher time.
_____
_____

Home Situations Problems:
  Number of Situations _____ 13
  Average Severity _____ Mild to moderate
School Situations Problems:
  Number of Situations _____ 10
  Average Severity _____ Mild
Parent Social Skills: Type of Problems

1. Lacks social skills
2. Misses social cues
_____
_____

Teacher Social Skills: Type of Problems
1. Mildly disturbing
2. Misses social cues
_____
_____

Observation During Assessment
1. Calm, related well
2. Inconsistent, impulsive style
3. Cooperative
_____
_____
_____

PERSONALITY OR EMOTIONAL FACTORS
1. Impulsive, inattentive style
2. Aware of problems
3. Limited self-awareness
_____
_____

WECHSLER

Verbal	S.S.	Performance	S.S.
Information	15	Picture Completion	9
Similarities	14	Picture Arrangement	9
Arithmetic	8	Block Design	13
Vocabulary	16	Object Assembly	11
Comprehension	13	Coding	8
Digit Span	9	Mazes	11
Verbal I.Q.	119	Performance I.Q.	100
	Full Scale I.Q.	111	

MOTOR SKILLS

Purdue Pegboard: Preferred Hand _____ 1st %ile
                  Non-preferred hand _____ 1st %ile
                  Both hands _____ 1st %ile
                  Assembly _____ 1st %ile
Developmental Test of Visual Motor
  Integration _____ %ile
Bender Visual Motor Gestalt Test _____ 5th %ile
Benton Visual Retention Test _____ %ile
Detroit Test:
  Auditory Attention Span _____ 7 yr 6 mo
  Visual Attention Span _____ 8 yr 0 mo
  Notes on Performance _____
_____

Matching Familiar Figures Test:
  Errors _____ 94th %ile
  Completion Time _____ 12th %ile
Peabody Picture Vocabulary Test _____ %ile
Trail Making Test: Completion Time _____ %ile
                   Errors _____ %ile
Progressive Figures Test _____ %ile
Rapidly Recurring Target Figures:
  592: Completion Time _____ 98th %ile
       Errors _____ 86th %ile
  Diamond: Completion Time _____ 95th %ile
           Errors _____ 50th %ile
Motor Free Visual Perception Test _____ %ile
Hand Preference _____ XX _____ Left _____ Right

ACADEMICS

Test	Grade	%ile
WRAT-Reading		37th %ile
WRAT-Math		21st %ile

OTHER TESTS OR QUESTIONNAIRES

Test	Score or %ile
Test of Non-Verbal Intell.	26th %ile
Wepman Auditory Discrimination	5 errors

ADHD Diagnostic Checklist Criteria

I	Yes	III	Yes
II	Yes	IV	Yes
		V	Yes

Figure 7.6 ADHD and mild perceptual learning disability: The case of D. B.

unremarkable. Parental history suggested that D. B. was a difficult child from birth. As an infant, D. B. was irritable, did not fit routines well, had difficulty sleeping and was overactive. As soon as he was mobile, he was constantly into things. He had difficulty benefiting from his experiences. Toilet training was difficult, and D. B. experienced problems with encopresis up through six years of age. Despite above-average intelligence, D. B. had difficulty following directions and benefiting from discipline. The family history was positive for attention problems on both sides. D. B. exhibited attention and arousal-level problems as soon as he entered kindergarten. He continued to display a pattern of high activity level, along with poor fine and large motor skills. He was managing to function in the lower academic groups in the first-grade classroom. Previous assessment two years earlier in a learning problems clinic resulted in a diagnosis of ADHD, encopresis and oppositional problems. Despite D. B.'s difficulty, his parents described him quite positively as a warm, loveable child accepted by his siblings.

Parent and teacher questionnaires revealed significant problems with attention span and arousal level. D. B.'s teacher appeared extremely well organized and effective in managing D. B.'s problems in the classroom. Although the history did not reflect problems with helplessness or depression, parental response suggested that at times D.B. was overly emotional and insecure. A consistent pattern of mild to moderate problems was noted in most home situations, with mild problems observed in all school situations. D. B.'s parents and teachers noted a lack of social skills and difficulty reading social cues, which resulted in D. B. having problems with high incidence, low impact behavior.

During assessment, D. B. appeared healthy. He was generally calm and related well to the examiner. Although he was somewhat fidgety, he was cooperative and attempted all tasks presented. His approach to most test tasks was inconsistent and reflected his impulsive style.

Assessment data suggested a child with a significant discrepancy between higher verbal skills and lower perceptual skills. D. B.'s impulsive style also resulted in a significant degree of intratest scatter, suggesting that his intellectual skills were even better than test measures indicated. Significant fine motor and visual perception difficulty was observed in D. B.'s test performance. Despite an exceptionally good fund of information, vocabulary and comprehension, D. B. struggled with tasks of reflection, divided attention, vigilance and persistence. Although on some tasks D. B. was able to remain working a longer amount of time than the average for his age, his approach was quite disorganized, and the additional work time did not result in improved performance. Brief screening of word-reading and arithmetical skills suggested lower average academic achievement, well below expectation based on D. B.'s overall intellect but within expectation given his perceptual problems.

D. B.'s history and behavior met the DSM-III-R diagnostic criteria for ADHD. Consistent situational and behavioral problems reflecting attention and arousal difficulty were noted on questionnaires. Objective data also reflected D. B.'s problems with attentional skills. The history suggested that problems were observed long before D. B. entered school. His perceptual difficulty appeared to be causing delay in academic achievement but did not appear to be causing significant frustration. Of concern were parents' observations that at times D. B. appeared helpless and insecure. Over the past two years, D. B. had not shown significant oppositional behavior or a reoccurrence of encopresis. Diagnoses of ADHD and developmental learning disorder were made.

UNDIFFERENTIATED ATTENTION DISORDER AND LEARNING DISABILITY:
THE CASE OF G. A.

G. A., an almost 12-year-old fifth grader, was referred by his pediatrician as a result of a long-standing and increasing pattern of school problems characterized by delayed achievement, inattention and seemingly poor motivation. The pediatrician's evaluation did not identify a specific medical cause of these problems. G. A.'s parents noted that there was an extended family history of attention difficulty. They described G. A. as having an uneventful childhood before entering school. They noted, however, that he had always had problems following through with directions. He did not create significant behavioral problems at home but tended to repeat mistakes because of his apparent inattention and incompetence. G. A.'s parents noted that his independent attention span was approximately ten minutes. He did not become easily overaroused but could act impulsively. The effect of rewards was variable in changing G. A.'s behavior.

His parents were concerned about G. A.'s decreasing rate of academic progress. The parental history and interview suggested that these parents coped very well with their child's attentional disabilities.

Parent and teacher questionnaires reported moderate problems with inattention at home, but greater problems were noted at school. Situationally, G. A. did not present home difficulties and at school presented mild problems related only to work situations. Teachers noted that at times G. A. was socially isolated and appeared to lack self-esteem. They questioned his motivation. He was frequently off task but did not create discipline problems when he was not doing his work.

During assessment, he appeared healthy, but seemed uncomfortable in the assessment situation. He engaged in limited conversation and had an inconsistent approach to the test tasks that appeared to result from limited motivation and variable ability to focus concentration.

Assessment data indicated a child functioning in the lower average range of intellectual skill with fine motor speed and coordination problems. Significant difficulty was observed in vigilance and divided attention skill. G. A. was able to persist on task but frequently was disorganized, and the increased time did not result in improved performance. Academic achievement data suggested a significant delay resulting from a combination of lowered intellectual ability, weaknesses in visual skills and difficulty with sound/symbol association. Over time, G. A.'s inability to succeed at school and the increased pressure he received in response was resulting in increasing feelings of helplessness and poor motivation. This further compounded delays in achievement. G. A. presented as an immature child with no significant emotional problems. He was quite open in acknowledging that he disliked school

NAME _____ G.A. _____ D.O.B. _____ AGE 11 yr 10 mo DATE _____

HISTORY

Age of Onset ____6____
Average Independent Attention Span
  (Minutes) ____10____
Easily Overaroused ____No____
Impulsive ____Yes____
S'Not Effective ____Variable____
Other 1. Father had similar problems
2. Enuresis
3. Problems with directions
4. Not a significant behavior problem
5. Repeat offender-incompetent
6. Parents cope well with G.A.
7. Decreasing academic achievement

QUESTIONNAIRES

Parent Conners ____ 80th %ile
Teacher Conners ____ %ile
ACTeRS: Attention ____ 20th %ile
        Hyperactivity ____ 75th %ile
        Social Skills ____ 18th %ile
        Oppositional ____ 60th %ile
Parent Achenbach: Scales Above 98th %ile
  None _____ _____
       _____ _____
       _____ _____
       _____ _____

Teacher Achenbach: Scales Above 98th %ile
  Inattentive _____ _____
       _____ _____
       _____ _____
       _____ _____

Home Situations Problems:
  Number of Situations ____none____
  Average Severity _____
School Situations Problems:
  Number of Situations ____3____
  Average Severity ____Mild____
Parent Social Skills: Type of Problems
None _____
_____
_____
_____

Teacher Social Skills: Type of Problems
1. Socially isolated at times
2. Off task but not disruptive
3. Variable concentration
_____

Observation During Assessment
1. Seemed uncomfortable
2. Limited conversation
3. Variable concentration
_____
_____

PERSONALITY OR EMOTIONAL FACTORS
1. Immature but adequate emotional
   development
2. Pre-occupied by small stature
3. Lacks academic motivation
4. Helpless

WECHSLER

Verbal	S.S.	Performance	S.S.
Information	10	Picture Completion	7
Similarities	9	Picture Arrangement	9
Arithmetic	8	Block Design	10
Vocabulary	8	Object Assembly	6
Comprehension	7	Coding	8
Digit Span		Mazes	9
Verbal I.Q.	90	Performance I.Q.	86

Full Scale I.Q. ____87____

MOTOR SKILLS

Purdue Pegboard: Preferred Hand ____ 40th %ile
                 Non-preferred hand ____ 30th %ile
                 Both hands ____ 1st %ile
                 Assembly ____ 1st %ile
Developmental Test of Visual Motor
  Integration ____ %ile
Bender Visual Motor Gestalt Test ____ 20th %ile
Benton Visual Retention Test ____ %ile
Detroit Test:
  Auditory Attention Span ____ 4 yr 0 mo
  Visual Attention Span ____ 6 yr 9 mo
  Notes on Performance _____
  _____

Matching Familiar Figures Test:
  Errors ____ 25th %ile
  Completion Time ____ 52nd %ile
Peabody Picture Vocabulary Test ____ %ile
Trail Making Test: Completion Time ____ %ile
                   Errors ____ %ile
Progressive Figures Test ____ %ile
Rapidly Recurring Target Figures:
  592: Completion Time ____ 85th %ile
       Errors ____ 85th %ile
  Diamond: Completion Time ____ 85th %ile
           Errors ____ 16th %ile
Motor Free Visual Perception Test ____ %ile
Hand Preference ____ Left ____ XX Right

ACADEMICS

Test	Grade	%ile
WRAT-Reading		3rd %ile
WRAT-Spelling		2nd %ile
WRAT-Arithmetic		12th %ile

OTHER TESTS OR QUESTIONNAIRES

Test	Score or %ile
Visual Aural Digit Span	15th %ile

ADHD Diagnostic Checklist Criteria

I	Yes	III	Yes
II	Marginal	IV	Variable/No
	V	Yes	

Figure 7.7 Undifferentiated attention disorder and learning disability: The case of G. A.

and felt he was not as smart or as competent as the other children. He also appeared somewhat preoccupied with the fact that he was smaller than the other children in his class.

G. A.'s history and presentation met the DSM-III-R diagnosis for undifferentiated attention disorder. The practitioner must keep in mind that children with primary attention problems who do not have difficulty with arousal level, restlessness or reflection will not present significantly elevated attention-problem scales on the majority of attention-related questionnaires. The ACTeRS is the best questionnaire for separating attention and activity-level difficulty. Teacher responses suggested significant problems with attention but not activity level. Test data was consistent in supporting this conclusion. Situational problems were variable but not of significant occurrence or severity. Although G. A.'s problems appeared to be compounded by his lower intellect and a learning disability, attention difficulty was a primary problem for G. A. in all areas of his life. Diagnoses of undifferentiated attention disorder and developmental learning problems were made. A concern was also noted that G. A.'s emotional status suggested that he was at increasing risk to develop adjustment problems.

ADHD AND PERCEPTUAL ORGANIZATION LEARNING DISABILITY:
THE CASE OF J. C.

J. C., a 15½-year-old tenth grader, was referred by a family friend because of a long-standing pattern of inattention, impulsivity and emotional overarousal. Despite a fairly benign infancy, toddler and preschool period, complaints of attention difficulty were initially made by J. C.'s first grade teacher. J. C.'s average independent attention span presently was estimated by his parents to be 20 minutes. Within the home he was easily overaroused and impulsive and his behavior was not altered by rewards. Although he appeared to have a social network, J. C. was argumentative and disturbing to his friends. He also denied having problems. Stimulant medication was attempted by the family physician in eighth grade with some improvements noted. It was not continued because of J. C.'s resistance to taking medication. Problems within the home appeared to be increasing as the result of the parents' determination that the source of J. C.'s problems was a lack of effort. J. C. also had long-standing problems of mild to moderate difficulty with arithmetic at school.

Questionnaires suggested that J. C. experienced significant attention and arousal-related problems in the home, and three of J. C.'s academic teachers observed similar difficulty. Significant aggressive problems were observed only within the home. Teachers noted that J. C. talked excessively and at times disturbed his peers. Significant problems of mild to moderate severity were observed in both school and home situations.

J. C. was very pleasant during the assessment. He was cooperative and related well to the examiner. His approach, however, was inconsistent and quite disorganized. He demonstrated an impulsive work style. He appeared to have a positive self-image but excessively used denial as a psychological defense, repeatedly

NAME ___J.C._____ D.O.B. _____ AGE 15 yr 6 mo DATE _____

HISTORY	WECHSLER

HISTORY

Age of Onset _____7_____
Average Independent Attention Span
  (Minutes)   20
Easily Overaroused   Yes
Impulsive   Yes
S Not Effective   Yes
Other 1. Unremarkable infancy
2. Complaints of inattention in 1st grade
3. Has friends
4. Non-compliant
5. Temper outbursts
6. Denies problems 7. Ritalin helped
in 8th grade 8. Trouble with arithmetic

QUESTIONNAIRES

Parent Conners   98th %ile
Teacher Conners   98th %ile
ACTeRS: Attention   %ile
      Hyperactivity   %ile
      Social Skills   %ile
      Oppositional   %ile
Parent Achenbach: Scales Above 98th %ile
Hyperactivity _____ _____
Aggression _____ _____
_____ _____
_____ _____

Teacher Achenbach: Scales Above 98th %ile
_____ _____
_____ _____
_____ _____
_____ _____

Home Situations Problems:
  Number of Situations   8
  Average Severity Mild to moderate
School Situations Problems:
  Number of Situations   5
  Average Severity Moderate
Parent Social Skills: Type of Problems
1. Disturbs others
2. Argumentative
_____
_____
Teacher Social Skills: Type of Problems
1. Disturbs others
2. Talks too much
_____
_____
Observation During Assessment
1. Inconsistent in approach to tasks
2. Disorganized
3. Related well
_____
_____
_____
PERSONALITY OR EMOTIONAL FACTORS
1. Impulsive style
2. Positive self-image
3. Denial as defense
_____
_____

WECHSLER

Verbal	S.S.	Performance	S.S.
Information	13	Picture Completion	7
Similarities	14	Picture Arrangement	10
Arithmetic	11	Block Design	9
Vocabulary	10	Object Assembly	14
Comprehension	15	Coding	6
Digit Span	10	Mazes	7
Verbal I.Q.	115	Performance I.Q.	93
	Full Scale I.Q.	105	

MOTOR SKILLS

Purdue Pegboard: Preferred Hand   30th %ile
                 Non-preferred hand 20th %ile
                 Both hands   1st %ile
                 Assembly   15th %ile
Developmental Test of Visual Motor
  Integration   %ile
Bender Visual Motor Gestalt Test   %ile
Benton Visual Retention Test   30th %ile
Detroit Test:
  Auditory Attention Span   12 yr 6 mo
  Visual Attention Span   12 yr 3 mo
  Notes on Performance _____
_____

Matching Familiar Figures Test:
  Errors   %ile
  Completion Time   %ile
Peabody Picture Vocabulary Test   %ile
Trail Making Test: Completion Time 50th %ile
                  Errors   50th %ile
Progressive Figures Test   %ile
Rapidly Recurring Target Figures:
  592: Completion Time   %ile
      Errors   %ile
  Diamond: Completion Time   %ile
      Errors   %ile
Motor Free Visual Perception Test   %ile
Hand Preference _____ Left   X Right

ACADEMICS

Test	Grade	%ile
WRAT-Reading		58th %ile
WRAT-Math		27th %ile

OTHER TESTS OR QUESTIONNAIRES

Test	Score or %ile
Symbol Digit Modalities	50th %ile
Rey Figure Drawing	1st %ile

ADHD Diagnostic Checklist Criteria

I	Yes	III	Yes
II	Yes	IV	Yes
	V	Yes	

Figure 7.8 ADHD and perceptual organization learning disability: The case of J. C.

185

indicating that he was not experiencing any of the problems that his parents had reported.

Assessment data revealed an adolescent with significantly above-average verbal skills but below-average perceptual skills. Specific weaknesses were noted in tasks requiring reflection, vigilance and persistence. Auditory and visual attention span tested below J. C.'s chronological age. Brief academic assessment pointed to average reading skills with below-average arithmetic achievement. J. C.'s approach to visual tasks indicated a learning disability that appeared to reflect problems with perceptual organization. In all likelihood, the combination of J. C.'s inattentive style and perceptual organization difficulty accounted for his arithmetic problems.

The late referral of J. C.'s attention problems suggested the strong likelihood that the frustration he may have experienced in the early elementary school grades as the result of his perceptual organization and difficulty with work completion exacerbated problems with inattention and arousal level, leading to poor motivation. Present behavior across situations met the DSM-III-R diagnosis for ADHD. Objective assessment clearly reflected problems with inattention and impulsivity. A primary diagnosis of ADHD with secondary perceptual organization problems as a contributing factor was made. Parental rigidity in defining J. C.'s problems as stemming from poor motivation appeared to be primarily responsible for increasing problems observed within the home.

ADHD, INTELLECTUAL HANDICAP AND OPPOSITIONAL DISORDER: THE CASE OF S. A.

S. A., an almost 11-year-old third grader in a self-contained classroom for children with intellectual handicaps, was referred by her pediatrician because of an increasing pattern of inattention, overarousal and oppositional behavior. History suggested a child with a long-standing pattern of developmental delay beginning at birth. The divorce of S. A.'s parents five years prior resulted in part from the significant problems S. A. presented to her mother. S. A. was rejected by her mother and since that time had lived with her father, having minimal interaction with her mother. She exhibited sleep problems, enuresis and an increasing pattern of noncompliance within the home. Family history was negative for retardation but positive for attention disorder on both sides of the family. In addition to her pervasive developmental delay, S. A. presented in infancy with a pattern of irritability and overarousal. Speech and language skills had been significantly delayed. At home, S. A. had an attention span of approximately five minutes in an independent activity. She was impulsive and easily overaroused, and rewards had been ineffective in changing her behavior. S. A.'s appetite was reported as poor. The pediatrician reported that otherwise, however, she did not appear to be experiencing specific medical problems.

Parent and teacher data suggested that S. A. met the DSM-III-R diagnostic criteria for ADHD. Although the complication of her intellectual handicap must be considered, situational problems in both home and school ranged from moderate to severe and occurred in the majority of situational contexts. S. A. presented with

NAME _____ S.A. _____ D.O.B. _____ AGE 10 yr 10 moDATE _____

HISTORY		WECHSLER			

HISTORY

Age of Onset ___ Birth
Average Independent Attention Span
  (Minutes) ___ 5
Easily Overaroused ___ Yes
Impulsive ___ Yes
S Not Effective ___ Yes
Other 1. Divorce of parents
2. Rejected by mother
3. Sleep problems, enuresis
4. Delayed development
5. Intellectual handicapped classroom

QUESTIONNAIRES

Parent Conners ___ Above 99th %ile
Teacher Conners ___ %ile
ACTeRS: Attention ___ Below 1st %ile
  Hyperactivity ___ Below 1st %ile
  Social Skills ___ 10th %ile
  Oppositional ___ 5th %ile
Parent Achenbach: Scales Above 98th %ile
Hyperactivity _____ _____
Aggression _____ _____
_____ _____
_____ _____

Teacher Achenbach: Scales Above 98th %ile
_____ _____
_____ _____
_____ _____
_____ _____

Home Situations Problems:
  Number of Situations ___ 10
  Average Severity ___ Moderate
School Situations Problems:
  Number of Situations ___ 12
  Average Severity ___ Moderate
Parent Social Skills: Type of Problems
1. Lacks social skills
2. Negative, bossy, annoying
3. Disturbs others
_____

Teacher Social Skills: Type of Problems
1. Socially isolated
2. Negative, controlling
3. Rejected by peers
_____

Observation During Assessment
1. Nails bitten
2. Poor language skills
3. Poor concentration
4. Easily distracted
5. Impulsive, restless
_____

PERSONALITY OR EMOTIONAL FACTORS
1. Immature
2. Controlling
_____
_____
_____

WECHSLER

Verbal	S.S.	Performance	S.S.
Information	4	Picture Completion	7
Similarities	5	Picture Arrangement	3
Arithmetic	5	Block Design	1
Vocabulary	4	Object Assembly	6
Comprehension	4	Coding	8
Digit Span		Mazes	6
Verbal I.Q.	66	Performance I.Q.	67
	Full Scale I.Q.	64	

MOTOR SKILLS

below:
Purdue Pegboard: Preferred Hand ___ 1st %ile
  Non-preferred hand ___ 1st %ile
  Both hands ___ 1st %ile
  Assembly ___ 1st %ile
Developmental Test of Visual Motor
  Integration ___ %ile
Bender Visual Motor Gestalt Test ___ 1st %ile
Benton Visual Retention Test ___ %ile
Detroit Test:
  Auditory Attention Span ___ 4 yr old
  Visual Attention Span ___ 8 yr old
  Notes on Performance _____
_____

Matching Familiar Figures Test:
  Errors ___ 99th %ile
  Completion Time ___ 1st %ile
Peabody Picture Vocabulary Test ___ 1st %ile
Trail Making Test: Completion Time ___ %ile
  Errors ___ %ile
Progressive Figures Test ___ %ile
Rapidly Recurring Target Figures:
  592: Completion Time ___ %ile
  Errors ___ above 90th %ile
  Diamond: Completion Time ___ above 98th %ile
  Errors ___ 50th %ile
Motor Free Visual Perception ___ below 1st %ile
Hand Preference ___ Left ___ X Right

ACADEMICS

Test	Grade	%ile
WRAT-Reading		1st %ile
WRAT-Math		1st %ile

OTHER TESTS OR QUESTIONNAIRES

Test	Score or %ile
AAMD Adaptive Behavior Scale	Scores generally average for EMR population
Test of Non-Verbal Intell.	below 1st %ile

ADHD Diagnostic Checklist Criteria

I ___ Yes   III ___ Yes
II ___ Yes   IV ___ Yes
          V ___ Yes

Figure 7.9 ADHD, intellectual handicap and oppositional disorder: The case of S. A.

difficulty in public places and with noncompliance at home. Within the school setting, significant problems were noted during small group activities, class lectures and individual task work. S. A. was socially isolated, negative, bossy and annoying to her peers. An AAMD Adaptive Behavior Scale questionnaire completed by S. A.'s father suggested that her adaptive behavior was most similar to an average population of mildly intellectually handicapped children, but that her behavioral problems were significantly greater.

During assessment she was noted to be a child of average appearance, with poor language skills, difficulty with concentration, a tendency to be easily distracted, impulsivity and a significant degree of restlessness. S. A.'s nails were moderately bitten. She was immature and controlling during the evaluation and required a great deal of examiner structure, praise and encouragement to maintain on task.

Assessment data revealed a child functioning intellectually below the first percentile with overall cognitive skills and academic functioning equivalent to the average $6^{1}/_{2}$-year-old child. Relative to this level of functioning, significant difficulty was noted with auditory attention span and an impulsive work style. S. A.'s test performance also reflected her oppositional behavior and occasional unwillingness to use the attention and cognitive skills that she appeared to possess.

Based on history, test data and S. A.'s presentation, there appeared to be no doubt that she was an intellectually handicapped child. Her level of overarousal, attention difficulty and impulsivity suggested that she was experiencing greater problems with these skills than would be expected. Parent and teacher reports, as well as the examiner's observation, were in agreement that S. A. exhibited a pattern of negative, provocative and oppositional behavior. Diagnoses of mild mental retardation, ADHD and oppositional defiant disorder were made. The foundational problem for S. A. appeared to be her intellectual handicap. Her emotional problems had been exacerbated not only by her family history but by her pattern of overarousal and impulsivity.

ADHD, LEARNING DISABILITY AND COMPLEX EMOTIONAL PROBLEMS: THE CASE OF J. G.

J. G., a 7-year, 9-month-old second grader, was referred by the special education team at his elementary school. After one week at the elementary school, J. G. was presenting significant problems. He was impulsive, overactive, stubborn, provocative, aggressive and out of control. He appeared delayed in learning and language skills. J. G.'s history as provided by his mother was complex. His father died as a result of a drug overdose when J. G. was three years of age. Both parents had been drug and alcohol abusers. Shortly after the death of his father, J. G. was separated from his mother a number of times while she was hospitalized as the result of drug and alcohol problems. J. G. lived with various relatives. His older brother and younger sister went to live with two different families. J. G.'s mother subsequently relinquished custody of them, and they were adopted by these families. J. G. remained with his mother and moved numerous times to various

NAME _____ J.G. _____ D.O.B. _____ AGE 7 yr 9 mo DATE _____

HISTORY

Age of Onset _____ Infancy
Average Independent Attention Span
  (Minutes) _____ 10
Easily Overaroused _____ Yes
Impulsive _____ Yes
S Not Effective _____ Yes
Other 1. Father died of drug overdose
2. 2 siblings given up for adoption
   3 years ago
3. Mother remained & separated again
4. Delayed motor development
5. Early history of intervention

QUESTIONNAIRES

Parent Conners _____ Above 99th %ile
Teacher Conners _____ Above 99th %ile
ACTeRS: Attention _____ %ile
       Hyperactivity _____ %ile
       Social Skills _____ %ile
       Oppositional _____ %ile
Parent Achenbach: Scales Above 98th %ile
Depression _____ Delinquent
Uncommunicative
Social withdrawal
Hyperactive
Aggressive
Teacher Achenbach: Scales Above 98th %ile
_____ _____
_____ _____
_____ _____
_____ _____

Home Situations Problems:
  Number of Situations _____ 9
  Average Severity _____ Severe
School Situations Problems:
  Number of Situations _____ 10
  Average Severity _____ Severe
Parent Social Skills: Type of Problems
_____
_____
_____
_____

Teacher Social Skills: Type of Problems
_____
_____
_____
_____

Observation During Assessment
1. Friendly and cooperative
2. Impulsive
3. Positive mood
4. Related well to examiner
_____
_____

PERSONALITY OR EMOTIONAL FACTORS
1. Express unhappiness
2. Expresses concern about father's
   death and loss of siblings
3. Aggressive problem solving
4. Poor self-image

WECHSLER

Verbal	S.S.	Performance	S.S.
Information	10	Picture Completion	9
Similarities	13	Picture Arrangement	11
Arithmetic	6	Block Design	9
Vocabulary	11	Object Assembly	11
Comprehension	10	Coding	8
Digit Span		Mazes	7
Verbal I.Q.	100	Performance I.Q.	96
	Full Scale I.Q.	98	

MOTOR SKILLS

Purdue Pegboard: Preferred Hand _____ %ile
              Non-preferred hand _____ %ile
              Both hands _____ %ile
              Assembly _____ %ile
Developmental Test of Visual Motor
  Integration _____ %ile
Bender Visual Motor Gestalt Test _____ %ile
Benton Visual Retention Test _____ 46th %ile
Detroit Test:
  Auditory Attention Span _____
  Visual Attention Span _____
  Notes on Performance _____
_____
_____

Matching Familiar Figures Test:
  Errors _____ %ile
  Completion Time _____ %ile
Peabody Picture Vocabulary Test _____ %ile
Trail Making Test: Completion Time _____ %ile
                Errors _____ %ile
Progressive Figures Test _____ %ile
Rapidly Recurring Target Figures:
  592: Completion Time _____ %ile
     Errors _____ %ile
  Diamond: Completion Time _____ %ile
     Errors _____ %ile
Motor Free Visual Perception Test _____ %ile
Hand Preference _____ Left _____ Right

ACADEMICS

Test	Grade	%ile
Woodcock-Johnson Psychoeducational		
Battery:		
_____	Reading	5th %ile
_____	Math	55th %ile
_____	Written Lang.	9th %ile

OTHER TESTS OR QUESTIONNAIRES

Test	Score or %ile
_____	_____
_____	_____
_____	_____
_____	_____

ADHD Diagnostic Checklist Criteria

I _____ Yes   III _____ Yes
II _____ Yes   IV _____ Yes
        V _____ Complex

Figure 7.10 ADHD, learning disability and complex emotional problems: The case of J. G.

parts of the country. She remarried for two years and again moved numerous times. In his short elementary-school experience, J. G. had attended six different schools.

J. G.'s mother noted that he was an extremely difficult infant. At three years of age he was evaluated and treated for a number of months at a preschool, child psychiatric day treatment facility. J. G.'s mother noted that when the family lived in another state, J. G. was evaluated and placed in a self-contained educational program for children with significant behavioral and learning problems. He was reportedly classified as having multiple handicaps.

Parent questionnaires identified attention and arousal-level problems and difficulty with internalizing behaviors such as depression and poor communication and externalizing problems such as aggression. A severe level of difficulty was noted in many home situations. J. G. had been at his elementary school for only a brief period of time, reducing the validity of teacher questionnaires; however, teachers noted a similar level of attention and overarousal problems. J. G. appeared to have severe difficulty in almost all school situations.

During assessment, J. G. was surprisingly friendly and cooperative. He had a positive mood and related well to the examiner. It was very clear, however, that he had an extremely impulsive, disorganized work style.

Assessment data revealed a child with average intellectual skill but relative problems with reflection, vigilance and persistence. Because his parents did not follow through, complete assessment data was not collected. Educational screening suggested significant problems with reading and written language that may have resulted from mild perceptual delay but more likely resulted from lack of consistent educational experience. J. G. was able to express his unhappiness with himself and his life. He expressed significant concern about the loss of his father and the fact that he had no idea where his brother and sister were. His social perception appeared limited, and he exhibited an aggressive approach to problem solution.

J. G.'s history and presentation met the DSM-III-R diagnostic criteria for ADHD. Parent and teacher questionnaires suggested significant attention and arousal-level problems that occurred in multiple situations. Objective assessment data also reflected difficulty with attention-related skills. Medical evaluation was unremarkable. J. G.'s emotional history, however, was complex. His pattern of stubbornness, violation of rules, temper problems and provocative behavior suggested that he also met the diagnostic criteria for oppositional defiant disorder. The number and severity of stressors J. G. experienced in his short lifetime appeared significant. He was initially exposed to an environment with violent and substance-abusing parents. His father died, and J. G. continued to experience unresolved issues with respect to that separation. He was then separated repeatedly from his mother and lost his siblings. He moved repeatedly from school to school, and his mother apparently continued to experience drug and alcohol problems. J. G.'s history suggested that there was a strong likelihood that many of the other behaviors he was presenting resulted secondarily from this history. J. G. was referred to an inpatient child psychiatric program to allow more in-depth assessment, observation, diagnosis and treatment planning.

ADHD, Complex Language and Learning Problems: The Case of R. J.

R.J., a 9½-year-old fourth grader, was initially referred at 6 years, 3 months of age by a pediatric neurologist. R. J. was seen for a history of apparent seizures that proved negative. The neurologist was concerned by R. J.'s significant attention and language problems. However, no specific medical problems were identified by the neurologist. When evaluated initially, R. J. was diagnosed as experiencing ADD-H and developmental problems. Concerns were raised about his helpless, unhappy behavior as well. At the time of re-evaluation, R. J. was in a regular classroom with two hours a day of special education support. The services appeared inadequate, and the educational team was preparing to place R. J. in a self-contained program for children with significant learning problems. R. J. was receiving a regime of 15 mg. of Ritalin® in the morning and 10 mg. of Ritalin in the afternoon. Continued social and self-image problems were noted by R. J.'s parents. Developmental history indicated a very difficult birth and mildly delayed development. There was a positive family history for attention disorder.

Questionnaire data suggested that even with stimulant medication, R. J. was continuing to present with significant attention problems. Pre- and post-medication questionnaire data suggested that medication was effective in reducing problems with excessive activity level. However, parents and teachers noted continued problems with attention span. Mild situational difficulty was observed consistently at home and mild to moderate problems noted primarily in work-related situations at school. Parents and teachers reported that R. J. appeared socially isolated, lacked social skills and was shy. Teachers observed that he appeared overanxious and was frequently a target of other children's taunts.

During assessment, R. J. appeared physically to be a normal child. He received stimulant medication one hour before the evaluation. He presented as mildly anxious and clearly immature. He was easily distracted and appeared to lack self-confidence. He frequently made self-deprecatory statements. Receptive and expressive language problems were readily apparent.

Assessment data suggested that R. J. had maintained steady intellectual growth and was functioning in the average range of intellectual skill. Despite the ability to persist on task, his approach to many tasks was quite disorganized. Stimulants improved persistence, divided attention and vigilance. Significant language problems were noted, including R. J.'s delayed response when attempting to think of words, word substitutions, spontaneous revisions of his speech and syntax problems. Academic screening suggested that his skills were significantly impaired. R. J. was able to express his unhappiness but appeared pessimistic and helpless. He acknowledged an awareness of his current problems. He expressed concern that other children did not like him and made fun of him. He noted that this had occurred all of his life and would probably continue to occur for the remainder of his life. R. J. was unable to speak positively about himself or any of his accomplishments. He denied being interested in any extracurricular activities or finding pleasure in any of the activities of his life. It appeared that R. J.'s academic achievement was impaired because of a language-based learning disability.

NAME _____R.J._____ D.O.B. _____ AGE 9 yr 5 mo DATE _____

HISTORY

Age of Onset _____ Birth
Average Independent Attention Span
  (Minutes) _____ 2
Easily Overaroused _____ Yes
Impulsive _____ Yes
S'Not Effective _____ Yes
Other 1. Trauma at birth
2. Delayed development
3. Epilepsy suspected
4. Helplessness
5. Previous evaluation CA 6 yr 3 mo
6. Ritalin has helped

QUESTIONNAIRES
  * With Ritalin
*Parent Conners _____ 95th %ile
*Teacher Conners _____ %ile
*ACTeRS: Attention _____ 5th %ile
         Hyperactivity _____ 50th %ile
         Social Skills below 1st %ile
         Oppositional _____ 50th %ile
Parent Achenbach: Scales Above 98th %ile
Hyperactivity _____
Social Withdrawal _____

_____ _____
_____ _____

Teacher Achenbach: Scales Above 98th %ile

_____ _____
_____ _____
_____ _____

_____ _____

*Home Situations Problems:
  Number of Situations _____ 8
  Average Severity _____ Mild
School Situations Problems:
  Number of Situations _____ 6
  Average Severity _____ Mild-Moderate
Parent Social Skills: Type of Problems

1. Socially isolated
2. Shy
3. Lacks social skills

Teacher Social Skills: Type of Problems
1. Socially isolated
2. Lacks social skills
3. Overanxious
4. Made fun of

Observation During Assessment
1. Received Ritalin
2. Language problems
3. Mildly anxious
4. Immature
5. Easily distracted
6. Poor self-confidence

PERSONALITY OR EMOTIONAL FACTORS
1. Unhappy
2. Aware of problems
3. Pessimistic
4. Helpless
5. Concerned about social problems

WECHSLER

Verbal	S.S.	Performance	S.S.
Information	7	Picture Completion	6
Similarities	12	Picture Arrangement	14
Arithmetic	8	Block Design	12
Vocabulary	10	Object Assembly	14
Comprehension	13	Coding	7
Digit Span		Mazes	
Verbal I.Q.	100	Performance I.Q.	104

Full Scale I.Q. _____ 101

MOTOR SKILLS

Purdue Pegboard: Preferred Hand _____ %ile
                 Non-preferred hand _____ %ile
                 Both hands _____ %ile
                 Assembly _____ %ile
Developmental Test of Visual Motor
  Integration _____ %ile
Bender Visual Motor Gestalt Test _____ 50th %ile
Benton Visual Retention Test _____ %ile
Detroit Test:
  Auditory Attention Span _____ 10 yr 9 mo
  Visual Attention Span _____ 11 yr 3 mo
  Notes on Performance _____

Matching Familiar Figures Test:
  Errors _____ 75th %ile
  Completion Time _____ 28th %ile
Peabody Picture Vocabulary Test _____ %ile
Trail Making Test: Completion Time _____ %ile
                   Errors _____ %ile
Progressive Figures Test _____ %ile
Rapidly Recurring Target Figures:
  592: Completion Time _____ 98th %ile
       Errors _____ 86th %ile
  Diamond: Completion Time _____ 90th %ile
           Errors _____ 40th %ile
Motor Free Visual Perception Test _____ %ile
Hand Preference _____ Left ___X___ Right

ACADEMICS

Test	Grade	%ile
WRAT-Reading		1st %ile
Spelling		below 1st
Arithmetic		3rd %ile
Mirror image reversals		

OTHER TESTS OR QUESTIONNAIRES

Test	Score or %ile
Word Finding survey	significant problems
Auditory Discrimination Test	2 errors
Visual Aural Digit Span Test	25th %ile

ADHD Diagnostic Criteria Criteria

I	Yes	III	Yes
II	Yes	IV	Yes
		V	Yes

Figure 7.11 ADHD, complex language and learning problems: The case of R. J.

R. J.'s history and current functioning continued to meet the DSM-III-R diagnostic criteria for ADHD and multiple developmental problems. The long-standing pattern of his unhappiness and lack of success strongly raised concerns that he was experiencing a dysthymic disorder. Although receiving fairly intensive special education intervention at school, R. J. was continuing to experience significant academic delays and severe language problems, despite adequate intellect. The frustration of these difficulties, combined with R. J.'s lack of success socially, appeared to be leading to increased feelings of helplessness and unhappiness.

Concerns were raised that although stimulant medication appeared to be helping some of R. J.'s attention-related difficulties, his developmental problems were causing further lack of motivation, which had a negative impact on his willingness to persist on school tasks. Diagnoses of ADHD, developmental, expressive and receptive language disorders and a dysthymic disorder were made.

ADHD, Oppositional Defiant Disorder and Dysthymia: The Case of J. B.

J. B., a 9½-year-old fourth grader, was referred by his family physician because of ongoing and increasing problems with attention span, arousal level, schoolwork completion and oppositional behavior. Medical evaluation did not identify a remediable medical problem. Despite trials of both Ritalin® and Dexedrine®, J. B.'s problems continued to be severe. The family physician raised the question as to whether he was attempting to treat nonmedication problems with stimulants. Parental history reflected an only child born out of wedlock whose parents had been separated for the previous six years. J. B. lived with his mother and saw his father rarely. Two months before the evaluation he had seen his father for the first time in three years. During this and previous visits his father always promised to see him more often and then never returned. J. B.'s behavior since this last visit had deteriorated. His mother appeared overwhelmed and expressed her frustration about being unable to control J. B.'s behavior.

Developmental history included sleep problems in infancy but a fairly benign toddler and preschool period. Problems with attention span and aggression were immediately observed when J. B. entered kindergarten. Stimulant medication was started in first grade with a positive response noted. By second grade, medication did not appear effective. A child psychiatrist was consulted, and J. B. was placed on a different stimulant. There was an immediate improvement in his behavior, but during the past year behavioral problems had gradually increased despite attempts at increasing stimulant medication. J. B.'s mother noted that although he had significant behavioral problems at home, when he did not take medication his problems were worse. With medication he appeared to have a 30-minute independent attention span. Even with medication he was easily overaroused and impulsive, and rewards were not effective in changing his behavior.

Parent and teacher questionnaires reflected a child experiencing significant attention, arousal and aggressive problems, even when receiving stimulant medication. Situational problems were mostly of mild severity in the home and of strong severity

NAME   J.B.   D.O.B. _____ AGE 9 yr 6 mo DATE _____

HISTORY

Age of Onset   5
Average Independent Attention Span
    (Minutes)   30 with medication
Easily Overaroused   Yes
Impulsive   Yes
S Not Effective   Yes
Other 1. Parents separated 6 years
2. Rarely sees father
3. Problems wtih sleep in infancy
4. Problems immediately observed in kinder.
5. Stimulants tried w/mixed reaction
6. Mother overwhelmed 7. Temper outbursts
8. Sleep problems persistent

QUESTIONNAIRES
    * With Ritalin

*Parent Conners   Above 99th %ile
Teacher Conners   _____ %ile
*ACTeRS: Attention   Below 1st %ile
        Hyperactivity Below 1st %ile
        Social Skills Below 1st %ile
        Oppositional   40th %ile
*Parent Achenbach: Scales Above 98th %ile
Hyperactivity   _____
Aggression   _____
Obsessive-Compulsive   _____

*Teacher Achenbach: Scales Above 98th %ile
Unpopular   _____
Inattentive   _____
Nervous-Overactive   _____
Aggressive   _____

*Home Situations Problems:
    Number of Situations   9
    Average Severity   Mild
*School Situations Problems:
    Number of Situations   11
    Average Severity   Severe
*Parent Social Skills: Type of Problems

1. Negative w/peers
2. Argumentative
3. Aggressive

*Teacher Social Skills: Type of Problems
1. Socially isolated
2. Lacks social skills
3. Negative, bossy, aggressive

Observation During Assessment
1. Wouldn't remove coat
2. Avoids eye contact
3. Rarey spoke
4. Poor cooperation
5. Tried to control session
6. No medication today

PERSONALITY OR EMOTIONAL FACTORS
1. Control issues
2. Undifferentiated anger
3. Denial concerning father
4. Poor social perception
5. Poor self-image
6. Aggressive

WECHSLER

Verbal	S.S.	Performance	S.S.
Information		Picture Completion	
Similarities		Picture Arrangement	
Arithmetic	9	Block Design	
Vocabulary		Object Assembly	
Comprehension		Coding	2
Digit Span	13	Mazes	9
Verbal I.Q.		Performance I.Q.	
	Full Scale I.Q.		

MOTOR SKILLS

Purdue Pegboard: Preferred Hand   BN %ile
                  Non-preferred hand 50th %ile
                  Both hands   1st %ile
                  Assembly   10th %ile
Developmental Test of Visual Motor
    Integration   _____ %ile
Bender Visual Motor Gestalt Test   40th %ile
Benton Visual Retention Test   _____ %ile
Detroit Test:
    Auditory Attention Span   9 yr 0 mo
    Visual Attention Span   9 yr 9 mo
    Notes on Performance   _____

Matching Familiar Figures Test:
    Errors   60th %ile
    Completion Time   10th %ile
Peabody Picture Vocabulary Test   _____ %ile
Trail Making Test: Completion Time 50th %ile
                    Errors   50th %ile
Progressive Figures Test   _____ %ile
Rapidly Recurring Target Figures:
    592: Completion Time   86th %ile
         Errors   16th %ile
    Diamond: Completion Time   98th %ile
             Errors   16th %ile
Motor Free Visual Perception Test   _____ %ile
Hand Preference   _____ Left   X Right

ACADEMICS

	Test	Grade	* %ile
SAT:	Reading		15th %ile
	Math		22nd %ile
	Listening		36th %ile
Total Battery			29th %ile

    (decreasing levels over past 3 years)
                * National Sample

OTHER TESTS OR QUESTIONNAIRES

Test	Score or %ile
10/86 Slosson Intelligence Test	124

ADHD Diagnostic Checklist Criteria

I	Yes	III	No/Mixed
II	Yes	IV	Yes
	V	Complex Emotional History	

Figure 7.12 ADHD, oppositional defiant disorder and dysthymia: The case of J. B.

within the school. Both mother and teachers described J. B. as socially isloated, argumentative, negative, bossy and aggressive with his peers.

For the first hour of the evaluation J. B. would not remove his coat and avoided eye contact. He rarely initiated conversation and his cooperation was poor. He appeared interested in controlling the assessment session. Past assessment data from the school suggested that J. B. was functioning in the lower average range academically with a consistent pattern of decreasing achievement over the past three years. Prior intellectual assessment indicated that J. B. was of at least higher average to superior intelligence.

As a result of J. B.'s passive, at times creative opposition, assessment data clearly reflected less than his capabilities. J. B.'s test performance reflected mild fine motor difficulties but adequate ability to reflect, sustain and persist. J. B. appeared able to focus divided attention and persist on task. His responses to the clinical interview revealed a child experiencing a significant degree of undifferentiated anger and a strong need to control. J. B. denied any negative feelings about his father and defended his absence by explaining that his father had to work. J. B. exhibited aggressive problem solutions, poor social perception and a poor self-image.

J. B.'s history and behavior appeared to meet the DSM-III-R criteria for ADHD. Questionnaire data indicated problems with opposition and aggression that overshadowed difficulties with attention span and arousal level. His history suggested a mother with limited parenting skills and a poor social support system. J. B.'s problems were further compounded by an absent father who appeared just often enough to keep J. B. angry, frustrated and possibly involved in a grief process. Objective data did not support the view that J.B. experienced problems with attention and reflection skills. Situationally, he appeared to have more problems of greater severity within the school. The complex history and assessment data suggested a child experiencing primarily a significant degree of oppositional behavior problems, possible dysthymia and symptoms of ADHD that may or may not be secondary to other behavioral difficulty. The increasing spiral in the use of medication with good short-term but poor long-term response raised questions as to the primacy of J. B.'s attentional problems. Inpatient child psychiatric hospitalization was recommended in an effort to provide more opportunity for observation and assessment.

ADHD AND DEPRESSION: THE CASE OF N. W.

N. W., an almost 10-year-old fourth grader, was referred by her pediatrician. She presented an increasing pattern over the past three months of moody, depressed behavior marked by feelings of helplessness, increased inattentive behavior at school and a lack of schoolwork completion. Parents observed a similar set of problems at home. Increased social isolation was observed. Medical evaluation was unremarkable. The history suggested no significant parental concerns of attention deficit before first grade; however, her parents reported that N. W. had never paid attention as well as her siblings. Her parents noted a positive family history on

NAME _____ N.W. _____ D.O.B. _____ AGE 9 yr 11 mo DATE _____

HISTORY

Age of Onset _____ 6 _____
Average Independent Attention Span
  (Minutes) _____ 15 _____
Easily Overaroused _____ Yes _____
Impulsive _____ Sometimes _____
S Not Effective _____ Yes _____
Other 1. Increasingly moody _____
2. Concerned with weight and appearance
3. No special education _____
_____
_____

QUESTIONNAIRES

Parent Conners _____ Over 99th %ile
Teacher Conners _____ %ile
ACTeRS: Attention ___ Below 15th %ile
    Hyperactivity ___ 60th ___ %ile
    Social Skills ___ 10th ___ %ile
    Oppositional ___ 15th ___ %ile
Parent Achenbach: Scales Above 98th %ile
Depression _____
Social withdrawal _____
Hyperactivity _____
Aggression _____

Teacher Achenbach: Scales Above 98th %ile
_____ _____
_____ _____
_____ _____

Home Situations Problems:
  Number of Situations ___ 11 ___
  Average Severity ___ Moderate ___
School Situations Problems:
  Number of Situations ___ 3 ___
  Average Severity ___ Moderate ___
Parent Social Skills: Type of Problems
  Socially isolated _____
_____
_____
_____

Teacher Social Skills: Type of Problems
1. Socially isolated _____
2. Shy, timid _____
3. Negative, bossy, annoying when she
   interacts _____

Observation During Assessment
1. No spontaneous conversation _____
2. Distrusts abilities _____
3. Anxious but denies _____
4. Lack of effort at times _____
_____
_____

PERSONALITY OR EMOTIONAL FACTORS
1. Thoughts of suicide _____
2. Wants more friends _____
3. Insecure _____
4. Feelings of inadequacy _____
5. Can't fall asleep _____
6. Excessive worrying

WECHSLER

Verbal	S.S.	Performance	S.S.
Information	13	Picture Completion	12
Similarities	12	Picture Arrangement	13
Arithmetic	7	Block Design	15
Vocabulary	12	Object Assembly	12
Comprehension	11	Coding	8
Digit Span	12	Mazes	8
Verbal I.Q.	106	Performance I.Q.	114

Full Scale I.Q. ___ 110 ___

MOTOR SKILLS

Purdue Pegboard: Preferred Hand ___ 40th %ile
            Non-preferred hand ___ 50th %ile
            Both hands ___ 10th %ile
            Assembly ___ 35th %ile
Developmental Test of Visual Motor
  Integration _____ %ile
Bender Visual Motor Gestalt Test ___ 50th %ile
Benton Visual Retention Test _____ %ile
Detroit Test:
  Auditory Attention Span ___ 9 yr 6 mo
  Visual Attention Span ___ 6 yr 9 mo
  Notes on Performance _____
_____

Matching Familiar Figures Test:
  Errors ___ 90th %ile
  Completion Time ___ 6th %ile
Peabody Picture Vocabulary Test _____ %ile
Trail Making Test: Completion Time ___ 50th %ile
            Errors ___ 10th %ile
Progressive Figures Test _____ %ile
Rapidly Recurring Target Figures:
  592: Completion Time ___ 16th %ile
    Errors ___ 50th %ile
  Diamond: Completion Time ___ 16th %ile
    Errors ___ 50th %ile
Motor Free Visual Perception Test _____ %ile
Hand Preference ___ X ___ Left _____ Right

ACADEMICS

	Test	Grade	%ile
SAT			Average to above
			in all areas

OTHER TESTS OR QUESTIONNAIRES

Test	Score or %ile
1. Test of Non-Verbal	
Intelligence	57th %ile
2. Children's Depression	
Inventory	Average

ADHD Diagnostic Checklist Criteria

I	Yes	III	Yes
II	Yes	IV	Yes
		V	Yes

Figure 7.13 ADHD and depression: The case of N. W.

the father's side of the family for attention deficit, and they also observed that N. W. was having increasing difficulty falling asleep at night and was making self-deprecatory statements.

Parent and teacher reports yielded data meeting DSM-III-R criteria for ADHD. Situational problems were significant within the home but primarily limited to work situations in the school. Problems with inattention appeared greater than problems with motor restlessness. Social skills questionnaires yielded a consistent pattern of social isolation, shyness and timidity. When N. W. interacted with peers, a pattern of negative, bossy and annoying behavior was observed.

During assessment, N. W. appeared anxious and distrustful of her abilities. She did not engage in spontaneous conversation and at times lacked effort. She acknowledged previous thoughts of suicide, feelings of inadequacy and insecurity. Difficulty falling asleep and excessive worrying, as well as a desire for more friends, were also acknowledged.

Assessment data portrayed a bright child with academic achievement slightly below expectation based on intellect. Significant problems with vigilance, persistence, sustained attention and reflection were observed. A relative weakness in the dominant left hand was observed. Data also suggested that N. W. appeared to have persistence and attention skills that she was not using because of her emotional status.

Based on the history, current behavior and assessment data, there appeared to be sufficient justification to make diagnoses of both major depression and ADHD. It additionally appeared that the depression was exacerbating what historically had been mild to moderate problems with attention span.

ADHD, TOURETTE'S SYNDROME AND ADJUSTMENT DIFFICULTY: THE CASE OF K. H.

K. H., a 9-year-old third grader, was referred by a child neurologist. She had been placed by her pediatrician on increasingly larger doses of Ritalin for attention problems. At the time of referral she was prescribed 25 mg. of Ritalin twice daily. During the six-month period prior to the neurologist's evaluation, K. H. developed a series of severe vocal and motor tics. The pediatrician maintained the dose of Ritalin and added 5 mg. of Haldol®. Tics were reduced but continued to be present, most noticeably a facial tic. K. H. continued to experience significant social, achievement and behavioral problems both at home and at school.

Parental history noted toxemia during the pregnancy but an uneventful infancy, toddler and preschool period. Her parents had no major concerns about K. H. before kindergarten, but problems with attention span and work completion were immediately observed in kindergarten. Problems escalated until second grade when K. H. was initially placed on stimulant medication.

Stimulants appeared to help, but after a short time K. H.'s behavior deteriorated and increasingly larger doses of stimulant medication were prescribed by the pediatrician with positive response observed each time. Parents reported a pill-rolling behavior that K. H. exhibited before being placed on stimulant medication.

NAME _____ K.H. _____ D.O.B. _____ AGE 9 yr 1 mo DATE _____

HISTORY

Age of Onset _____ 5 _____
Average Independent Attention Span
  (Minutes) _____ 5 _____
Easily Overaroused _____ Yes _____
Impulsive _____ Yes _____
S Not Effective _____ Yes _____
Other 1. Toxemia during pregnancy
2. No major concerns prior to kinder.
3. Problems immediately seen in kinder.
4. Multiple tics developed in response
   to Ritalin
5. Poor self control 6. Obsessive
7. Anxious

QUESTIONNAIRES
  * With Ritalin and Haldol

| Parent Conners | Above 99th %ile |
| Teacher Conners | %ile |

*ACTeRS: Attention   Above 5th %ile
         Hyperactivity   10th %ile
         Social Skills   5th %ile
         Oppositional   Below 5th %ile

*Parent Achenbach: Scales Above 98th %ile

Depression	Sex problems
Social Withdrawal	Delinquent
Somatic Complaints	Aggressive
Schizoid	Cruel
Hyperactive	

*Teacher Achenbach: Scales Above 98th %ile
Anxious
Social Withdrawal
Unpopular
Inattentive
Nervous-Overactive

*Home Situations Problems:
  Number of Situations _____ 14
  Average Severity _____ Moderate
School Situations Problems:
  Number of Situations _____ 5
  Average Severity _____ Moderate
Parent Social Skills: Type of Problems

1. Socially isolated
2. Strikes out with angry behavior
3. Lacks social skills

*Teacher Social Skills: Type of Problems
1. Shy, timid, isolated often
2. Bossy or disturbing
3. Argumentative
4. Aggressive

Observation During Assessment
1. Multiple facial tics
2. Easily distracted
3. Anxious, picking at fingers
4. Cooperative
5. No medication today

PERSONALITY OR EMOTIONAL FACTORS
1. Inhibited and anxious when
   unstructured
2. Aware of tics
3. Helpless feelings
4. Poor self-image
5. Poor self-perspective

WECHSLER

Verbal	S.S.	Performance	S.S.
Information	11	Picture Completion	4
Similarities	9	Picture Arrangement	5
Arithmetic	6	Block Design	8
Vocabulary	8	Object Assembly	7
Comprehension	6	Coding	1
Digit Span	8	Mazes	6
Verbal I.Q.	87	Performance I.Q.	68
	Full Scale I.Q.	76	

MOTOR SKILLS

Purdue Pegboard:	Preferred Hand	10th %ile
	Non-preferred hand	10th %ile
	Both hands	1st %ile
	Assembly	1st %ile

Developmental Test of Visual Motor
  Integration _____ %ile
Bender Visual Motor Gestalt Test ___ 2nd %ile
Benton Visual Retention Test _____ %ile
Detroit Test:
  Auditory Attention Span   Below 3 Yr
  Visual Attention Span   Below 3 Yr
  Notes on Performance Struggled but tried

Matching Familiar Figures Test:
  Errors   Above 99th %ile
  Completion Time   Below 1st %ile
Peabody Picture Vocabulary Test _____ %ile
Trail Making: Completion Time   Below 1st %ile
              Errors   50th %ile
Progressive Figures Test _____ %ile
Rapidly Recurring Target Figures:
  592: Completion Time   98th %ile
       Errors   98th %ile
  Diamond: Completion Time   90th %ile
           Errors   98th %ile
Motor Free Visual Perception Test _____ %ile
Hand Preference   X Left ____ Right

ACADEMICS

Test	Grade	%ile
WRAT-Reading		47th %ile
WRAT-Math		16th %ile

OTHER TESTS OR QUESTIONNAIRES

Test	Score or %ile
Wepman Auditory Discrimination	Significant
	5 errors

ADHD Diagnostic Checklist Criteria

I	Yes	III	Yes
II	Yes	IV	Yes
	V Complex Problems		

Figure 7.14 ADHD, Tourette's syndrome and adjustment difficulty: The case of K. H.

Tics that developed included flipping of the head, picking at her lips, barking, smelling things excessively, continued pill rolling, picking at her thumb, chewing at her fingernails, eye blinking and facial grimacing. Parents also noted that K. H. had a very strong need for perfection and appeared anxious under any sort of stress. Family history was negative for psychiatric problems. K. H.'s parents noted that she became overaroused easily and was impulsive. Rewards did not appear effective. Her average independent attention span was estimated to be five minutes.

Parent and teacher questionnaires reflected a child experiencing significant externalizing and internalizing problems. Even with stimulant medication, significant problems with attention span and overarousal were observed in both the home and the school. Moderate problems were observed in almost all home situations, with moderate problems observed primarily in any classroom work-related situations. K. H. appeared socially isolated. When she interacted with others, she would be angry, argumentative or aggressive.

Observation during assessment reflected a cooperative child of normal physical appearance. K. H. exhibited multiple complex facial tics, approximately two or three per minute. These consisted of eye blinking and tightening of the facial muscles. K. H. appeared aware of the tics and able to control them for brief periods. K. H. denied anxiety, but her presentation to the examiner suggested that she was experiencing some degree of anxiety and compulsive behavior. She frequently commented that her performance on various assessment instruments was inadequate. Her impulsive style appeared to have a negative impact on test performance.

Assessment suggested a child functioning in the borderline range of intellectual skill with a significant relative weakness in perceptual ability. Motor speed and coordination were impaired. Objective data reflected problems with reflection, organization, divided attention, vigilance and persistence capacity. K. H. appeared to have the ability to persist on task, but even when doing so, she was extremely disorganized. Brief screening of academic skills suggested adequate word-reading ability but difficulty with arithmetic. Assessment data also indicated problems with auditory discrimination, strongly raising the possibility that K. H. experienced additional auditory processing difficulty as well. K. H.'s responses during the clinical interview reflected an inhibited, anxious child. She appeared to foster feelings of helplessness and a poor self-image. She did not appear to have an adequate perspective of the difficulty she was experiencing. Denial and projection appeared to be her primary psychological defenses. K. H. was aware of her tics and expressed frustration in being unable to control them.

History, present functioning and assessment data suggested that K.H. presented behavior meeting the DSM-III-R diagnostic criteria for ADHD and Tourette's Syndrome. Consistent situational problems related to attention difficulty, anxiety and oppositional behavior were noted on questionnaires and, in part, during the evaluation. Consistent problems with attentional skills were observed during objective assessment. The complexity of K. H.'s problems made it difficult to include or rule out other specific diagnostic problems with anxiety, oppositional behavior or depression. Attention problems appeared to be one of the primary foundations upon which K. H.'s other difficulties developed. Referral to an inpatient child psychiatric setting was recommended to provide additional observation, assessment and treatment.

ADHD AND COMPLEX PSYCHOLOGICAL PROBLEMS: THE CASE OF K. B.

K. B., a 9-year-old fourth grader, was referred by his pediatrician when medical evaluation did not provide an explanation for K. B.'s increasing pattern of oppositional, defiant and overaroused behavior. K. B. had been treated over the past two years with stimulant medication for attention problems. His history was complex. His parents had separated six years before. K. B. initially remained with his mother. She evidently neglected him, and his father was awarded custody of K. B. and his older sister. Over the past six years K. B. had seen his mother infrequently. She had an unstable history and would arrive and leave without warning. For a period of time, K. B. and his sister were cared for by their maternal grandmother. She did not set or enforce behavioral limits. When K. B. was four years old, his father obtained an apartment of his own and took the children.

The family history was positive for both psychiatric problems and attention disorder. The pregnancy was complicated by blood loss and alcohol consumption. His father recalled that K. B. was strong-minded and busy as an infant. He was constantly into things as soon as he was mobile. He was nocturnally enuretic until six years of age. Despite these problems, K. B.'s father was not concerned about K. B.'s ability to function in kindergarten. Immediately upon entering school, K. B. was unruly and nonconforming. During first grade, Resource services were initiated. Toward the end of first grade, a trial of stimulant medication was attempted with some positive response. Socialization and behavioral problems, however, continued to escalate over the next two years.

K. B.'s father remarried when K. B. was eight years old, and K. B. worked to create conflicts in the marriage. He refused to respond to limits set by his stepmother. He had recently begun seeing his natural mother again, and she had, through her comments to him, increased his behavioral problems within the home, particularly his oppositional behavior toward his stepmother. Additionally, K. B.'s father and stepmother disagreed on disciplinary procedures. Parenting and group counseling intervention through a local mental health center over the past year had not been successful in reducing problems. Both K. B.'s father and stepmother felt that K. B. was extremely angry. They described his independent attention span as ten minutes. He became overaroused easily and was impulsive. Reinforcement had not been effective in changing his behavior. Most recently, K. B. had been receiving a 20 mg Ritalin spansule in the morning with an occasional 10 mg standard dose given at home in the afternoon.

Parent and teacher questionnaires were consistent in reporting significant attention and arousal-level problems, even with the use of stimulant medication. Additionally, both parents and teachers observed significant problems with aggression, social withdrawal and poor communication. Moderate to severe problems were consistently observed in almost all home and school situations. Both parent

NAME _____ K.B. _____ D.O.B. _____ AGE 9 yr 1 mo DATE _____

HISTORY

Age of Onset _____ 2
Average Independent Attention Span
  (Minutes) _____ 10
Easily Overaroused _____ Yes
Impulsive _____ Yes
S Not Effective _____ Yes
Other 1. History of significant family
  problems
2. Absent mother
3. Paternal grandmother created more
  problems   4. Angry
5. Father remarried - blended family
  problems

QUESTIONNAIRES
  * With Ritalin
*Parent Conners _____ 99th %ile
*Teacher Conners _____ 98th %ile
ACTeRS: Attention _____ %ile
  Hyperactivity _____ %ile
  Social Skills _____ %ile
  Oppositional _____ %ile
*Parent Achenbach: Scales Above 98th %ile
  Hyperactivity   Social Withdrawal
  Aggression
  Delinquency
  Depression
  Poor Communication
*Teacher Achenbach: Scales Above 98th %ile
  Unpopular
  Self-destructive
  Inattentive
  Overactive
  Aggressive
*Home Situations Problems:
  Number of Situations _____ 13
  Average Severity   Moderate-severe
School Situations Problems:
  Number of Situations _____ 8
  Average Severity   Moderate
Parent Social Skills: Type of Problems

1. Lacks social skills
2. Negative, bossy
3. Aggressive

*Teacher Social Skills: Type of Problems
1. Aggressive
2. Somewhat isolated

Observation During Assessment
1. Related well to examiner
2. No medication on day of evaluation
3. Some fidgeting

PERSONALITY OR EMOTIONAL FACTORS
1. Unresolved divorce issues
2. Unhappy with father's marriage
3. Poorly motivated academically
4. Angry
5. Unhappy
6. Pessimistic

WECHSLER

Verbal	S.S.	Performance	S.S.
Information	11	Picture Completion	10
Similarities	10	Picture Arrangement	15
Arithmetic	8	Block Design	12
Vocabulary	10	Object Assembly	11
Comprehension	6	Coding	12
Digit Span	8	Mazes	7
Verbal I.Q.	94	Performance I.Q.	114

Full Scale I.Q. _____ 102

MOTOR SKILLS

Purdue Pegboard:	Preferred Hand	90th %ile
	Non-preferred hand	20th %ile
	Both hands	25th %ile
	Assembly	90th %ile
Developmental Test of Visual Motor		
Integration		%ile
Bender Visual Motor Gestalt Test		50th %ile
Benton Visual Retention Test		%ile
Detroit Test:		
Auditory Attention Span		7 yr 3 mo
Visual Attention Span		9 yr 0 mo
Notes on Performance		

Matching Familiar Figures Test:		
Errors		75th %ile
Completion Time		30th %ile
Peabody Picture Vocabulary Test		%ile
Trail Making Test: Completion Time		10th %ile
Errors		50th %ile
Progressive Figures Test		%ile
Rapidly Recurring Target Figures:		
592: Completion Time		30th %ile
Errors		86th %ile
Diamond: Completion Time		35th %ile
Errors		86th %ile
Motor Free Visual Perception Test		%ile
Hand Preference	X Left	Right

ACADEMICS

Test	Grade	* %ile
SAT - Reading		37th %ile
Math		48th %ile
Language		20th %ile
Listening		71st %ile

* National Sample

OTHER TESTS OR QUESTIONNAIRES

Test	Score or %ile
Visual Aural Digit Span Test	10th %ile

ADHD Diagnostic Checklist Criteria

I	Yes	III	Yes
II	Yes	IV	Yes
		V	Yes

Figure 7.15 ADHD and complex psychological problems: The case of K. B.

and teachers noted that when K. B. interacted with other children he was negative, bossy and aggressive.

During assessment, K. B. related well to the examiner. He had not received stimulant medication on the day of the evaluation. Some fidgeting was observed, and his affect also appeared somewhat constricted. Assessment data revealed a child functioning in the average range of intellectual skill with a significant relative weakness in verbal ability. Left-brain problems were further reflected in measures of laterality. Auditory attention skills appeared significantly weaker than visual skills.

Data suggested problems with reflection, divided attention and vigilance. Problems appeared inconsistent, which may have resulted from K. B.'s emotional status. Academic achievement tests completed three months prior documented lower average academic skills with a relative weakness in language ability. K. B. presented as an unhappy, pessimistic, angry child. He was able to talk about his active attempts to disrupt his parent's marriage, his unhappiness with his mother's absence and his poor academic motivation. He was unable to speak positively of himself or perceive that anything was going to happen to make his life better.

K. B.'s history and questionnaire data suggested that he met the DSM-III-R diagnostic criteria for ADHD. Assessment data further reflected attentional problems with situational difficulty noted fairly consistently both at home and at school. His psychological history, however, was extremely complex, suggesting that a major component of K. B.'s problems stemmed from this history. The history, present functioning and assessment data were not sufficient to clearly determine whether symptoms of attention problems, restlessness and arousal were secondary to K. B.'s noncompliance and depression. In addition, assessment data indicated that K. B. displayed relatively greater problems with verbal/linguistic skills and auditory attention, suggesting that he may experience an auditory processing disorder. Assessment by an audiologist supported this hypothesis. Provisional diagnoses of oppositional defiant disorder, major depression and ADHD were made. K. B. was referred to an inpatient child psychiatric setting to allow closer observation and intensive treatment intervention.

ADHD SECONDARY TO EPILEPTIC SYNDROME: THE CASE OF B. J.

B. J., a 5½-year-old kindergartener, was referred by a pediatric neurologist because of a pattern of impulsive, inattentive and overaroused behavior. B. J.'s thought processes at times also appeared somewhat tangential. B. J. had been treated by the neurologist for a year as the result of Lennox-Gastaut syndrome. The syndrome consists of akinetic myoclonic, absence and generalized tonic-clonic seizures. Cognitive functioning is usually impaired in children experiencing this syndrome (Aicardi, 1988). During the year in which seizures were brought under control, B. J. appeared to slow in development and exhibited increasing problems of inattention and overarousal. Following periods of seizures, B. J. would regress and then during seizure-free periods appeared to make progress. After previous medical evaluation, the neurologist had placed B. J. on 20 mg of methylphenidate

NAME _____B.J._____ D.O.B. _____ AGE 5 yr 8 mo   DATE _____

HISTORY

Age of Onset _____5_____
Average Independent Attention Span
  (Minutes) _____3_____
Easily Overaroused ____Yes____
Impulsive _____Yes____
S'Not Effective _____Yes____
Other 1. Uneventful pregnancy
2. Difficult infancy
3. Milestones initially adequate
4. Development slowed after seizures
5. Impulsive and inattentive

QUESTIONNAIRES

Parent Conners   Above 98th %ile
Teacher Conners   Above 98th %ile
ACTeRS: Attention _____ %ile
      Hyperactivity _____ %ile
      Social Skills _____ %ile
      Oppositional _____ %ile
Parent Achenbach: Scales Above 98th %ile
Depression _____ _____
Anxious _____
Social Withdrawal _____
Hyperactive _____

Teacher Achenbach: Scales Above 98th %ile
_____ _____
_____ _____
_____ _____
_____ _____

Home Situations Problems:
  Number of Situations _____8_____
  Average Severity ___Moderate___
School Situations Problems:
  Number of Situations _____5_____
  Average Severity ___Moderate___
Parent Social Skills: Type of Problems
_____
_____
_____
_____

Teacher Social Skills: Type of Problems
_____
_____
_____
_____

Observation During Assessment
_____
_____
_____
_____
_____

PERSONALITY OR EMOTIONAL FACTORS
_____
_____
_____
_____

WECHSLER

Verbal	S.S.	Performance	S.S.
Information		Picture Completion	
Similarities		Picture Arrangement	
Arithmetic		Block Design	
Vocabulary		Object Assembly	
Comprehension		Coding	
Digit Span		Mazes	
Verbal I.Q.		Performance I.Q.	
	Full Scale I.Q.		

MOTOR SKILLS

Purdue Pegboard: Preferred Hand   10th %ile
               Non-preferred hand 10th %ile
               Both hands   10th %ile
               Assembly   15th %ile
Developmental Test of Visual Motor
  Integration _____ %ile
Bender Visual Motor Gestalt Test   40th %ile
Benton Visual Retention Test   30th %ile
Detroit Test:
  Auditory Attention Span   4 yr 3 mo
  Visual Attention Span _____
  Notes on Performance _____
_____
_____

Matching Familiar Figures Test:
  Errors _____ %ile
  Completion Time _____ %ile
Peabody Picture Vocabulary Test ____ %ile
Trail Making Test: Completion Time __ %ile
           Errors _____ %ile
Progressive Figures Test _____ %ile
Rapidly Recurring Target Figures:
  592: Completion Time _____ %ile
     Errors _____ %ile
  Diamond: Completion Time   2nd %ile
     Errors   98th %ile
Motor Free Visual Perception Test ___ %ile
Hand Preference _____ Left   X Right

VINELAND ADAPTIVE BEHAVIOR SCALES

Test	Standard Score	Age
Communication	79	4 yr 4 mo
Daily Living	91	4 yr 11 mo
Socialization	86	4 yr 6 mo
Motor Skills	73	5 yr 11 mo
Maladaptive Behavior	Elevated	

OTHER TESTS OR QUESTIONNAIRES

Test	Score or %ile
Stanford-Binet	40th %ile
Detroit Oral Commissions	4 yr 9 mo
Detroit Oral Directors	Below norms
Frostig Eye Motor	4 yr 6 mo

ADHD Diagnostic Checklist Criteria

I _____ Yes _____   III _____ Some _____
II _____ Yes _____   IV _____ Yes _____
        V _Complex Medical_

Figure 7.16 ADHD secondary to epileptic syndrome: The case of B. J.

in addition to her anticonvulsants. Methylphenidate appeared to reduce inattentive, overaroused behavior without increasing seizure episodes.

Parental history indicated that B. J. became overaroused easily, was impulsive, and rewards were not effective in changing her behavior. Her independent attention span presently was approximately three minutes. She was the product of an uncomplicated pregnancy but was a somewhat irritable, overactive infant. Her developmental milestones were initially reached within normal limits. At the time of referral, she appeared impulsive, inattentive and at times tangential in her verbalizations.

Parent and teacher questionnaires suggested significant attention and arousal level problems. Difficulty with anxiety and social withdrawal were also observed by the parents. A moderate degree of problems were noted in many home situations, with moderate problems noted primarily in work-related situations in the kindergarten classroom. Parents and teachers noted that B. J. was socially isolated, at times disoriented and awkward in her behavior. She did not appear socially accepted and was having difficulty relating to her siblings.

During assessment, B. J. related easily to the examiner but had poor eye contact, was distractible, inattentive and fidgeted excessively. She was disorganized in her approach to the testing tasks, had poor speech skills and at times made odd, irrelevant comments. She appeared immature, and at times her thought processes lacked a reality orientation.

B. J. was only marginally cooperative in completing testing tasks. She appeared to function in the lower average range of intellectual skill with significant language and auditory problems. Fine motor skills were delayed. B. J.'s approach to many test items was impulsive and disorganized. B. J.'s adaptive behavior appeared approximately one year delayed in communication, daily living and socialization skills. She appeared to have significant maladaptive behaviors in comparison to children of her chronological age.

B. J.'s current presentation met the DSM-III-R diagnostic criteria for ADHD. Etiology appeared primarily a function of brain injury associated with an epileptic syndrome usually characterized by deteriorating cognitive and behavioral functioning. Parent and teacher questionnaires reflected significant attention and arousal-level problems in the majority of home and school situations. Assessment data suggested difficulty with attention span, but assessment was complicated by the significant auditory and linguistic problems B. J. presented. Given the complexity of B. J.'s problems and an etiology based on a medical disorder, a diagnosis of organic brain syndrome was made.

ADHD SECONDARY TO BRAIN TRAUMA IN A YOUNG CHILD: THE CASE OF K. A.

K. A., a 2½-year-old, was referred by his pediatric neurologist. At birth K. A. sustained an occipital depressed skull fracture with subarachnoid hemorrhage, bleeding from the right ear, a large soft hematoma over the right ear and marked right-side paralysis. Facial palsy presented and resolved at 12 months of age. Seizures developed within the first hour of life. A diagnosis of hydrocephalus was

NAME _____K.A._____ D.O.B. _____ AGE 2 yr 5 mo DATE _____

HISTORY

Age of Onset ____Birth_____
Average Independent Attention Span
  (Minutes) ____2_____
Easily Overaroused ___Yes___
Impulsive ___Yes___
S Not Effective ___Yes___
Other 1. Brain injury at birth
2. Delayed development
3. Good progress over past 7 months
4. Incrasing discipline problems
_____

QUESTIONNAIRES

Parent Conners _____%ile
Teacher Conners _____%ile
ACTeRS: Attention _____%ile
      Hyperactivity _____%ile
      Social Skills _____%ile
      Oppositional _____%ile
Parent Achenbach: Scales Above 98th %ile
Social Withdrawal _____
Sleep problems _____
Aggressive _____
Destructive _____

Teacher Achenbach: Scales Above 98th %ile
_____ _____
_____ _____
_____ _____
_____ _____

Home Situations Problems:
Number of Situations ___11___
Average Severity ___Severe___
School Situations Problems:
Number of Situations _____
Average Severity _____
Parent Social Skills: Type of Problems
Parallel play _____
Can be aggressive _____
_____
_____

Teacher Social Skills: Type of Problems
_____
_____
_____
_____

Observation During Assessment
1. Good eye contact
2. Imitates verbally
3. Delayed receptive and expressive
   language
4. Worked for one half hour well
5. Oppositional but controllable with
   limits

PERSONALITY OR EMOTIONAL FACTORS
1. Interacted with examiner
2. Testing
3. Related adequate to examiner
4. Regresses behaviorally when task
   complexity increases

WECHSLER

Verbal	S.S.	Performance	S.S.
Information	___	Picture Completion	___
Similarities	___	Picture Arrangement	___
Arithmetic	___	Block Design	___
Vocabulary	___	Object Assembly	___
Comprehension	___	Coding	___
Digit Span	___	Mazes	___
Verbal I.Q.	___	Performance I.Q.	___
	Full Scale I.Q.	___	

MOTOR SKILLS

Purdue Pegboard: Preferred Hand _____%ile
             Non-preferred hand _____%ile
             Both hands _____%ile
             Assembly _____%ile
Developmental Test of Visual Motor
  Integration _____50th %ile
Bender Visual Motor Gestalt Test _____%ile
Benton Visual Retention Test _____%ile
Detroit Test:
  Auditory Attention Span _____
  Visual Attention Span _____
  Notes on Performance _____
_____

Matching Familiar Figures Test:
  Errors _____%ile
  Completion Time _____%ile
Peabody Picture Vocabulary Test _____%ile
Trail Making Test: Completion Time ___23rd %ile
            Errors _____%ile
Progressive Figures Test _____%ile
Rapidly Recurring Target Figures:
  592: Completion Time _____%ile
     Errors _____%ile
  Diamond: Completion Time _____%ile
        Errors _____%ile
Motor Free Visual Perception Test _____%ile
Hand Preference ___X__ Left _____ Right
          Simian Grip Limited use of
                 right hand

ACADEMICS

Test	Grade	%ile
_____	_____	_____
_____	_____	_____
_____	_____	_____
_____	_____	_____

OTHER TESTS OR QUESTIONNAIRES

Test	Score or %ile
Stanford-Binet	97th %ile
Receptive-Expressive Emergent	
Language Scale:	
Receptive	18–20 mo.
Expressive	16–18 mo.

ADHD Diagnostic Checklist Criteria

I	Yes	III	Untestable
II	Yes	IV	Yes
		V	Complex

Figure 7.17 ADHD secondary to brain trauma in a young child: The case of K. A.

made, and a ventricular peritoneal shunt was placed to control intracranial pressure. K.A.'s early development was significantly delayed. Evaluation at 24 months of age noted no spontaneous vocalization, limited cooperation and poor motor skills. K. A. was subsequently placed in a five-day-a-week, intensive child development program. At the time of evaluation, K. A.'s parents reported that his independent attention span was two minutes. He was easily overaroused and impulsive, and rewards had not been effective in changing his behavior. Although he made very good progress in the child development program, his parents were concerned by an increasing pattern of inattention, emotionality and noncompliant behavior at home.

Information from parent questionnaires suggested that K. A. was approximately 10 to 12 months delayed in receptive and expressive language with an overall 6 month delay in general development. Behavioral difficulties with socialization, adaptation to routines, destruction and aggression were observed. Severe problems were noted in almost all home situations. His parents observed that K. A. would engage in parallel play with other children. When he interacted, frequently he was aggressive. Child development staff noted marked improvements in K. A.'s ability to follow routines and participate in their program. Inattention and restless behavior were observed.

During the evaluation, K. A. related well to the examiner. He was able to remain seated, working for a half-hour period. He made good eye contact and could imitate verbally. He was clearly delayed in receptive and expressive language skills. When tasks became more difficult, he tested limits and became oppositional or regressed in his behavior and became silly. When clear-cut limits were set, he improved very quickly.

Standardized assessment data was surprisingly good. K. A. appeared to have average intellectual skill despite significant language impairments. The data strongly raised the possibility that K. A. possessed better intellectual potential. During the play session, K. A. interacted appropriately with the examiner and related well. There were a number of times when he attempted to test limits, but once the examiner set a limit he responded appropriately. His overall presentation and behavior demonstrated marked improvement from assessment six months previously.

A component of K. A.'s attention and arousal-level problems was clearly physiologically based. Other significant components of these problems appeared to be K. A.'s inability to deal effectively with his environment, frustration from receptive and expressive language problems and, as is characteristic for many two-year-olds, the increasing awareness that he could exert control over his environment. A primary diagnosis of brain injury with behavioral problems was made. Subsequent follow-up when K. A. was five years of age revealed higher average to superior intellectual skills with no significant attention or arousal-level problems. K. A. appeared mildly delayed in academic achievement relative to his chronological age and significantly delayed relative to his intellect. Concerns were raised that once he left the child development program and began kindergarten, his inability to perform academically could result in increasing stress and again create significant arousal and attention problems.

ADHD SECONDARY TO BRAIN INJURY: THE CASE OF D. E.

D. E., a 6½-year-old first grader, was referred by his neurosurgeon two years after an automobile/pedestrian accident in which D. E. was hit by an automobile and thrown 50 feet. He was unconscious for approximately two hours and suffered a basilar skull fracture. In the weeks after the accident, D. E. became extremely aggressive, oppositional and destructive. These symptoms did not remit within a year, and D. E. was referred for further evaluation. D. E.'s mother was single and raising D. E. while living in her mother's home. There was no family history of attention or psychiatric problems. D. E.'s mother was employed by an airline. Prior to the injury, D. E. presented with a normal developmental history. His mother noted that he was beginning to read just prior to the injury. In addition to behavioral changes following the injury, D. E. appeared to have lost the reading skills he had acquired and was struggling with reading achievement. Of the attention and arousal problems that were immediately apparent after the injury, only D. E.'s level of aggression had responded to behavioral intervention.

Parent and teacher questionnaires reported significant problems with attention span and arousal-level. D. E. also appeared socially isolated. When he interacted with peers, he was bossy, annoying and at times aggressive. Situational problems of moderate severity were noted in both the home and school. The severity of home problems had been reduced following his mother's participation in a parenting class on behavioral management. D. E.'s preschool teacher recalled that there was a dramatic decrease in his behavior and achievement capabilities following his return to school after the injury.

D. E. appeared to be a healthy child. He was somewhat inhibited during the assessment session. He spoke at a low volume and was mildly constricted in the range and tone of his emotions. He fidgeted excessively and exhibited an impulsive work style.

Assessment suggested a child functioning in the average range of intelligence who was generally capable of focusing and who displayed age-appropriate attention and reflection skills. Academic achievement tests showed significant reading problems with at least average to above-average arithmetic ability. The test data did not reveal a clear pattern of skill deficits that could account for D. E.'s reading achievement problems. During the clinical interview, D. E. was clearly somewhat constricted and had difficulty expressing himself. He was aware of the problems he was presently experiencing at home and at school. It appeared clear that he was having some difficulty adjusting to the changes in himself and the reactions his behavior was now eliciting from others.

The accumulated data for D. E. reflected a child experiencing problems with arousal level and aggression secondary to head trauma. Objective assessment data further suggested that he possessed attentional skills that he was often unable to use effectively in his home or classroom. Although D. E.'s current presentation met the DSM-III-R diagnostic criteria for ADHD, a diagnosis of brain injury with associated arousal and attention problems appeared to better define D. E.'s current problems.

NAME _____ D.E. _____ D.O.B. _____ AGE 6 yr 7 mo DATE _____

HISTORY

Age of Onset _____ 5 _____
Average Independent Attention Span
  (Minutes) _____ 5 _____
Easily Overaroused ____ Yes ____
Impulsive ____ Yes ____
S'Not Effective ____ Yes ____
Other 1. Head trauma
2. Dramatic change
3. Normal previous development
4. Attention and arousal problems
5. Delayed achievement
6. Previously very aggressive

QUESTIONNAIRES

Parent Conners ____ Above 98th ____ %ile
Teacher Conners _____ %ile
ACTeRS: Attention ____ Below 5th ____ %ile
  Hyperactivity ____ Below 5th ____ %ile
  Social Skills ____ Below 5th ____ %ile
  Oppositional _____ 5th ____ %ile
Parent Achenbach: Scales Above 98th %ile
Social Withdrawal _____
Aggression _____
Hyperactivity _____
_____

Teacher Achenbach: Scales Above 98th %ile
Social Withdrawal _____
Inattentive _____
Nervous-Overactive _____
_____

Home Situations Problems:
  Number of Situations ____ 6 ____
  Average Severity ____ Moderate ____
School Situations Problems:
  Number of Situations ____ 6 ____
  Average Severity ____ Moderate ____
Parent Social Skills: Type of Problems

1. Isolated at times
2. Bossy, annoying
3. Can be aggressive
_____

Teacher Social Skills: Type of Problems
1. Shy
2. Can be aggressive if provoked
3. Doesn't contribute
_____

Observation During Assessment
1. Spoke in low volume
2. Impulsive style
3. Fidgeting
4. Somewhat distant
_____
_____

PERSONALITY OR EMOTIONAL FACTORS
1. Somewhat constricted
2. Aware of problems
3. No significant problems observed
_____
_____

WECHSLER

Verbal	S.S.	Performance	S.S.
Information	11	Picture Completion	14
Similarities	12	Picture Arrangement	7
Arithmetic	10	Block Design	11
Vocabulary	11	Object Assembly	9
Comprehension	10	Coding	10
Digit Span	8	Mazes	8
Verbal I.Q.	105	Performance I.Q.	101

Full Scale I.Q. ____ 102 ____

MOTOR SKILLS

Purdue Pegboard: Preferred Hand ____ 45th %ile
  Non-preferred hand ____ 50th %ile
  Both hands ____ 50th %ile
  Assembly ____ 40th %ile
Developmental Test of Visual Motor
  Integration _____ %ile
Bender Visual Motor Gestalt Test ____ 50th %ile
Benton Visual Retention Test _____ %ile
Detroit Test:
  Auditory Attention Span ____ 6 yr 3 mo
  Visual Attention Span ____ 7 yr 3 mo
  Notes on Performance _____
_____
_____

Matching Familiar Figures Test:
  Errors ____ 21st %ile
  Completion Time ____ 80th %ile
Peabody Picture Vocabulary Test ____ 37th %ile
Trail Making Test: Completion Time ____ %ile
  Errors ____ %ile
Progressive Figures Test ____ 40th %ile
Rapidly Recurring Target Figures:
  592: Completion Time ____ %ile
  Errors ____ %ile
  Diamond: Completion Time ____ 50th %ile
  Errors ____ 20th %ile
Motor Free Visual Perception Test ____ 70th %ile
Hand Preference ____ Left ____ X ____ Right

ACADEMICS

Test	Grade	%ile
Woodcock-Johnson:		
Reading		27th %ile
Arithmetic		83rd %ile
WRAT-Reading		12th %ile
Arithmetic		50th

OTHER TESTS OR QUESTIONNAIRES

Test	Score or %ile
Halstead Category Test	Average errors
Wepman Auditory Discrimination	
Test	Above average errors
Visual Aural Digit Span Test	10th %ile

ADHD Diagnostic Checklist Criteria

I	Yes	III	Marginal
II	Yes	IV	Yes

V Medical Factors

Figure 7.18 ADHD secondary to brain injury: The case of D. E.

THE WRITTEN REPORT

It is essential for the practitioner to organize, present and summarize all of the data collected in the process of evaluation. The depth and format of the written report is a matter of individual preference. The report should include a summary of the developmental history, analysis of parent and teacher questionnaires, presentation and interpretation of objective assessment data, a synthesis of the accumulated data in a diagnostic impression and finally, a list of recommendations. For some practitioners, this results in a report of two to three pages, while for others the report runs eight to ten pages. Although longer reports may not be read carefully by other practitioners, for those who do read them, the data presented often facilitates insight into the child's history and functioning and the process by which the practitioner drew diagnostic conclusions and made recommendations. Regardless of the length of the report, it is this document which the practitioner uses to explain and transmit his impressions to parents, teachers and other professionals. It is this document that will remain as a record of the evaluation and a standard against which to compare the child's future functioning.

Some practitioners provide lengthy treatment recommendations. Often these recommendations, because of their specificity, may be unwanted by other professionals or teachers. For example, classroom recommendations that do not fit within a particular teacher's style and classroom structure stand little chance of being implemented. It is recommended that the practitioner make general recommendations but communicate to parents and other professionals the willingness to provide specific assistance if that assistance is requested and if the practitioner is given an understanding of the system in which those recommendations will be implemented.

It is recommended that parents be provided with a copy of the evaluation report. Practitioners must be willing to share with parents the majority of information and impressions they relay to other professionals. Additionally, in some situations parents may wish to have certain information deleted from the evaluation report before granting permission for it to be released to schools or other community agencies. Given our increasingly litigious society, it is also recommended that the practitioner verbally communicate those clinical impressions that he or she does not wish to share with parents but believes are important to share with other professionals involved with the child. However, permission for verbal communication with other professionals must first be obtained from the parents.

EXPLAINING THE DATA TO PARENTS

Making the diagnosis is an important part of the evaluation. Helping parents understand the specific problems the child is experiencing and the implications of the diagnosis is an even more important part. Helping parents see the world through their child's eyes and understand the reasons and causes for the child's difficulties facilitates the process of beginning treatment. It allows the parents to play an active role and helps them make appropriate treatment decisions for their child.

The practitioner may find it helpful to explain the test data to parents by placing the child in specific situations and explaining how the child's weaknesses may then compromise his ability to function in, and meet the demands of, that setting. For descriptive purposes, the hypothetical example of Allen will be presented below. The example describes the impact Allen's disabilities are having upon his ability to function at school.

> The assessment data has revealed that Allen is extremely intelligent and was able to initially use his intelligence to compensate for his inattention and lack of persistence in kindergarten. He began having increasing problems in first and second grade. The assessment data we collected suggests that Allen has difficulty with vigilance, which means he has trouble waiting or being ready for the teacher to present important information. He also has trouble with selective attention and even after a task is presented he may have difficulty selecting this task as important and settling down to work. He also has problems with persistence and does not stick to tasks until they are completed. We have also discovered that he has difficulty effectively manipulating a pencil. Even when he pays attention and knows what to do and gets down to task it is harder for him to write his work on the paper neatly and efficiently. During a spelling test for example, even when he is paying attention to the teacher, knows what word is to be spelled, and how to spell the word, it takes him longer to get it written down on the paper. By that time the teacher may have gone to another word or Allen may become frustrated and not finish spelling the word correctly. He also appears somewhat impulsive and in a situation where choices must be made he tends to choose the path that is going to involve least effort and the choice that initially seems most attractive. He does not stop and use his intelligence to carefully consider each choice and make the best choice.
>
> Socially, Allen's inability to plan, difficulty compromising, and his inability to stop and think about the consequences that his behavior may have upon his peers has resulted in delayed development of social skills and over time, social isolation. A pattern of negative reinforcement has resulted in Allen not only having difficulty remaining on task due to his temperament but also being reinforced for beginning tasks but not for completing them. Given these attention and arousal level problems, it is not surprising that despite adequate intellect and ability to learn, Allen is experiencing significant difficulty fitting into the school setting.

Such a description not only helps parents understand the extent and nature of the child's problems but ties those problems to specific situations (i.e., social interaction or completing class work), which then allows the practitioner to describe specific interventions and components of a treatment plan.

SUMMARY

This chapter synthesized and integrated a model for collecting data and considering the important factors for making a diagnosis of ADHD. The practitioner is directed to use a multifaceted diagnostic procedure including the DSM-III-R criteria, data from behavioral and situational questionnaires and objective assessment. The practitioner must also consider emotional, developmental, cognitive and medical factors as alternative causes of attention and arousal-level problems. The ADHD Diagnostic Checklist is provided to summarize and facilitate the diagnostic process. This diagnostic process is recommended for a number of reasons, including the complexity of ADHD behavior problems, the occurrence of many of these behavioral problems as the result of other disorders of childhood and the likelihood that the use of a single type of data will result in a high number of false positive diagnoses. This chapter also presented case examples for the purpose of helping the practitioner understand the model used in making the diagnosis of ADHD and sensitizing the practitioner to the interaction of ADHD with other disorders of childhood.

PART 3

Intervention

It is critical for the process of evaluation and diagnosis to closely involve the child's parents at all steps. Educating parents to the impact and effect their child's attention and arousal problems are having helps parents understand the need for intervention and assists them in understanding specifically the need for multiple interventions. Educating parents about the nature of the disorder is the first step in the intervention process. The evaluation not only makes the diagnosis of ADHD but specifically defines skill deficits and specific areas of the child's life in which those deficits are having negative impact. An evaluative product of this sort facilitates the development of treatment intervention. Treatment can be designed to meet each child's specific needs.

ADHD is a disorder that is managed, not cured. Each of the child's specific problems, whether they are behavioral, cognitive or psychological, must be identified and treated. Some problems are treated effectively with medication; others with psychotherapy, behavior management or skill building. Parents and professionals must understand that with this disorder it is rare for an effective management or treatment plan to consist of only one intervention. The ADHD child, parents, siblings, teachers and other professionals must be active participants in the treatment program. It is essential that all involved develop sensitivity to the complex and pervasive impact attention and arousal–level problems have on a day–in and day–out basis in compromising the child's ability to meet the expectations of his world. These problems potentially have a negative impact psychologically, academically, interpersonally and vocationally on a long–term basis.

Chapter 8 provides an overview of the research literature investigating both single treatments and combinations of treatments with ADHD children. It is important for the practitioner to understand the research data and the research–based rationale for using a multitreatment intervention with ADHD children.

Chapters 9 through 13 review the research literature and provide practical suggestions for implementing the basic treatments for the problems ADHD children experience. Chapter 9 reviews medications and their use with this population of children. Chapter 10 presents cognitive-mediational interventions and reviews text and software materials that practitioners can use as part of the treatment process. Chapter 11 reviews the school–based research on ADHD and provides in–depth explanations for classroom interventions. Chapter 12 explains the myriad of social problems ADHD children experience, reviews commercially available social skills programs and provides definitions of basic social skills and ways to teach those skills to ADHD children. Finally, Chapter 13 provides a parenting model and specific recommendations to help parents deal with the ADHD child's behavior and the problems frequently encountered in the home.

CHAPTER 8

The Multidisciplinary/
Multitreatment Model

Providing a specific treatment for a specific symptom or skill deficit associated with ADHD may not reduce ADHD symptoms caused by different skill deficits. Common sense dictates that many problems and skill deficits the ADHD child experiences must be approached from a multidisciplinary/multitreatment perspective. This chapter will provide a brief overview concerning single treatments and combinations of treatments that have been reported with ADHD children. The chapter will also present an approach for parents that will help them understand the need for multiple treatments in response to the multiple problems ADHD children experience.

SINGLE TREATMENTS

Medication

Medication continues to be the most common method of treatment for ADHD children. Over ten years ago it was suggested that at least 500,000 children in the United States were being treated with stimulant medication for attention deficit (Sprague & Sleator, 1977). More recent studies have suggested that in some areas of the country the number of children receiving stimulant medication has increased at such a significant rate that currently even more children are receiving stimulant medication than ten years ago (Safer & Krager, 1983).

The continued and widespread use of medications, specifically stimulants, in the treatment of attention disorder is a result of both cost efficiency and a large volume of research demonstrating significant short-term positive effects (Ross & Ross, 1982). However, despite their effectiveness, medications have had their disadvantages. These include: reports of a lack of effectiveness in a small but significant percentage of inattentive children (Barkley, 1977; Rapport, DuPaul, Stoner & Jones, 1986); unwanted side effects including potentially irreversible problems with tics (Lowe, Cohen, Detlor, Kremenitzer & Shaywitz, 1982); anorexia, insomnia and irritability (Barkley, 1977); and a lack of consistent positive impact in improving academic performance, social behavior and emotional development (Ross & Ross, 1982). At this point, medications have not been found to contribute significantly to a positive outcome as this population grows into adulthood. The combination of the limitations of medication in solving the multiple problems of the ADHD child, medication-related side effects and a large volume of studies demonstrating the effectiveness of nonmedication treatments has lead to increasing interest in the clinical use of nonmedication treatments for this disorder. It must be noted that researchers and clinicians have been using other nonmedication treatments and combination treatments for this disorder during the past 20 years.

Parent Training

The second most widely used treatment for ADHD is parent training. It has long been recognized that increasing parental competence has a positive effect on children's behavior. The majority of parent training programs suggested for attention-deficient children are based upon learning theory principles (Patterson, 1974; Barkley, 1981a). Parents are taught techniques for manipulating the environment in an organized fashion to reduce the probability of noncompliant behavior and increase the probability of compliant behavior. In some studies, parent training programs have demonstrated short-term positive results (Graziano, 1983; Moreland, Schwebel, Beck & Wells, 1982) but have not been effective in precipitating long-term change in the management of the attention-disordered child (Phillips & Ray, 1980; Gittelman-Klein, Abikoff, Pollack, Klein, Katz & Mattes, 1980). Barkley (1981b) suggested that the ADHD child has a coercively more powerful effect on parents than vice versa.

It has been demonstrated that hyperactive children are more likely than learning-disabled or normal children to be noncompliant (Campbell, 1985). When observed in a playroom setting, mothers of hyperactive boys gave more commands, were less responsive, and responded more negatively than mothers of normal boys (Barkley & Cunningham, 1980). Although these studies may suggest that parental behavior causes child misbehavior, researchers have demonstrated, again in a playroom setting, that reducing children's attention, arousal and hyperactivity problems with stimulant medication has a significant effect in producing more normal parent-child interactions (Humphries, Kinsbourne & Swanson, 1978). Normalization of parental behavior was achieved specifically by the reduction of excessive negative child behaviors. As Barkley (1981a) points out, ". . . the child's behavior exerts a great deal of control over parental responses" (p. 60).

Conners and Wells (1986) noted that a decrease in negative parent behaviors as the result of a reduction in impulsive, inattentive and hyperactive child behaviors is not always accompanied by a corresponding increase in positive parent behaviors. Barkley and Cunningham (1979) and Cunningham and Barkley (1978b) consistently demonstrated that stimulant medication did not increase positive maternal social initiation or maternal reward for child compliance and free play. Pollard, Ward and Barkley (1983) also demonstrated that stimulant medication did not consistently increase the total amount of reward and social reinforcement provided by mothers during a structured task with their children. From an interactional perspective, this data makes sense. The medicated ADHD child's increased compliance may frequently result in the parent's perception of less need for negative, controlling behavior; however, parents of such children have frequently not had the opportunity to develop a repertoire of positive interactional skills. In such situations, the data suggests that parents' behavior becomes neither negative nor positive, but benign. This data argues for a combination of medication and parent training to improve basic communication and interactional style between parents and ADHD children.

Behavioral Techniques

Researchers have also attempted to develop learning and behavioral models that are directed at teaching the child to be his own change agent (Rapport 1988). These models, an outgrowth of the work of Luria (1961), have as their basic premise that the ADHD child lacks effective cognitive or mediational skills. These models attempt to teach such skills through a variety of techniques. For example, teaching the child to accurately monitor and record his behavior is an example of a cognitive technique. Although positive results have been noted in laboratory settings, the inattentive child has difficulty generalizing and using these strategies in the environment (Abikoff & Gittelman, 1985). This may result from either the child's impulsive, inattentive style or a history of behavioral contingencies in the environment that elicit and maintain the learned component of the ADHD child's maladaptive behavior (Abikoff, 1985; Abikoff & Gittelman, 1985).

Increasingly, attempts are being made to apply behavioral and cognitive techniques in the classroom (Coleman, 1988; Goldstein & Goldstein, 1987). Many of the techniques taught to parents have been adapted for use by classroom teachers. It is recognized that while stimulant medication can be very effective in the classroom, increasing teacher competence to understand, anticipate and manage the ADHD child's problems leads to more effective intervention.

MULTITREATMENT APPROACHES

Multitreatment approaches have included various combinations of specific interventions: (1) medication and behavioral management at home and school (Pelham, Schnedler, Miller, Ronnei, Paluchowski, Budrow, Marx, Nilsson & Bender, 1986; Gittelman-Klein et al., 1980; Wolraich, Drummond, Salomon, O'Brien, and Sivage (1978); (2) medication and self-control training (Horn, Chatoor & Conners, 1983); (3) parent management and self-control training (Horn, Ialongo, Popovich & Peradotto, 1987); and (4) medication, self-control training and teacher and parent behavioral management (Satterfield et al., 1981; Pelham, Schnedler, Bologna & Contreras, 1980). In reviewing 18 treatment studies, including a combination of medication, behavioral and social treatments, Horn and Ialongo (1988) found that medication enhanced the efficacy of the behavioral and social interventions in 12 studies. Investigators have not examined the effects on treatment outcome of educating parents concerning various aspects of attention disorder. It is our experience that the parent knowledgeable about the causes and ramifications of ADHD responds better to treatment interventions. Parents able to attribute the ADHD child's problems to incompetence as opposed to purposeful noncompliance are more motivated, less threatened and overall less angry in their dealings with the child. It has also been suggested by Horn and Ialongo (1988) that a combination of parent– and child–centered behavioral treatments has an additive effect in improving behavior, resulting in lower doses of stimulant medications being required.

In an excellent review of the status of multimodal treatment for attention disorders in children, Horn and Ialongo (1988) make a strong case that single-modality treatment is generally not effective in dealing with the wide range of problems experienced by ADHD children. These authors conclude that the failure of some researchers to find positive additive effects of stimulant medication and behavioral treatments (Abikoff & Gittelman, 1985; Brown, Borden, Wynne, Schleser & Clingerman, 1986) may result from the exclusion of either the parent or child therapeutic component. Based on our experience, it also appears that the child therapy component must include not only training in self-control and cognitive strategies but a counseling or therapeutic component that helps the child to understand the reasons for her difficulties, to accept a benign or nonblaming attribution for problems and to work through frustrations and negative feelings. Similarly, the parent training component must include education to help parents understand cause, reattribute problems benignly and incorporate positive behavioral techniques and strategies. Studies that have included medication and this combination of parent and child interventions have consistently reported statistically positive results from treatment (Horn et al., 1988; Satterfield et al., 1981).

Based on concerns that intensive six- to eight-week summer intervention programs for ADHD children do not afford sufficient opportunity for maintenance and generalization of effects after treatment, Swanson (1988) extended the program developed by Whalen, Henker, and Hinshaw (1985). The length of treatment was extended from eight weeks to one year and included planned generalization training on a daily basis in the classroom and on the playground. This multimodality program included direct intervention on a daily basis in the classroom, daily social skill and cognitive training sessions in small groups, interactions with parents approximately three to five hours per week, and a careful assessment in the use of medication with each child. Swanson notes that "as these interventions mature, they will require a long-term perspective follow-up of treated and untreated cases to document effectiveness" (p. 545).

Horn and Ialongo (1988) have also suggested that there may be a "sleeper effect" in which the combination of behavioral parent training and child therapy results in improvement that is not easily observed or measured until six to eight months after treatment. The authors also stated, based on parental reports, that the combination of these two interventions reduced the severity of ADHD problems in the home significantly. Problems at school, however, remained high. These authors have theorized about which type and situational manifestations of ADHD problems might best be addressed by a particular treatment. They suggested that problems with attention span appear to be dealt with most effectively through the use of stimulant medication; problems with impulse control, however, require medication intervention and behavioral training; academic achievement problems in ADHD children may require both of these components and educational intervention as well. These recommendations are logical when viewed from the perspective of the model presented in this text, which hypothesizes: (1) that difficulty with attention span is primarily a physiological modulation problem; (2) that difficulty with impulse control results from a combination of inattention and a lack of effective higher cerebral problem–solving skills; and (3) that inattention and impulsivity can create or compound difficulties with scholastic achievement resulting, over time, in a lack of basic academic foundations upon which to build further achievement.

It appears at this time that the multimodal treatment model offers a combination of interventions that provide promise of effective management for the wide range of problems ADHD children experience. It is clear that the combination of suggested treatments does not provide a cure; it is yet to be demonstrated that this combination of treatments will lead to significantly better outcome as individuals with ADHD move into adulthood. It has been our experience, however, that over the short term the suggested combination of treatments offers more thorough, effective intervention and the promise of greater therapeutic progress than the use of any one treatment alone.

IMPLICATIONS FOR PARENTS

The ADHD child's parents must be included in each step of the process of evaluation and diagnosis. The concept of a number of specific skill deficits causing varied and multiple problems in most if not all areas of the ADHD child's interaction with the environment facilitates parents' ability to understand the need for multiple interventions.

The following story may assist parents to understand the need for multiple treatments. It is the story of Tom, a second–grade child with a history of attention and overarousal problems. As Tom began second grade, he very much desired to succeed. His attention problems resulted in unfinished school work. Impulsivity had also interfered with the development of appropriate social interaction skills. The combination of these two problems led to Tom being identified as the family problem. In response to all of these difficulties, Tom began to develop a pattern of increasing helplessness, frustration and angry, oppositional behavior. Out of frustration, he impulsively picked up a rock and threw it at a car as an expression of anger. Assessment by the pediatrician, based on a simple medical model, resulted in a diagnosis of ADHD and initiation of stimulant medication as the treatment plan. Medication was effective in assisting Tom to sit still and remain on task, which resulted in schoolwork being attempted more consistently. Unfortunately, Tom was also experiencing some degree of learning disability, and the quality of his work did not increase significantly. His approach to his work continued to be disorganized because study skills must be learned rather than ingested. On the playground, Tom did not frustrate quite as easily but continued to lack effective social and problem-solving skills. Within the home, his siblings continued to identify him as the family problem even in situations where he was not at fault.

Medication had little impact on changing this pattern of family behavior. Finally, the stimulant medication allowed Tom to be somewhat more reflective and not act as impulsively. Instead of picking up the first rock he saw, he could now look around for a nice large one. He was also able to delay gratification and wait until a bus came by before throwing the rock.

The point of this story, as explained to parents, is that *pills will not substitute for skills*. Parents must be helped to understand and accept the premise that ADHD is a disorder that is managed, not cured.

SUMMARY

This chapter briefly reviewed the current state of single and multiple treatments for attention and hyperactivity disorders in childhood. Practitioners are increasingly aware that the multiproblem, multiskill deficits of ADHD children require a well-organized, multiple treatment plan. A plan must include treatments that have demonstrated success for specific ADHD problems such as parent education, medication, parent and teacher behavior management training, cognitive-mediational training, social skills training and academic support. Although questions have been raised concerning the additive benefits of multiple treatments, research has demonstrated that providing an appropriate combination of treatments as needed will result in improved functioning for the child over the short term.

The practitioner must assist parents to understand the need for multiple treatment modalities to deal with multi-faceted problems. The treatment section of this text provides the practitioner with a basic overview and specific recommendations concerning the treatments currently used with ADHD children.

CHAPTER 9

Medication Intervention

Medication intervention is a widely used treatment for ADHD. Safer and Krager (1988) reported that in 1987, 5.96% of public elementary students, 3.68% of public middle-school students and 0.4% of public senior high-school students in Baltimore County were taking medication for hyperactivity and inattention. The highest incidence occurred in the second and third grade. (See Figure 9.1.)

Discussions of medication intervention, however, rarely present clear guidelines to help determine which children should be placed on medication. Shaywitz and Shaywitz (1988) noted that of the myriad influences both biological and environmental that contribute to school failure, only ADHD can be ameliorated using treatment programs incorporating stimulant medication. While practitioners can be cautioned not to use medication in children who do not fit the ADHD diagnostic criteria (such as those with only learning disabilities), there is no consensus on the criteria to apply to decide which children should receive medication for ADHD symptoms.

This chapter will present principles that can be applied to help with the decision to use medication intervention for ADHD treatment of individual children. Benefits of medication intervention are presented and compared with risks of and alternatives to medication intervention.

In a wide range of medical situations, the decision to proceed with an intervention is based on comparison of the risks, benefits and intervention alternatives. The potential for a negative outcome resulting from treatment is compared with the natural course of the disease process. Different alternatives for intervention can be compared to see which has either decreased risk or increased benefit. The risks of treatment are also compared with the risk of no treatment. If the natural course of a disease process is likely to result in severe injury, a high risk is acceptable. But risk is acceptable only if the treatment is likely to work. The treatment of Attention-deficit can be considered along these lines. First the likelihood of side effects is considered, including the possibility of permanent injury. How likely are mild or severe side effects? Are they likely to be temporary or permanent? What can be accomplished by the medication intervention? How likely is a dramatic positive response? Finally, the alternatives must be understood. For ADHD symptoms, the alternatives include different medications as well as the alternative of not undertaking medication intervention at all. What will happen without medication intervention? Using this approach, the decision to undertake medication intervention in each individual will be based upon evaluation of the risks, benefits and alternatives.

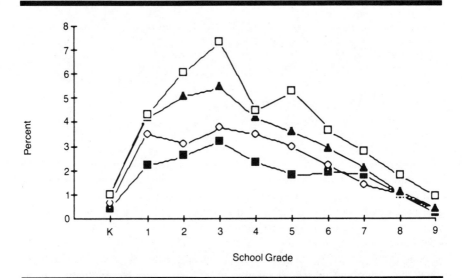

Percent of students receiving medication for hyperactivity by school grade. Special classes or special schools not included. Solid square indicates year 1981; open circle, 1983; solid triangle, 1985; and open square, 1987.

Figure 9.1 Percent of Students Receiving Medication for Hyperactivity. From D. J. Safer and J. M. Krager. Survey of Medication Treatment for Hyperactive/Inattentive Students. Copyright 1988 by the American Medical Association. Used by permission of the publishers.

METHYLPHENIDATE

Methylphenidate is by far the most common chemical substance used for medication intervention. Ritalin is the brand name of methylphenidate. Surveys of nurses in public and private schools in Baltimore County revealed that 93% of medication used to treat hyperactivity and inattention was methylphenidate (Safer & Krager, 1988). In addition, a survey mailed to 800 randomly selected members of the American Academy of Pediatrics revealed that 84% of the pediatricians responding used methylphenidate (Copeland, Wolraich, Lindgren, Milich & Woolson, 1987). Because of the prevalent use of methylphenidate, we will consider its risks and benefits as well as alternative interventions. Other medications will then be considered in comparison with methylphenidate.

Risks of Methylphenidate Intervention

Assessing the risks of methylphenidate is not always a simple task. Side effects are often presented in long lists that are difficult to apply to an individual patient. The *Physician's Desk Reference* (PDR, 1989) contains contraindications, warnings, precautions and adverse reactions for the Ritalin brand of methylphenidate (see Figure 9.2).

Contraindications
Marked anxiety, tension, and agitation are contraindications to Ritalin, since the drug may aggravate these symptoms. Ritalin is contraindicated also in patients known to be hypertensive to the drug, in patients with glaucoma, and in patients with motor tics or with a family history or diagnosis of Tourette's syndrome.

Warnings
Ritalin should not be used in children under six years, since safety and efficacy in this age group have not been established.

Sufficient data on safety and efficacy of long-term use of Ritalin in children are not yet available. Although a casual relationship has not been established, suppression of growth (i.e., weight gain, and/or height) has been reported with the long-term use of stimulants in children. Therefore, patients requiring long-term therapy should be carefully monitored. Ritalin should not be used for severe depression of either exogenous or endogenous origin. Clinical experience suggests that in psychotic children, administration of Ritalin may exacerbate symptoms of behavior disturbance and thought disorder.

Ritalin should not be used for the prevention or treatment of normal fatigue states.

There is some clinical evidence that Ritalin may lower the convulsive threshold in patients with prior history of seizures, with prior EEG abnormalities in absence of seizures, and, very rarely, in absence of history of seizures and no prior EEG evidence of seizures. Safe concomitant use of anticonvulsants and Ritalin has not been established. In the presence of seizures, the drug should be discontinued. Use cautiously in patients with hypertension. Blood pressure should be monitored at appropriate intervals in all patients. Symptoms of visual disturbances have been encountered in rare cases. Difficulties with accommodation and blurring of vision have been reported.

Drug Interactions
Ritalin may decrease the hypotensive effect of guanethidine. Use cautiously with pressor agents and MAO inhibitors.

Human pharmacologic studies have shown that Ritalin may inhibit the metabolism of coumarin anticoagulants, anticonvulsants (phenobarbital, diphenylhydantoin, primidone), phenylbutazone, and tricyclic antidepressants (imipramine, desipramine). Downward dosage adjustments of these drugs may be required when given concomitantly with Ritalin.

Usage in Pregnancy
Adequate animal reproduction studies to establish safe use of Ritalin during pregnancy have not been conducted. Therefore, until more information is available, Ritalin should not be prescribed for women of childbearing age unless, in the opinion of the physician, the potential benefits outweigh the possible risks.

Drug Dependence
Ritalin should be given cautiously to emotionally unstable patients, such as those with a history of drug dependence or alcoholism, because such patients may increase dosage on their own initiative.

Figure 9.2 Physician's Desk Reference/Ritalin. From *Physician's Desk Reference*, 1989, 856–857. Printed with permission of the publisher.

Chronically abusive use can lead to marked tolerance and psychic dependence with varying degrees of abnormal behavior. Frank psychotic episodes can occur, especially with parenteral abuse. Careful supervision is required during drug withdrawal, since severe depression as well as the effects of chronic overactivity can be unmasked. Long-term follow-up may be required because of the patient's basic personality disturbances.

Precautions
Patients with an element of agitation may react adversely, discontinue therapy if necessary. Periodic CBC, differential, and platelet counts are advised during prolonged therapy.

Drug treatment is not indicated in all cases of this behavioral syndrome and should be considered only in light of the complete history and evaluation of the child. The decision to prescribe Ritalin should depend on the physician's assessment of the chronicity and severity of the child's symptoms and their appropriateness for his/her age. Prescription should not depend solely on the presence of one or more of the behavioral characteristics.

When these symptoms are associated with acute stress reactions, treatment with Ritalin is usually not indicated. Long-term effects of Ritalin in children have not been well established.

Adverse Reactions
Nervousness and insomnia are the most common adverse reactions but are usually controlled by reducing dosage and omitting the drug in the afternoon or evening. Other reactions include hypersensitivity (including skin rash, urticaria, fever, arthralgia, exfoliative dermatitis, erythema, multiforme with histopathological findings of necrotizing vasculitis, and thrombocytopenic purpura); anorexia; nausea; dizziness; palpitations; headaches; dyskinesia; drowsiness; blood pressure and pulse changes, both up and down; tachycardia; angina; cardiac arrhythmia; abdominal pain; weight loss during prolonged therapy. There have been rare reports of Tourette's syndrome. Toxic psychosis has been reported. Although a definite causal relationship has not been established, the following have been reported in patients taking this drug: leukopenia and/or anemia; a few instances of scalp hair loss.

In children, loss of appetite, abdominal pain, weight loss during prolonged therapy, insomnia, and tachycardia may occur more frequently, however, any of the other adverse reactions listed above may also occur (PDR, 1989, 856-857).

Figure 9.2 (continued)

It is difficult to assess the risks to an individual patient from the list of reported side effects. An emphasis on side effects without a broader perspective was a concern discussed by Russell Barkley (1988a). He considers that there is "a national campaign against the labeling of children with a diagnosis of Attention-deficit Hyperactivity Disorder and especially its treatment with stimulant medication such as Ritalin" (p. 1). This is a conclusion that has also been drawn by other respected practitioners and researchers (Cowart, 1988a, 1988b). Barkley presented this campaign as a product of the Church of Scientology through its psychiatric "watch dog," the Committee Concerned for Human Rights (CCHR). According to Barkley, the CCHR put out a "set of exaggerated claims" (that) "these drugs are highly addictive, can often lead to suicide and permanent severe emotional disturbance as a common consequence, in some instances have led to murder by children treated with Ritalin, significantly increased the risk of criminal behavior and substance abuse among children so treated, and are prescribed excessively as a straight jacket for the mind creating a zombie-like state in order to subdue children" (p. 2).

Even well-meaning school programs, the purpose of which are to decrease illicit drug use, may emphasize the risks of methylphenidate and imply that the use of stimulant medications, even for medical treatment of ADHD, is "wrong" and will produce substantial injury. An 11-year-old related to the authors that a report presented in her classroom program to discourage wrong use of drugs stated that Ritalin was harmful. Children in the class who were taking such medication were asked by the teacher to identify themselves. These children became the subject of peer pressure to stop using medication. One child responded by refusing to take her medication, which resulted in recurrence of her ADHD symptoms. She continued to refuse medication despite deterioration in her academic performance and relationship with friends.

A physician may respond to the concern over drug abuse and lists of potential side effects by rejecting medication intervention for most, if not all, ADHD children. A physician may respond to false exaggeration of some medication-related problems by ignoring the potential side effects and advocating medication intervention on a "trial basis", for every child with a school, social or family problem, possibly telling the child and family that the medication "can't hurt and it might help." Blanket rejection of medication overlooks an effective treatment, and unselected medication intervention results in increased risk of potentially harmful side effects. Only with an understanding of the true risks of medication can medication intervention be appropriately evaluated.

Mild Side Effects

As a result of a review of 110 studies including more than 4200 hyperactive children, Barkley (1976) concluded that the primary side effects noted for the stimulants were insomnia, anorexia or loss of appetite, weight loss and irritability. These and other side effects were reported to be transitory and to disappear with a reduction in drug dosage. Ross and Ross (1982) agree that "the most frequent short-term side effects of the stimulants are anorexia and insomnia, both of which are usually of short duration" (p. 190). Other mild but less common side effects included sadness, depression, fearfulness, social withdrawal, sleepiness, headaches, nail biting, stomach upset and weight loss. These are reported to resolve spontaneously with decrease in dosage, or considered acceptable side effects in light of clinical improvement. These side effects are mild, but they occur in 20% to 50% of children treated with stimulant medication.

Side Effects of Placebo

Most reports of medication side effects focus on problems reported by children who are taking medication. Studies involving comparisons of medication and placebo reveal that children taking placebo also suffer significant numbers of problems. Barkley (1989) studied 82 ADHD children taking placebo and 2 doses of Ritalin (0.3 and 0.5 mg/kg, twice daily). He found that side effects, including irritability, sadness and excessive staring were essentially the same among the placebo group as the medication-related group. Barkley related that "many of the purported side effects are actually pre-existing behavioral or emotional problems in an ADHD population" (p. 2). It is important to understand that many of these symptoms may be reported by patients taking medication but not be the result of medication ingestion.

Toxic Psychosis

Barkley (1976) referenced seven reports of toxic psychosis associated with stimulant medications. Four were associated with methylphenidate and three with amphetamine. Psychotic episodes began after the administration of the stimulant with symptoms of visual and tactile hallucinations. Hallucinations subsided in each case once drug treatment had been discontinued. Bloom, Russell, Weisskopf and Blackerby (1988) reported a methylphenidate-induced delusional disorder in a child with Attention-deficit Hyperactivity Disorder and concluded that "it is strongly recommended that children undergoing stimulant therapy receive careful monitoring of their behavior and emotional status" (p. 89). These reports suggest that psychosis, though rare, can be induced by stimulant medications. While the symptoms resolved when the medication was discontinued, the risk of toxic psychosis must be considered when the determination is made whether to use medication intervention.

Seizures

The *PDR* suggests that the use of methylphenidate carries with it a risk of epileptic seizures. Adequate information is not available to allow accurate determination of the likelihood of seizures resulting from treatment of ADHD symptoms with commonly used dosages of medication or to assess what increased risk is present, if any, in children with a history of epilepsy, family history of epilepsy or abnormal EEG. It should be noted, however, that seizures were not a side effect noted in the review by Barkley (1976) of over 2000 reported cases of children with hyperkinetic symptoms treated with stimulant medications. It is difficult for the medical practitioner and family of the child with ADHD to be certain of the risk of seizures resulting from treatment with stimulant medication. However, the available information indicates that the risk of epileptic seizures resulting from medication intervention for ADHD must be quite low.

Tourette's Syndrome

Gilles de la Tourette's syndrome is a combination of recurrent, involuntary, repetitive, rapid, purposeless motor movements (tics). Multiple purposeless vocalizations (vocal tics) are also present (APA, 1980). Age at onset is between 2 and 15 years, and the tics must be present for more than one year before the diagnosis can be made (APA, 1980). The peak onset of the disorder is at age five, with the age at onset usually between ages four and nine (McDaniel, 1986). Severity of the disease is variable. Vocal outbursts and coprolalia characterize some of the more severe cases.

More than 50% of children with Tourette's syndrome manifest behaviors of inattention and hyperactivity (Golden, 1977; Shapiro, 1981). These symptoms may be more prominent than the other symptoms of Tourette's and/or may appear before the tics. As a result, many children with Tourette's have been treated with stimulant medications. Barkley (1976) commented on several children treated with dextroamphetamine and methylphenidate who developed "tics." Possibly the most extensive study of tics associated with methylphenidate is reported by Denckla, Bemporad and MacKay (1976). Of the 1520 children treated with methylphenidate studied, tics occurred in 20 cases, or 1.3%. Only 1 of the 20 developed Tourette's syndrome. Tics resolved completely when medication was withdrawn in the other 19. This data suggest, roughly, a 1% risk of the development of motor tics and .05% risk of the development of Tourette's syndrome with methylphenidate treatment for ADHD symptoms. Onset of Tourette's has also been associated with another stimulant, pemoline (Mitchell & Matthews, 1980; Bachman, 1981).

In an effort to understand the relationship of Tourette's to stimulant medication, Erenberg, Cruse, and Rothmer (1985) studied 200 children with Tourette's syndrome. Of the 200 children studied, 48 had received stimulant medication at some time. Nine had been treated with stimulants before the onset of the tics, but only 4 were still receiving stimulants when tics began. Therefore, only these 4 had their first symptoms of Tourette's occur while they were taking stimulant medications. Thirty-nine of the children had tics before their treatment with stimulant medication. Of these 39 children, 11 had worsening of tics on stimulant medication, 26 had no change in their tics when treated with stimulants, and 2 actually experienced improvement. While they found it difficult to be certain whether some patients develop Tourette's syndrome only and entirely as a result of stimulant medication, Erenberg et al. (1985) stated, "We believe that exposure to stimulants causes the premature onset of GTS in patients who would have developed their symptoms spontaneously at a later age" (p. 1347). They recommended that close observation and caution is also necessary when siblings of children with Tourette's syndrome are treated with stimulant medications. The authors also recommended that in patients who develop tics or whose prior tics worsen, medication should be discontinued.

The studies presented suggest that stimulant medication can bring out latent symptoms of Tourette's syndrome in children who might eventually develop these symptoms without stimulant medication. It is virtually impossible to prove that medication is never a primary cause of Tourette's. Therefore, it may be more prudent to summarize the available information by stating that stimulant medication is rarely, if ever, a primary cause of Tourette's syndrome.

Growth Suppression

The question of the effect of stimulant medication on height and weight was first raised by Safer, Allen and Barr (1972) and Safer and Allen (1973). They studied 49 children taking dextroamphetamine or methylphenidate and 14 children used as controls. The children were compared with standard growth percentiles as published by Vaughn (1969). The 29 children taking dextroamphetamine had an average loss of 20 percentile points in weight and 13 points in height over an average of 2.9 years. The 20 children on methylphenidate showed smaller losses of 6 percentile points in weight and 5 in height. The 14 hyperactive controls not on medication showed small percentile increases during the 4.2 years that the growth was followed. Dextroamphetamine produced a statistically significant weight percentile loss that was greater than any other group. They concluded that "the long-term use of dextroamphetamine depresses growth to a significantly greater degree than does methylphenidate" and that "the greater growth suppressant effect of dextroamphetamine lies clearly in favor of the use of methylphenidate for hyperactive children" (Safer & Allen, 1973, p. 666).

Safer et al. (1972) also suggested that discontinuation of medication over the summer might allow for increasd weight and height gain. Through the statistical procedure of analysis of variance, summer disuse of medication was evaluated. There was a significant increase in height without medication over the summer for the methylphenidate group but not for the dextroamphetamine group. Eliminating medication over the summer did not produce a significant weight gain for either group. The authors concluded that stimulants cause growth suppression and that this growth suppression can be ameliorated by drug holidays. The evidence, however, for this now popular belief was very limited. Only dextroamphetamine (not methylphenidate) was found to significantly decrease height and weight growth. In addition, the significant rebound growth with methylphenidate drug holiday over the summer was not replicated in a later study (Safer & Allen, 1973).

Belief that stimulants cause long-term growth suppression has been difficult to disprove. Gross (1976) reported the growth status of 100 children followed for 5.8 years versus the 3.0 years for Safer and Allen. Sixty were treated with methylphenidate, 24 were given dextroamphetamine and 16 were given antidepressants, either imipramine or desipramine. Dosage of daily medication (34 mg methylphenidate, 16.5 mg dextroamphetamine) was higher than that used by Safer and Allen. Decreased weight percentiles were seen with both methylphenidate and dextroamphetamine for the first three years. This was consistent with Safer and Allen's work. However, as the years progressed, the rate of weight gain increased so that at final follow-up after the seventh year there was an increase in weight percentile of 16% for dextroamphetamine and 11% for methylphenidate. Safer and Allen had followed their children only an average of three years. A significant increase in the weight percentile in children taking stimulants means that children treated with methylphenidate and dextroamphentamine were heavier than predicted by their weight prior to receiving medication.

The authors discussed several possible reasons why the children might have grown more than predicted, but whatever the reason, the important finding was no long-term suppression of height or weight. A child with Attention-deficit symptoms treated with methylphenidate or dextroamphetamine could expect, on the average, to be in a higher percentile for height and weight after an average of 5.8 years than he or she was prior to treatment. For the first three years, however, he or she would be at the same or a lower percentile. This data was not related to the duration or the dosage of treatment. It is also important to note that the dosages of medications used were in the "high" group by Safer and Allen's terminology and children were taking medication on a daily basis without weekend or vacation holidays. Attempts to understand the metabolic basis of these changes was reported by Shaywitz et al. (1982). They studied release of growth hormone as measured by blood levels and found that a low dose of methylphenidate increases the release of growth hormone at two hours after the ingestion of medication.

Other long-term studies of stimulant effect on growth have demonstrated similar results. No significant changes in growth were noted when McNutt, Ballard and Boileau (1976) studied 23 normal and 20 hyperactive children on daily doses of 0.67 mg/kg of methylphenidate for one year. Kalachnik, Sprague, Sleator, Cohen and Ullmann (1982) studied 26 hyperactive children. Dosages of methylphenidate up to 0.8 mg/kg per day were used, and predicted stature was measured at zero, one, two and three years of therapy. No significant differences were found for any dosage at any time during the study. The authors concluded, "This study indicates that stature suppression does not occur in male children below thirteen years of age when methylphenidate is used up to 0.8 mg/kg per day for one or two years and up to 0.6 mg/kg per day for three years" (p. 593).

The American Academy of Pediatrics Committee on Drugs Report (1987) summarized this information and reported, "There was fear that stimulant medications would lead to growth retardation; however, growth suppression is only minimally related to stimulant dosage. Results of a study indicate that no growth suppression occurred in doses of methylphenidate up to 0.8 mg/kg during a prolonged period" (p. 759).

Nevertheless, there appears to be a common misconception that stimulant medications can and regularly do cause growth suppression, and that discontinuation of medication over the summer will prevent the presumed growth suppression. Children treated with stimulant medications (especially dextroamphetamine) may have a transient decrease in weight and may have a period lasting two to three years of slight slowing of growth. This must be taken into consideration when deciding whether to undertake medication intervention. However, studies do not show a risk of long-term effect on height or weight. The decision to use stimulant medication intervention for ADHD symptoms should not be affected by the incorrect hypothesis that stimulant medication results in a long-term decrease in height or weight of the child.

Drug Abuse

There has been concern that medication intervention with a controlled substance such as methylphenidate could increase the likelihood of future drug abuse. Stimulant use as a recreational activity by some adolescents and young adults encourages this perception. Research has not provided a clear answer to this question. Arguing in favor of the risk of drug abuse are studies suggesting: (1) an increased likelihood that children may take more than their prescribed medication to "get high" (Goyer, Davis & Rapoport, 1979); (2) hyperactive adolescents, because of their histories of poor achievement and difficulty with social interaction, are at greater risk for drug abuse (Loney, 1980b); and (3) many hyperactive children and adolescents are rewarded for taking their medication (Whalen & Henker, 1980).

Arguing against increased risk for potential drug abuse are a number of studies, including one by Beck, Langford, MacKay and Sum (1975). These authors compared 30 adolescents previously medicated with 30 similar nonmedicated controls. No difference in drug abuse was found. Further, it has been suggested that the stigma associated with having to take a medication on a regular basis decreased the likelihood that this population of children would be willing to take or abuse other drugs (Collins, Whalen & Henker, 1980). Although the ADHD group of adolescents, because of their history of impulsive behavior and social failure, may be at greater risk to abuse drugs, there does not appear to be available data at this time to suggest that taking stimulant medication for medical reasons increases the likelihood of drug abuse (Gittelman, et al., 1985; Weiss & Hechtman, 1986).

Higher Risk Situations

Are there identifiable situations where a higher risk of side effects can be predicted? Younger children (under the age of six) and children with autism, psychosis, tics or a family history of these problems have been suggested to be more likely to encounter side effects. Some families have difficulty following through with instructions and nonmedication intervention. If children in these situations are more likely to encounter side effects, physicians should be more reluctant to undertake medication intervention.

AUTISTIC CHILDREN.   Autistic children may be at higher risk for adverse side effects. Cantwell and Baker (1987) suggested that some retarded and autistic children have symptoms similar to ADHD. "However, when treated with stimulant medication these children experience a further narrowing of an already fixed narrow attention span" (p. 170). This was disputed by Strayhorn, Rapp, Donina and Strain (1988), who presented a case of a six-year-old autistic boy and concluded that negative effects on mood and tantrums seemed to be outweighed by positive effects on attention and activity, destructive behavior and stereotyped movements. They concluded that this result failed to support past statements that stimulants are contraindicated with autistic children.

Improvement in autistic children was also reported by Birmaher, Quintana and Greenhill (1988). They studied methylphenidate in hyperactive autistic children, ages 4 to 16. Methylphenidate was used in doses ranging from 10 to 15 mg per day. Eight of the nine children showed significant improvement on all ratings scales. No major side effects or worsening of stereotyped movements were seen. These reports suggest that methylphenidate may be helpful in children with autism and ADHD. Studies on the effect of stimulants on children with autism and ADHD are limited, however. One cannot be certain of the frequency or severity of side effects, or of positive effects, in this group of children.

INTELLECTUALLY HANDICAPPED CHILDREN.   Intellectually handicapped children have been considered candidates for stimulant medication in an effort to improve both cognitive functioning and behavior. Early studies focusing on the effects of stimulants on cognitive functioning did not yield positive results (Cutler, Little & Strauss, 1940). More recent research has attempted to evaluate the effects of stimulant medication on a select population of intellectually handicapped individuals who also exhibit significant symptoms of attention deficit (Helsel, Hersen & Lubetsky, 1989). These authors report, however, an idiosyncratic response to dosage level and negative changes in social behavior resulting in increased social isolation. The authors suggest that this idiosyncratic response may reflect their difficulty in accurately differentiating attention-deficit from other deficit problems in intellectually handicapped individuals or may simply reflect the fact that stimulants are not as beneficial, even for specific target behaviors, for this population of individuals. Clearly, further research is needed.

YOUNGER CHILDREN.   Younger children are sometimes considered to have a higher incidence of side effects and a lower incidence of positive response to methylphenidate. Conners (1975b) and Schleifer et al. (1975) found the effectiveness of methylphenidate relative to placebo in attention-disordered preschool children was not as dramatic, consistent or positive as the results usually obtained with older children. Conners (1975b) did not report significant or serious side effects of the methylphenidate. This data, combined with the observation of some improvement in behavior, resulted in Conners suggesting that methylphenidate may be an effective treatment for preschoolers. Schleifer et al. (1975), however, observed more significant side effects, including irritability and solitary play, leading these authors to recommend that methylphenidate should not be considered an effective treatment for preschoolers.

A more recent study by Speltz, Varley, Peterson, and Beilke (1988) evaluated the effect of dextroamphetamine on a four-year-old and concluded that while there was improvement of tantrums and other behavioral measures, there was a tendency for increased social isolation. Even more careful supervision may be needed in this age group because of subtle changes that may occur, such as increase in solitary play. The use of stimulants in children under the age of six has not been well studied. One cannot state with certainty the likelihood of positive effects or negative side effects in this age group. Further studies are needed to produce additional information for this age group. Campbell (1985) cautions that the use of stimulants or other psychotropic medications with preschoolers should be considered in extreme cases with careful monitoring and close supportive work with the child's family.

OTHER SITUATIONS.   Many other situations suggest higher risk. History of psychosis or tics might alert the physician to the potential for medication side effects such as toxic psychosis, worsening of tics or exaggeration of Tourette's syndrome. Even the presence of tics or Tourette's syndrome in other family members might signal increased risk of these medication side effects and should be taken into consideration when determining whether medication intervention is appropriate.

Findings on examination can indicate higher risk situations. Cardiovascular side effects should be considered if the initial examination suggests hypertension or other cardiovascular abnormality. Follow-up examination, including cardiovascular evaluation, is generally recommended as part of the routine reevaluation process. A child with brain injury may be at higher risk but may also benefit from medication intervention. Kelly, Sonis, Fialkov, Kazdin and Matson (1986) present a six-year-old girl who experienced frontal-lobe damage. Her positive response to methylphenidate without side effects suggests that children with brain injury may be candidates for medication intervention without undue side effects. Further research is being conducted.

Management and Evaluation of Risks

Counseling the family concerning the short-term side effects, such as irritability, sleeplessness, anorexia and possible disturbance of weight and height gains, may minimize the disruptiveness of these usually mild symptoms and alert the medical practitioner to a situation where the child's individual reaction is beyond that normally expected. The family should be alerted to the possibility of a hypersensitivity reaction (rash, etc.) and the possibility of developing tics or psychosis so that these symptoms can be promptly reported to the medical practitioner and the medication probably discontinued.

Reevaluation is an important part of the medical program to identify and minimize the risk of medication intervention. Failure to obtain adequate follow-up evaluation can increase the risks of medication intervention. An assessment of the family's willingness and ability to participate in a follow-up evaluation program, therefore, is an important factor in determining the risk of medication intervention. If the child does not return for follow-up evaluation, side effects may continue and the child will be at increased risk for medication-related problems.

Although some practitioners may advocate medication as the initial treatment of choice for ADHD, behavioral or nonmedication intervention is an important part of the treatment of ADHD. These interventions may be sufficient for control of ADHD symptoms. Many children with ADHD symptoms will not need medication intervention if nonmedication intervention is used appropriately. The expected benefits of medication intervention cannot be adequately assessed until the effect of nonmedication intervention is known. For this reason, the assessment of expected benefits of medication usually cannot be completed until after a trial of nonmedication intervention.

An adequate evaluation, both to determine the presence or absence of ADHD and also to determine the presence or absence of other risk factors such as mental retardation, psychosis, autism and depression, will help to assess and control medication risks. The incidence of serious problems with stimulant medications is low. Even the child with an inadequate evaluation is not likely to develop a serious reaction to stimulant medication. Nevertheless, complete evaluation prior to initiation of medication intervention can decrease the likelihood of a high-risk child taking medication and, therefore, decrease the risk for the development of serious medication-related side effects. The increased risk of incomplete evaluation must be taken into consideration when deciding whether medication intervention is appropriate.

Medication may change a child's performance on tests, may change the child's appearance and behaviors during evaluation and may effect the parent's recollection of details. Once medication intervention has already begun, it is difficult to sort out medication effects from natural course. Double-blind studies show that improvement of symptoms may be unrelated to the actual effect of medication. At times, response to medication may be used as information assisting in the diagnosis, but the placebo response suggests that the response to medication alone cannot be used to diagnose or exclude attention deficit.

A sudden crisis may make deciding on medication intervention an emergency decision. As medication can be started quickly and has a rapid onset of action, the temptation may be present to begin medication intervention before completion of the diagnostic evaluation in hope of alleviating the crisis. It is exactly in those situations where a complete evaluation before medication intervention may be most important. After the crisis it may be more difficult to piece together everything needed for a complete diagnostic evaluation. As a crisis situation may involve symptoms of ADHD in combination with other problems, the additional difficulties are often obscured by the initial response to stimulant medication. Additional assessment and lost time may eventually result. A request by a family to start medication before the evaluation may be a sign that they are not willing to undertake the complete evaluation and follow through with nonmedication interventions. The family may want to "just give him something" to alleviate the problems. Treatment of attention deficit with a multidisciplinary approach includes nonmedication intervention. The families that are the most anxious to start medication before completion of the evaluation may benefit the most from postponing medication intervention until the entire evaluation is completed and the plans for nonmedication interventions have been established.

Benefits of Methylphenidate Intervention

The dramatic effect of stimulant medication on children with attention deficit was described by Conners and Wells (1986).

> Without doubt the single most striking phenomenon of hyperkinetic children is their response to stimulant drugs. The effect is both immediate and obvious. Often within the first hour after treatment a perceptible change in handwriting, talking, motility, attending, planfulness and perception may be observed. Classroom teachers may notice improvement in deportment and academic productivity after a single dose. Parents will frequently report a marked reduction in troublesome sibling interactions, inappropriate activity, and non-compliance. Even peers can identify the calmer, more organizing, cooperative behavior of stimulant treated children. (p. 97)

Stimulant medication for ADHD children has been demonstrated to lead to a dramatic reduction in negative behaviors with a concomitant increase in classroom on-task behaviors. This finding is supported by a study of ADHD children by Pelham, Bender, Caddell, Booth and Moorer (1985a). As the dosage of stimulant medication increased, on-task behavior increased and negative behaviors decreased. Pelham (1987) stated, "medicated children make fewer, impulsive responses to non-target stimuli, they maintain attention and miss fewer targets. These effects are most pronounced during the later portion of the task" (p. 101). Other effects include that children receiving stimulants are less likely "to (a) talk out inappropriately in class; (b) to bother peers who are working; (c) to violate classroom rules or engage in other behaviors that require teacher attention; and (d) to interact aggressively and otherwise inappropriately with peers" (p. 101).

By 1977, the progress of nearly 2000 children treated with stimulant medications for symptoms of hyperactivity had been studied. The review by Barkley (1977) presented data on 915 children treated with amphetamines and judged by 18 observers in 15 studies. On amphetamines 74% showed improvement; 26% did not improve or were worse. In a total of 14 studies, 77% of 866 methylphenidate-treated children improved. Two studies found a mean improvement rate of 73% in 105 children treated with premoline. In 8 studies, of 417 children given a placebo, 39% showed significant improvement. The overall average of these studies was 75% showing improvement with stimulant medications and 25% remaining unchanged or worse. Since 39% improved with placebo, Barkley concluded that future studies will have only limited value if they fail to employ a placebo condition.

It has been suggested that stimulant medication therapy alone may be the most effective form of therapy. Brown, Wynne and Medenis (1985), studied hyperactive boys using a three-month period of cognitive training, stimulant drug therapy (methylphenidate) or the two treatments combined. They concluded that, in their study, the combined medication and cognitive therapy condition was not any more effective than medication alone. This issue was discussed in depth in Chapter 8.

The most widely held opinion concerning medication, however, is reflected in a study by Hinshaw, Henker and Whalen (1984b). Based on a comparison study of methylphenidate, placebo and cognitive-behavioral intervention investigating social behavior, these authors concluded "that medication is not a sufficient treatment for hyperactivity and that alternatives or adjuncts are required" (p. 746). The American Academy of Pediatrics (1987) concurs with Hinshaw et al. (1984b) and states "Medication for children with attention deficit disorder should never be used as an isolated treatment. Proper classroom placement, physical education, programs for behavior modification, counseling, and provision of structure should be used before a trial of pharmacotherapy is attempted. This integrated approach should continue once the medication is begun" (p. 758).

Effect on Peer Relationships

The effect of medication is readily apparent to the child's peers. Whalen, Henker, Castro and Granger (1987) studied the reaction of normal fourth-and sixth-grade children to videotapes of students diagnosed as hyperactive. The children easily distinguished the medication responders on the basis of a broad range of behaviors. Observed differences between the medicated hyperactive boys and normal boys were rare. The authors described their results as systematic evidence that school-age youngsters detect the effects of methylphenidate in hyperactive peers.

Adult observers felt the changes occurring with medication represented improvement. Whalen et al. (1987) studied dose-related medication effects on social behaviors in a "natural context." The children, as a group, were judged to have improved their social interactions as a result of methylphenidate. The authors concluded that disruptive behaviors can be reduced successfully without decreasing overall sociability using methylphenidate. Additional social skills research will be reviewed in Chapter 12.

Effect on Family Relationships

Relationships between inattentive children and their families have been shown to improve with medication treatment. Schachar, Taylor, Wieselberg, Thorley and Rutter (1987) reported a study of family relationships in relation to methylphenidate. A group of 35 boys with ADD and other problems was treated with methylphenidate. In the eighteen boys found to be ritalin responders, interaction between the ADD child and his siblings and mother demonstrated increased maternal warmth, decreased maternal criticism, greater frequency of maternal contact, and fewer negative encounters with siblings. These positive changes were not observed in the non-methylphenidate responders. In contrast, no significant changes occurred in the frequency of paternal contact, parental ability to cope with a wide range of problems, or interparental consistency. The methylphenidate responders also did not appear to present an increased frequency of isolation within the family as previously reported by Barkley and Cunningham (1979). The finding of increased maternal warmth and contact, increased positive encounters with siblings and decreased maternal criticism in the families of children who responded positively to methylphenidate led the authors to conclude that "methylphenidate treatment of the hyperactive child may be a useful means of initiating improvement in a functional family system and that families of children who respond to methylphenidate might be more amenable to other types of intervention than before this treatment" (p. 731).

Similar improvement in interactions between inattentive children and their mothers was reported by Barkley, Karlsson, Strzelecki and Murphy (1984) and Barkley (1988b). In the first study, Barkley et. al. (1984) found that "mothers decrease their control and negative behavior towards children during high dose conditions" (p. 750), which resulted in improved mother-child interactions. The effect was not related to the age of the child. Conners and Wells (1986) reported, however, that in many instances decreased negative parenting behavior was not associated with an increase in positive parenting behaviors in a playroom setting. Barkley (1988) reported that 27 preschool ADHD children "decreased their off task and non-compliant behavior and significantly increased their rates of compliance as well as the length of sustained compliance with maternal commands" while taking methylphenidate (p. 336). These studies suggest that medication intervention consistantly decreases negative parent behaviors and in some settings may lead to an increase in positive parent behaviors.

Effect on Self-Esteem

Intervention that includes medication has been shown to increase self-esteem for preadolescents with attention deficit. Kelly, Cohen, Walker, Caskey and Atkinson (1989) studied 21 children, age 8 to 12, diagnosed ADD by DSM-III criteria. Multimodal management, including 5 to 10 mg of methylphenidate, was used twice daily for treatment. Improved general as well as academic self-esteem, as measured by the Culture Free Self-Esteem Inventory for Children, was seen for the 12 children followed in the long-term (average 16 months) follow-up group. No significant improvement in self-esteem was seen after only one month, however. The authors conclude that long-term multimodal management that includes methylphenidate does appear to improve self-esteem in ADD children.

Effect on Academic Achievement

Attempts to demonstrate effects of medication intervention on learning have had difficulty separating improved performance secondary to improved attention and concentration from primary effect. There is general agreement that classroom behavior is improved by stimulant medication. For example, Wallander, Schroeder, Michelli and Gualitieri (1987) in a double–blind placebo controlled trial with methylphenidate found that there were improvements in medicated children's oppositional, off-task and on-task behavior consistent with previous studies. At the most effective dose (0.6 mg/kg) Pelham, Bender, Caddell, Booth and Moorer (1985b) found a lesser effect on reading comprehension than on arithmetic. A previous study by Gittelman, Klein, and Feingold (1983) using similar dosage schedules showed improvement on some measures of reading without improvement on others. After reviewing over 200 reports on methylphenidate, Murray (1987) concluded, among other observations, that "the attention and concentration of ADHD children seems to benefit from treatment with methylphenidate, but except for contribution of improved attentional control, school work appears to not be facilitated by the drug" (p. 325).

Some authors argue that methylphenidate is effective at improving reading ability. Increased output, accuracy and efficiency and improved learning acquisition were reported by Douglas, Barr, O'Neil and Britton (1986) for ADHD children treated with 0.3 mg/kg methylphenidate. The authors described evidence of increased effort and self-correcting behavior and concluded that previous studies may have underestimated the potential of stimulants to improve the performance of ADHD children in academic learning and cognitive tasks.

Methylphenidate was found effective for inattentive reading-disabled children by Richardson, Kupietz, Winsberg, Maitinsky and Mendell (1988) and Kupietz, Winsberg, Richardson, Maitinsky and Mendell (1988). Various dosages were studied, but the major conclusion was that methylphenidate had a positive effect on reading, which the authors believe was mediated through both the behavioral control and also through a direct effect on learning ability. They concluded that: "(1) successful methylphenidate treatment of behavioral symptoms of ADHD is associated with improvement in academic learning; (2) this effect is primarily mediated by the behavioral change itself and is likely to be strongest in the early phases of treatment; and (3) methylphenidate has a direct positive effect on retrieval mechanisms involved in word recognition but more research is required to understand fully the extent and nature of this effect" (p. 86). Years earlier, Conners (1972) reported that methylphenidate, dextroamphetamine and pemoline treatment produced substantial improvements on a number of academic measures as well as behavioral improvement.

One of the factors contributing to the controversy about the effect of stimulant medication on learning ability is medication dose. Is the best dose for academic improvement different from the best dose for behavior? Sprague and Sleator (1977) reported that maximal effect on learning occurred at methylphenidate doses of 0.3 mg/kg, whereas maximal effects on behavior occurred at higher dosages up to 1 mg/kg. However, other studies have found that the best dose for behavior is the same as the best dose for learning.

Ullmann and Sleator (1985) studied 86 children diagnosed as ADD and ADHD (diagnostic criteria not described). Using a teacher questionnaire they had previously developed, attention, hyperactivity, social skills and oppositional behavior were evaluated on baseline, placebo and 0.3, 0.5 and 0.8 mg/kg of methylphenidate. A linear progression of improvements in all areas was seen with increasing doses of medication. However, the improvement in attention and hyper-activity was substantially greater than for social skills and oppositional behavior, leading the authors to conclude that methylphenidate has a major effect in improv-ing attention, that it is helpful in decreasing activity level, but that it often has only a minor effect on deficient social skills and oppositional (aggressive) behavior.

Elementary school age children with histories of academic achievement prob-lems treated with medication alone demonstrated marked improvements in Scholas-tic Achievement Test math and reading scores (Abikoff, Ganeles, Reiter, Blum, Foley & Klein, 1988). Based on this study the authors suggested that controlled investigations of the long-term efficacy of stimulant treatment on achievement should seriously be considered. Results of this study further suggested that cogni-tive training and academic tutoring may improve aspects of academic achievement that are not facilitated by stimulant medication treatment alone.

The effect of methylphenidate on reading grade level in ADHD children was studied by Winsberg, Maitinsky, Richardson and Kupietz (1988). They evaluated 42 children diagnosed by DSM-III criteria as displaying ADHD and a developmen-tal reading disorder with behavioral ratings from parents and teachers and achieve-ment test scores. Using methylphenidate doses from 0.3 to 0.7 mg/kg, a positive correlation between improved reading grade level and rating–scale improvement of ADHD symptoms was noted. Richardson, Kupietz and Maitinsky (1987) reported similar findings that the effective treatment of inattentive and hyperactive symp-toms appeared to produce dramatic improvement in reading ability. Children who demonstrated better behavioral response to Ritalin also demonstrated greater gains in reading grade level (see Figure 9.3). Since the reading grade level did not improve without improvement in rating scales of ADHD symptoms, Winsberg et al. (1988) concluded that physicians "can expect that when ADHD symptoms are effec-tively controlled, a positive response to reading instruction will follow. However, the latter qualification to this assertion is important. Unless children with learning

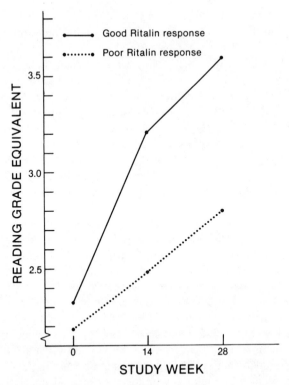

Figure 9.3 Reading grade scores of good and poor Ritalin responders. From E. Richardson, S. Kupietz and S. Maitinsky. What is the role of Academic Intervention in the Treatment of Hyperactive Children with Reading Disorders? In J. Loney (Ed.) *The Young Hyperactive Child: Answers to Questions about Diagnosis, Prognosis and Treatment.* Copyright 1987 by Haworth Press. Printed with permission from the publisher.

difficulties are provided with effective remedial instruction, methylphenidate is not likely to have either a positive or negative effect on achievement" (p. 241). These authors also discussed the finding of Sprague and Sleator (1977) that increasing dosage to 1 mg/kg resulted in decreased performance and mentioned several studies where individual doses as high as 0.8 mg/kg did not produce a decrease in learning performance. They also commented that their dose of 0.7 mg/kg was not quite as high as the Sprague & Sleator dose.

   Measures of reading and math ability improve in some children with adminis-tration of methylphenidate. There is disagreement whether this represents a direct effect of methylphenidate on reading and math ability or reflects improved con-centration and attention. With a few exceptions, the best dose for reading and math has been found to be the same as the best dose for behavior. Children are much less likely to experience a dramatic improvement in academic skills than in behavior. Nevertheless, there is ample experimental evidence to conclude that many ADHD children will improve their reading ability directly or indirectly as a result of stimulant medication treatment.

Medication Effect and Dosage Time Course of Medication Activity

The effect of medication varies with time after ingestion. Initially after medication is ingested, there will be a time where it is partly effective. It will then have a time of full effectiveness. Following the period of full effectiveness there is a period when the medication still has some effect but is decreasing in its effectiveness. At a later time, the medication will have ceased to become effective, and observed changes in behavior will not be related to the effect of medication but to the effect of the medication's dissipation or "wearing off." Finally, a return to baseline function will be seen. Observers of behavior must note the amount of time after medication ingestion so that an observed effect can be related to the time course. Medication given before a child goes to school may have its effect during the school hours. When a parent sees the child at home after school, rebound from medication rather than medication effect may be present, and the parent's observations that the child was either improved or worsened while taking medication may reflect the response of the child during the withdrawal period rather than to the medication response period.

Swanson, Kinsbourne, Roberts and Zucker (1978) determined that the "behavioral half-life" (the time taken for a 50% decline from maximum effect) of methylphenidate was four hours and its maximum effect was reached in two hours by studying 48 patients' ability to learn eight successive word lists. The dosage of methylphenidate ranged from 5 to 20 mg with an average of 12 mg. The behavioral half-life was independent of the dosage. The authors found that increasing the maximum effective dose resulted in decreased learning performance that followed the same time course as the positive performance rather than simply extending the time of positive medication effect. It is important to understand that medication effect varies with time from ingestion. The relationship between time and effect must be understood in order to manage medication effectively.

Optimal Dosage

Attempts to find the best dose of stimulant medication have looked at positive effects, such as improved learning and behavior, as well as side effects such as sleeplessness and irritability. Rapport, Stoner, DuPaul, Kelly, Tucker and Schoeler (1988) reported a dose-response relationship with methylphenidate in 20 ADHD children. These children were selected from a group meeting multiple criteria, including: (1) pediatrician and psychologist diagnosis using DSM–III criteria; (2) maternal history showing problems in at least 50% of home situations; (3) maternal rating of two standard deviations above the norm for age on the Weery-Weiss-Peters Activity Scale; (4) teacher rating on the Abbreviated Connors Teacher Rating Scale above 15; and (5) absence of any gross neurological sensory or motor impairment. Assessment for medication response included the Teacher's Self-Control Rating Scale (Humphrey, 1982), measures of on-task behavior and the Matching Familiar Figures Test. Placebo versus 5, 10, 15, and 20 mg dosage of methylphenidate was used. A linear relationship between dose and effect was uncovered, with increasing dose associated with improved effect. This is especially true between the 5-and 10-mg doses, with a significant improvement between 10 and 15 mg noted on the Teacher's Self-Control Rating Scale. Significant differences in the Matching Familiar Figures Test, however, were seen only between placebo and 15 mg or 20 mg. The 20-mg dose was significantly better than the 5-mg dose for all measures, and the 20-mg dose was significantly better than the 10-mg dose based on results from the Teacher's Self-Control Rating Scale. (See Figure 9.4.)

Rapport et al. (1988) argued in favor of a mg-per-dose schedule because this schedule reflects typical pediatric practice in the United States. They suggested, based on review of previous studies, that children's response to methylphenidate dosage manipulation has been shown to be independent of total body weight. They also noted that even at the highest dose of 20 mg (0.39 to 1.10 mg/kg) no significant deterioration in behavior was observed. The Teacher's Self-Control Rating Scale showed significant improvement when the 10-mg dose was increased to 15 or 20 mg. This careful work with a relatively small group of children strongly suggests that 15 to 20 mg of methylphenidate will improve some aspects of learning as well as behavior.

Dosage effect of methylphenidate on 29 children with attention deficit based on DSM-III criteria was studied by using a placebo controlled double-blind study of 0.15 mg/kg, 0.3 mg/kg and 0.6 mg/kg in a single dosage (Pelham, et al., 1985). Measures of academic performance including reading, arithmetic and spelling tasks were improved by methylphenidate. A dose of 0.6 mg/kg was more effective, especially on arithmetic tasks, than 0.3 mg/kg. No deterioration of behavior was discerned on the 0.6 mg/kg dose versus the others.

Some studies of maternal-child interaction (Barkley et at., 1984; Barkley, 1988b) suggested that a higher dosage of methylphenidate is more effective. The earlier study compared high-dose to low-dose therapy and concluded that mothers decrease their control and negative behavior towards the children during the high-dose conditions. This effect was not related to age. The higher dose also helped 27 preschool children with attention deficit hyperactivity "decrease their off task and non-compliant behavior and significantly increase their rates of compliance as well as the length of sustained compliance with maternal commands" (Barkley, 1988, p. 336).

A report by Sprague and Sleator (1977) sparked a controversy that still persists. They suggested that a higher dose of methylphenidate was more effective at controlling behavior but that a lower dose was more effective at improving learning skills. They reported an improvement in arithmetic scores with methylphenidate on a 0.3 mg/kg dose, but there was less improvement on a 0.6 mg/kg dose. The difference was not statistically significant, but the authors suggested that an even higher dose might have shown a significant decline in arithmetic skills. Even in their study, however, reading comprehension improved only with the 0.6 mg/kg dose and not with the 0.3 mg/kg dose. Other investigators have found that within a range of 0.3 to 0.8 mg/kg, performance on both behavioral and cognitive tasks improves in a dose-related fashion (Charles, Schain & Zelniker, 1981; Rapoport, Stoner, DuPaul, Birmingham and Tucker, 1985; Sebrechts, Shaywitz, Shaywitz, Jatlow, Anderson and Cohen 1986).

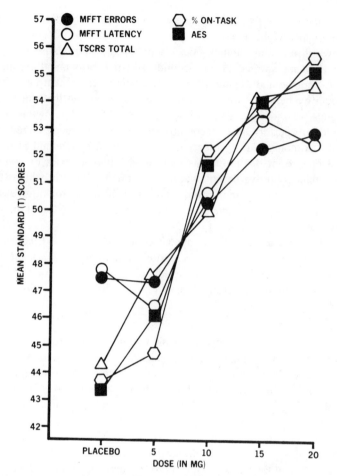

Figure 9.4 The effect of methyphenidate dose on five performance and behavior variables. From M. D. Rapport, G. Stoner, G. DuPaul, K. L. Kelly, S. B. Tucker and T. Schoeler. Attention Deficit Disorder and Methylphenidate: A Multilevel Analysis of Dose-Response Effects on Children's Impulsivity Across Settings. Copyright 1988 by the *American Academy of Child and Adolescent Psychiatry*. Printed with permission of the publisher.

Other studies have suggested a linear improvement in learning with dosage increases to 0.8 mg/kg. Pelham et al. (1985a) partly disagreed with the earlier study of Sprague and Sleator (1977). They felt that the 0.6 mg/kg dose was better for many cognitive functions and further expressed the opinion that their results suggested some beneficial effect of methylphenidate at doses as low as 0.15 mg/kg and as high as 0.6 mg/kg.

Effect of methylphenidate on disruptive behavior is seen to improve with medication dosage from 0.15 to 0.6 mg/kg (Cantwell and Carlson, 1978; Conners and Werry, 1979). Other researchers have found similar patterns (Winsberg, Kupietz, Sverd, Hungdung and Young, 1982). However, Pelham et al. (1985a) pointed out that 67% of the drug effect on negative behavior was accounted for by the 0.15 mg/kg dose of methylphenidate.

A review of previous studies concerning dosage and learning effects was reported by Pelham, Sturges, Hoza, Schmidt, Bijlsma, Milich and Moorer (1987). Referring to Sprague and Sleator's (1977) study, they related that laboratory measures of cognitive behavior were improved on 0.3 mg/kg but that improvement in teacher ratings was not apparent until the dose was 1.0 mg/kg. At this medication dosage, children's performance on cognitive tests was impaired relative to placebo. They stated, "Although most professionals agree with Sprague and Sleator's conclusion that classroom disruptiveness may require higher doses of stimulants to be corrected than cognitive deficits require, the precise point at which stimulants have adverse effects on cognition is not yet determined. Numerous studies that have administered the methylphenidate doses up to 0.75 mg/kg have found improvement on cognitive tasks" (pp. 102-103).

The results of these studies may appear contradictory and difficult to transfer to clinical practice. Taken in total, these studies demonstrate the need to closely monitor a number of variables, including schoolwork, socialization and behavioral compliance, as methylphenidate is titrated.

Medication and Age

Age also is a variable that affects medication response. The relationship between dose and response may change substantially at different ages. Whalen et al. (1987) found that the optimal dose for younger children was higher than for older children. They measured placebo against 0.3 mg/kg and 0.6mg/kg dosages of methylphenidate in effect on observed playground behavior during a seven-week summer program for 40 hyperactive children. Diagnosis was by referral, clinical evaluation by the project director and Connors Questionnaire. The authors studied dose-related medication effects on social behaviors in this "natural" context. The children, as a group, improved their social interactions as a result of methylphenidate. In younger children (age seven to eight), the higher dose was more effective than the lower dose. Other studies have not found age-related medication effect (Barkley, et al., 1984; Barkley, 1988b). With additional research, we may better understand the variation of medication benefits in relation to age.

Effect of Medication and Blood Levels

Blood-level evaluation of medications such as anticonvulsants, antidepressants, antibiotics and others have proven useful in adjusting these medications. Studies of methylphenidate, however, have not shown that plasma levels of this medication are likely to become part of the standard of treatment of ADHD. Winsberg, Maitinsky, Kupietz and Richardson (1987) studied oral dose in relation to plasma levels of methylphenidate and compared dose and blood level to behavioral response. They discovered that there is both a correlation between blood levels and response and a correlation between oral dose and blood levels. One can conclude from this data that titration of oral dose is equivalent to titration by blood levels. This would imply that changes in oral dose will result in proportional changes in blood level and that differences in dosage requirement reflect differences in blood-level requirement for optimal effect. Gualtieri, Hicks, Patrick, Schroeder and Breese (1984) did not find a relationship between serum levels of methylphenidate and either side effects (see Figure 9.5) or clinical response (Figure 9.6). Blood studies do not give additional assistance over clinical evaluation in maximizing benefits or decreasing risks of stimulant medication.

Long-Term Effects of Methylphenidate

Despite the dramatic short-term effects of methylphenidate treatment on symptoms of ADHD, it has been surprisingly difficult to demonstrate long-term effects. Riddle and Rapoport (1976) reported on a group of 72 hyperactive boys who had been followed for two years. They were able to follow 94% of an initial sample. Conners Questionnaires, among other measures, were used. The patient group continued to have academic difficulties, low peer status and depressive symptoms in comparison with a control group. A group consisting of 86% of the responders who were judged to be optimally medicated were compared with a group of dropouts from drug treatment. The authors concluded that the dropouts had almost identical academic achievement and social acceptance to that of the optimally medicated group. This report suggests limited effectiveness of medication intervention on long-term outcome.

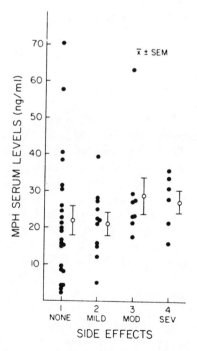

Figure 9.5 Methylphenidate serum levels and side effects. From Gualtieri et al, (1984). Printed with permission of the authors.

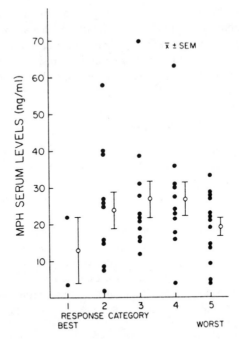

Figure 9.6 Methylphenidate serum levels and clinical response. From Gualtieri et al. (1984). Printed with permission of the authors.

A group of 20 children treated for hyperactivity for three years or longer were subjects of a ten-year follow-up study by Hechtman, Weiss and Perlman (1984). At an average age of 21.8 years, these patients were compared both with hyperactives who had not been treated by Ritalin®and with a control group of nonhyperactives. The treated hyperactives did not do as well as matched controls in areas such as schoolwork and personality disorders, but had fewer car accidents, a more positive view of childhood, less delinquency and better social skills and self-esteem than untreated hyperactives. They concluded that stimulant treatment for hyperactive children may not eliminate educational or personality difficulties but may result in less social ostracism and more positive feelings towards themselves and others.

Other studies have not shown much more positive effect on long-term outlook. Weiss, Kurger, Danielson and Elman (1975) presented a five-year follow-up of methylphenidate and no-treatment groups. They found that methylphenidate was helpful in making hyperactive children more manageable at home and at school but did not significantly affect the outcome after five years of treatment. Cantwell and Baker (1987) suggested that those in a multidisciplinary treatment program for three years or longer did show some long-term benefits of intervention.

When evaluating the benefits of medication intervention, one must accept that there is little evidence to support expectation of long-term benefits as the reason to undertake medication intervention. While medication intervention has many dramatic positive effects, it has been difficult to demonstrate long-term improvement as one of them.

MEDICATION INTERVENTION OTHER THAN METHYLPHENIDATE

Medication intervention was surveyed in the Baltimore School District on a biannual basis and reported by Safer and Krager (1983; 1988). In 1971, methylphenidate was used for medication intervention in approximately 40% of the patients, dextroamphetamine was used for 36%, pemoline in from 1% to 6% and nonstimulants (e.g., thioridazine and diphenhydromine) in approximately 24%. In 1987, the medications used for these very same problems had changed dramatically. Of the children receiving medications for hyperactivity approximately 91% were receiving methylphenidate. Only 4% were receiving dextroamphetamine and only 2% nonstimulant medications. Pemoline continued to be used in 1% to 6%. These alternate medications will be briefly presented, and suggestions will be made for their use.

Amphetamine

Bradley is often credited with the first report of the effect of a stimulant medication on inattentive and hyperactive symptoms as part of a study of the amphetamine Benzedrine® (Bradley, 1937). In 1950, Bradley was one of the first to compare the effect of different medications. He compared two chemically related amphetamines and decided there was no substantial difference between the two medications.

The relationship of attention-deficit symptoms and plasma levels of d-amphetamine was reported by Brown, Hunt, Ebert, Bunney and Kopin (1979). A single dose of dextroamphetamine of 0.45 mg/kg was administered. The plasma half-life was 6.8 hours, but the maximum effect occurred in one to two hours, which was the time of absorption of the dextroamphetamine. The authors speculated that this is the time of catecholamine release by medication. The time of most significant difference between placebo and amphetamine was at two hours after administration. The time of highest plasma level of d-amphetamine was at four hours. At five to six hours, no significant differences between placebo and amphetamine could be determined, but the blood level was still more than three-quarters of the maximal level. One can see from these results, as presented in Figures 9.7 and 9.8, that the clinical effect of dextroamphetamine follows a different time course from the plasma blood level. Blood levels, therefore, cannot be used to measure clinical effect of dextroamphetamine.

Measurements in the plasma concentration of the noradrenalin metabolite MHPG following methylphenidate and amphetamine suggest some difference in the mechanism of action of these two medications. Shaywitz, Shaywitz, Anderson, Jatlow, Gillespie, Sullivan, Riddle, Leckman and Cohen (1988) reported results

AMPHETAMINE BLOOD LEVELS AND MOTOR ACTIVITY

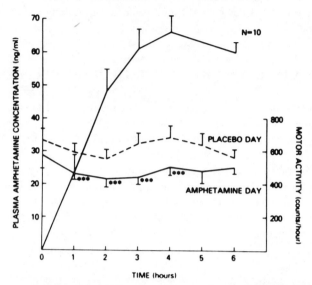

Hyperactive children ($n = 10$) were given a single oral mean ($\pm$ SEM) dose of 0.43 ± 0.02 mg kg d-amphetamine. The resulting mean ($\pm$ SEM) plasma levels are shown. Differences between motor activity as determined by a newly developed ambulatory motor monitor after placebo and after d-amphetamine were analyzed by one-tailed paired t-tests (••• $P < 0.005$)

Figure 9.7 Amphetamine blood levels and motor activity. From G. L. Brown, R. D. Hunt, M. H. Ebert, W. E. Bunney & I. J. Kopin, Plasma Levels of d-Amphetamine in Hyperactive Children. Copyright 1979 by *Psychopharmacology*. Printed with permission of the publisher.

of a study of 26 children with ADHD. They were treated daily for eight days with either 0.25 mg/kg of dextroamphetamine, 0.5 mg/kg methylphenidate or placebo. Significant differences in MHPG were noted with amphetamine treatment over four, five and six hours as compared with placebo and methylphenidate. Methylphenidate did not have the same effect on plasma MHPG concentration as amphetamine. Despite the possibility that changes in peripheral metabolism unrelated to brain metabolism could also affect plasma MHPG, the authors concluded that amphetamine and methylphenidate differ in their effects on brain catecholaminergic systems. They believed that amphetamine influences brain noradrenergic mechanisms, perhaps by reducing turnover of brain norepinepherine.

Dextroamphetamine is the only stimulant approved for children between the ages of three and six. The *Physician's Desk Reference* (1989), page 2047, describes Dexedrine®brand of dextroamphetamine as "not recommended" for children "under three years of age." The warning issued for methylphenidate, pemoline and even Desoxyn®(methamphetamine chemically similar to dextroamphetamine) suggests

AMPHETAMINE BLOOD LEVELS AND MOTOR ACTIVITY

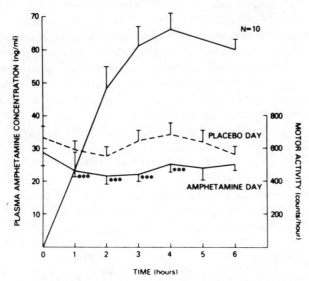

Hyperactive children ($n = 10$) were given a single oral mean ($\pm$ SEM) dose of 0.43 $\pm$ 0.02 mg kg d-amphetamine. The resulting mean ($\pm$ SEM) plasma levels are shown. Differences between motor activity as determined by a newly developed ambulatory motor monitor after placebo and after d-amphetamine were analyzed by one-tailed paired t-tests (*** $P < 0.005$)

Figure 9.8 Amphetamine blood levels and behavior. From Brown et al., Plasma Levels of d-Amphetamine in Hyperactive Children. Copyright 1979 by *Psychopharmacology*. Printed with permission of the publisher.

these medications should not be used for children younger than six years of age. A dosage schedule for dextroamphetamine is listed for children from three to five years of age but suggests the medication should not be used for children under three years of age. A starting daily dose of 2.5 mg (tablets or elixir) is suggested, with 1.5 mg increments weekly until optimal response is obtained.

Dextroamphetamine optimal dosage is often 5 to 10 mg per dose, almost one-half that of methylphenidate. Dextroamphetamine is available in tablets of 5 mg, spansules of 5, 10 and 15 mg and elixir with a concentration of 5 mg per 5 ml. While the *PDR* (1989) relates that peak blood level of radioactive-labeled dextroamphetamine contained in the spansule was, on the average, eight to ten hours post administration as opposed to the peak blood level at two hours for regular tablets, it remains to be shown that the spansules have significant clinical advantage over the regular tablets.

In an extensive review by Barkley (1977), studies of dextroamphetamine, methylphenidate and pemoline were presented. No significant differences between percentage of responders or percentage of nonresponders was shown. No significant differences in the types, severity or frequency of side effects was noted. Safer, Allen and Barr (1972) suggested that growth suppression was more pronounced with dextroamphetamine than with methylphenidate. Conners, Taylor, Meo, Kurtz and Fournier (1972) suggested that dextroamphetamine produced more "sadness" than pemoline. The growth suppression effect, however, of dextroamphetamine has been subsequently shown to remit spontaneously with time, and the depressant effects of dextroamphetamine were not considered severe nor did they require discontinuation of medication (Conners et al., 1972).

Pemoline

Pemoline (Cylert®) is a stimulant medication, as are dextroamphetamine and methylphenidate. One of the earliest studies to report the effectiveness of pemoline on hyperactive symptoms was reported by Conners et al. (1972). They studied 81 children with a diagnosis of minimal brain dysfunction based upon questionnaires, continuous performance tests and clinical evaluation. Both pemoline and dextroamphetamine were administered on a blind basis with one morning dose of pemoline and a morning and before-lunch dose of dextroamphetamine. At the end of the eight-week treatment period, both dextroamphetamine and pemoline appeared effective in improving symptoms. Approximately 96% of the dextroamphetamine patients and 77% of the pemoline patients were rated as improved or much improved. As in other studies, approximately 30% of the placebo patients were improved but none were much improved. Teacher ratings roughly paralleled the clinician's evaluation. Both medications produced similar side effects, although the incidence of insomnia and anorexia was slightly less with pemoline than with dextroamphetamine. One important difference was the time for onset of drug effect. At two weeks and at four weeks into the therapy, there was a significant difference between the effects of pemoline and dextroamphetamine. Dextroamphetamine was fully effective at the end of two weeks but pemoline was not fully effective until six weeks. At four weeks, dextroamphetamine was still significantly more effective than pemoline. By six weeks, the difference had disappeared and both were more effective than placebo. No changes in blood pressure or liver function studies were noted in these subjects. Conners et al. (1972) showed that pemoline was effective when used only once daily (an advantage over dextroamphetamine) but was not effective until it had been taken daily for four to six weeks.

Other studies of pemoline demonstrated positive effects and side effects similar to other stimulants (Pelham, Swanson, Bender & Wilson, (1980). Page, Bernstein, Janicki and Michelli (1974) reported a multiclinic trial of pemoline that included 238 patients. Parent and teacher questionnaires, global ratings and psychological tests, as well as physical and laboratory data, were evaluated. Evaluation was made at nine weeks of therapy. Side effects attributed to pemoline were insomnia and anorexia. Five of the patients had stomachache, mild depression, nausea, dizziness, headache or drowsiness requiring discontinuation of the medication. While side effects were more common in the pemoline group than in the placebo group, it might be noted that 33% of the side effects were noted in the placebo group. All observers, including physicians, parents, teachers and psychologists, noted a significant therapeutic benefit from pemoline when compared to placebo in this double-blind multiclinic trial. The authors noted that improvement with pemoline appears to be gradual, as reported by global ratings and individual questionnaire items. Significant benefit may not be evident until the third or fourth week of drug administration. Longer follow-up times also showed significant benefits and side effects much the same as for other stimulants.

Studies have also shown improvement in the intellectual functioning of children taking pemoline. Dykman, McGrew, and Ackerman (1974) studied 216 children taking pemoline over a nine-week period. Increase in performance was observed for I.Q. (WISC), reading and arithmetic (WRAT), auditory perception (Wepman), motor coordination involving complex left-right maneuvers (Lincoln-Oseretsky Factor II) and attention to details and organization (Draw-a-Man). The authors concluded that pemoline improves attention while decreasing distractibility and level of restlessness. Stevenson, Pelham, and Skinner (1984) studied methylphenidate and pemoline in comparison on paired associate learning tasks and spelling tasks in hyperactive children. They studied 36 children ages 5.8 to 11.6 who met the DSM–III criteria for a diagnosis of ADD. Maximum effect on learning occurred one hour after ingestion for methylphenidate (0.3 mg/kg) and two hours after ingestion for pemoline (1.9 mg/kg). Testing took place after two weeks on medication. Significant improvement in the paired associate learning task was seen. The authors believed that pemoline was superior to methylphenidate in some respects, especially in the paired associate learning task. However, they felt that this finding needed to be replicated.

Similar findings of four-to-eight week delayed onset of effectiveness for pemoline when compared to methylphenidate was reported by Conners and Taylor (1980) in a study of 60 hyperactive children. Children were selected on the basis of clinical evaluation, multiple psychological tests and parent and teacher ratings. Assessment of medication was determined on an individual basis. By the end of the treatment, approximately 88% of the pemoline and 90% of the methylphenidate groups were either improved or much improved, and 34% of the placebo group was improved. The authors related that, as in a previous study where pemoline was compared with dextroamphetamine, it seemed that the clinical effect of pemoline had a slower onset, with the major positive differences not appearing until between the fourth and the eighth weeks. Both drugs produced more side effects than placebo; however, it is notable that two-thirds of the patients had side effects from placebo. When medication was discontinued, the methylphenidate group immediately regressed, while the placebo group did not change. The pemoline group returned to baseline over several weeks, suggesting a longer lasting effect of pemoline than methylphenidate. Pemoline was found to be less effective than methylphenidate, but this difference was not significant. Side effects to pemoline were considered similar to other stimulants and included anorexia and insomnia.

The finding of a high degree of variability of pemoline metabolism has been suggested as a possible explanation of rare negative reactions such as psychosis or Tourette's. A 600% interindividual variation in elimination and a 300% variation in total body clearance of pemoline was discovered by Sallee, Stiller, Perel and Bates (1985) in a study of ten children, ages 5 to 12, diagnosed as hyperactive on the basis of Conners scores. The authors felt this finding may explain the unpredictable reactions of children to pemoline in some cases.

Possibly the greatest disadvantage of pemoline is the concern that it may cause liver failure. Prescription information for physicians in regard to Cylert®includes a warning about possible hepatic dysfunction or failure. "There have been reports of hepatic dysfunction including elevated liver enzymes, hepatitis and jaundice in patients taking Cylert®. The occurrence of elevated liver enzymes is not rare and these reactions appear to be reversible upon drug discontinuance. Most patients with elevated liver enzymes are asymptomatic. Although no causal relationship has been established, two hepatic-related fatalities have been reported involving patients taking Cylert" (PDR, 1989, p. 511). As a result, laboratory tests are recommended. "Liver function tests should be performed prior to and periodically during therapy with Cylert. The drug should be discontinued if abnormalities are revealed and confirmed by follow-up tests" (PDR, 1989, p. 510).

Jaffe (1989) obtained the FDA 1639 forms that contained the reports of the two pemoline-related deaths cited in the PDR (1989). The first was a ten-year-old who died in 1977. He had hypoplasia of extrahepatic ducts and biliary cirrhosis before taking pemoline. He developed jaundice three weeks after being placed on pemoline and died of liver failure 18 months later. The second was a twelve-year-old boy who died in 1981 after taking pemoline for three years. Data were limited to very high SGOT (liver enzyme) and bilirubin, as well as a negative test for infectious hepatitis A and B. The death was attributed to a toxic hepatitis secondary to overdose. The author "would interpret this information to indicate that liver function tests should be done before and periodically when using pemoline and that a history of liver disease/dysfunction should be a contraindication" (p. 458).

Page et al., (1974) studied 288 patients for as long as 77 weeks (most more than 50 weeks) in an open trial of pemoline at a dosage of 1.91 to 2.51 mg/kg/day. Nine of the 288 patients discontinued pemoline because of elevations of SGOT and/or SGPT liver enzymes. These elevations occurred after 250 days or more of continuous pemoline therapy and were discovered during routine testing procedure. There were no clinical signs or symptoms present in any patient demonstrating enzyme elevation. Bilirubin did not rise, and there was only inconsistent sporadic elevation of alkaline phosphatase in these patients. Drug administration was discontinued when elevations were noted, and the enzyme levels returned to normal. Two patients were rechallenged with pemoline, and the serum liver enzymes rose again. The authors believed that this represents an individual delayed hypersensitivity to pemoline that is reversible on discontinuation of the medication. They reported the overall incidence of this reaction in all studies as in the range of 1% to

2%. The authors did not find the problem of liver enzyme elevation a serious one, and no deaths or permanent liver failure were reported. Nevertheless, possible liver failure and need for frequent blood tests represent a significant disadvantage and may account, in part, for the lack of popularity of pemoline.

In two studies comparing placebo, pemoline and methylphenidate, Dykman, McGrew, Harris, Peters and Ackerman (1976) found that pemoline was less desirable than methylphenidate because of the eight-to-nine week delay in onset of full activity, an overall lower level of effectiveness compared to methylphenidate, and the finding that a smaller group of children responded better to pemoline than to methylphenidate. However, the fact remains that some children did respond better to pemoline.

Not all studies of pemoline have shown it to be effective on a once-a-day schedule. Collier, Soldin, Swanson, MacLeod, Weinberg and Rochefort (1985) found that after six months of treatment, most children were using Cylert on a morning and noon dosage schedule. In their study, 21 boys and 6 girls ages 5 to 12, diagnosed as ADD using DSM-III criteria, were followed for six months on pemoline with a clinically adjusted dosage. In 70% of the children, the medication was taken twice daily at breakfast and at noon. The other 30% took their medication only at breakfast. The authors were surprised that most (70%) of the children were judged on clinical evaluation to require twice-daily dosage.

Like the reports of psychosis from methylphenidate, there has been one report of a manic episode precipitated by Cylert®. Sternbach (1981) reported a case of a 20-year-old white female who within 24 hours of an increased dose of pemoline was noted to be euphoric, grandiose and hyperactive. She had pressured speech with flight of ideas. Pemoline was discontinued, and the manic episode was treated with lithium. The author presented this report to suggest that pemoline can induce mania in susceptable individuals. The scarcity of additional similar reports indicates that this occurrence is quite uncommon, if anything more than coincidental.

The effect of pemoline on growth was studied by Friedman, Carr, Elders, Ringdahal and Roache (1981). They studied the growth of a group of 22 children treated with pemoline for attention deficit disorder. The majority of children were followed for 4 years. At the study onset, the children ranged from age 6.5 to 11.8, with a mean age of 8.4 years. They were treated continuously for 12 months and then allowed drug "vacations." Dosage of pemoline was 56 to 150 mg per day during the first year of treatment. Both weight and height growth of treated children were found to lag significantly behind that which was expected from standard tables at 6 and 12 months. However, by 48 months, the treated group was essentially identical to expectation for height percentile and had actually surpassed expectation for weight. These results were strikingly similar to results observed with methylphenidate-treated children (American Academy of Pediatrics Committee on Drugs Report, 1987). Pemoline-treated children may experience short-term but not long-term deficits in weight and height growth.

The relationship between pemoline and Tourette's syndrome is similar to that of other stimulants (Mitchell & Matthews, 1980). Bachman (1981) reported a single case of Tourette's syndrome induced by pemoline. Tics immediately developed when the medication was started, but they did not resolve when medication was discontinued two months later. Subsequently, additional tics, including humming, panting and puppy-like sounds, developed. Improvement was seen for Tourette's after treatment with haloperidol.

Cylert is available in three dosage strengths: 18.75 mg, 37.5 mg, and 75 mg as well as chewable 37.5 mg tablets (*PDR*, 1989). Cylert has a recommended starting dose of 37.5 mg per day (*PDR*, 1989). The dose should be gradually increased by 18.75 mg at one-week intervals until the desired clinical response is obtained. The effective daily dose for most patients will range from 56.25 to 75 mg. The maximum recommended daily dose is 112.5 mg. Telephone prescriptions and refills for six months are allowed. This may be more convenient than methylphenidate, which can be prescribed for a maximum of only a 30-day supply with no refills.

Tricyclic Antidepressants

Tricyclic antidepressants such as imipramine (Tofranil®), the chemical structure of which is shown in Figure 9.9, have been shown to help ADHD symptoms. In an early study, Huessy and Wright (1970) suggested that tricyclic antidepressants were safe and effective based on clinical global impressions, objective measures of cognitive functioning and improvement in behavioral rating scales.

Garfinkel, Wender, Sloman and O'Neill (1983) used the tricyclic antidepressants imipramine and desipramine versus methylphenidate in a crossover, double-blind study of 12 male subjects who met the DSM-III criteria for ADD. Three-week periods in each treatment were used. The tricyclic antidepressants were more useful with affective symptoms and less likely to disturb sleep than methylphenidate, but behavior ratings by teachers and childcare workers indicated methylphenidate had a greater efficacy than the other drugs. They concluded that different medications could have differential effects on specific component symptoms of ADD.

Stimulant medications were judged superior to tricyclics for the treatment of attention-deficit symptoms by Pliszka (1987) as a result of a review of five quantitative studies of imipramine reported between 1972 and 1983. He discounted the conclusions of Huessy and Wright (1970) that imipramine was the drug of choice, citing what he described as poorly defined criteria in the Huessy and Wright study. Pliszka concluded that for children who do not respond to stimulants, imipramine or a similar tricyclic might be an appropriate second choice. While he concluded that children who were highly anxious or had mood disturbance might fair better with imipramine, children with aggression might deteriorate on imipramine. With regard to dosage, he concluded that low-dose tricyclics (50 mg per day or less), especially doses less than 1 mg/kg per day, had not been demonstrated to be effective. Most studies used a daily dose of 50 to 150 mg with 3 to 5 mg/kg on a weight-basis dosage. It was recommended that future studies control for blood levels and the presence of conduct and anxiety disorders in addition to clearly defining attention-deficit criteria.

Tricyclics were again advocated as the drug of choice for ADHD symptoms by

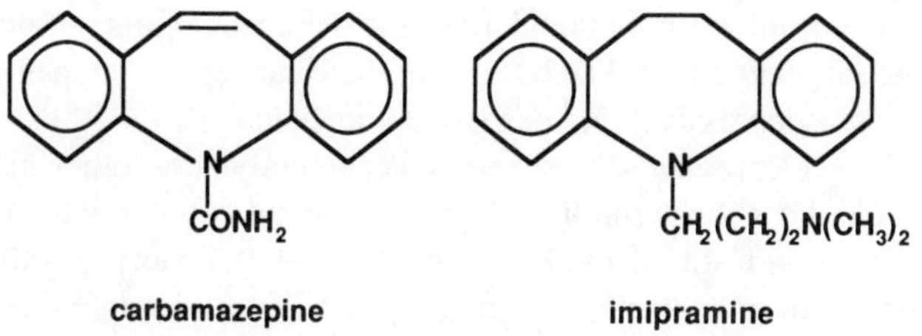

Figure 9.9 Structural comparisons of carbamazepine and imipramine. From R. R. Pleak, B. Birmaher, A. Gavrilescu, C. Abichandani & D. T. Williams, Mania and Neuropsychiatric Excitation Following Carbamazepine. Copyright 1988 by the *American Academy of Child and Adolescent Psychiatry*. Printed with permission of the publisher.

Huessy (1988), who reported that 90% of patients will respond to tricyclic antidepressants without side effects. For this reason, he argued that methylphenidate should be the drug of last resort. However, most authors would agree with Cowart (1988) that the scientific literature does not support Huessy's allegation that the tricyclic antidepressants are equal in efficacy over the long term to the sympathomimetics (methylphenidate, amphetamine, methamphetamine and pemoline). Cowart argues that tricyclics often take several weeks to reach full effectiveness. This slow response is a disadvantage in some patients and makes titration more difficult.

Side effects such as sleepiness, dryness of the mouth and constipation are common problems with tricyclic antidepressants but are usually mild and rarely require change of medication. Additional symptoms such as other gastrointestinal symptoms, blurred or double vision or other changes in mood are uncommon and usually mild in severity, rarely requiring alteration of dose or discontinuation of medication. Side effects can sometimes be minimized by beginning with a low dose (10 to 25 mg) and gradually increasing to an effective dose of 50 to 150 mg (3 to 5 mg/kg) in a single daily dose.

Preskorn, Bupp, Weller and Weller (1989) offer an alternate means of adjusting imipramine dosage to the therapeutic range based on the fact that individual blood levels are reproducible and linearly correlated with dose. These authors suggest that studies of major depression have found a therapeutic level of 125 to 250 mg/ml. The steady-state method of adjustment begins with an initial dose of 75 mg, followed by determination of the plasma blood level over a 7-to 10-day period. Using this 75-mg initial dose, only 12% of the children were found to have a high plasma level initially. The relationship between this initial 75-mg dose and the child's plasma level was then used to determine the optimal suggested dosage. This system resulted in plasma levels of imipramine and metabolites within the therapeutic range in 84% of the sample population. In the other 16%, further dosage adjustment was needed. Preskorn et.al., emphasized the importance of obtaining plasma levels to be certain that imipramine is not used in too high a dose. Use of plasma levels of imipramine will serve to help prevent side effects due to therapeutic overdosage.

In the absence of information that defines the therapeutic range of plasma levels for imipramine in treatment of ADHD, use of the established therapeutic range for treatment of major depressive disorder is recommended.

The tricyclic antidepressants are slower to act and probably somewhat less effective than stimulants for most children. Nevertheless, in children who are at higher risk for side effects with stimulant medication because of anxiety, psychosis or tics, imipramine or a similar tricyclic may produce satisfactory symptom resolution.

Antipsychotics

Thioridazine (Mellaril®), chlorpromazine (Thorazine®) and haloperidol (Haldol®) are major tranquilizers that are commonly used to control psychotic symptoms. They produce a decrease in activity and have also been used for treatment of children with ADHD symptoms. The major side effect of stiffness, sedation and possibly slower cognitive processing has proven a substantial disadvantage (Ross & Ross, 1982). They have also been implicated as causing tardive dyskinesia, a permanent movement disorder. Nevertheless, these medications have been considered effective by parents in some studies (Werry, Aman & Lampen, 1975; Gittelman-Klein, Klein, Katz, Saraf & Pollack, 1976), and are sometimes used in the treatment of hyperactive children (Ross & Ross, 1982). The average daily dosage of thioridazine for children ages 2 to 12 is 0.5 to 3.0 mg/kg (*PDR*, 1989, p. 1884); the dosage of haloperidol for ages 3 to 12 is 0.05 to 0.075 mg/kg (*PDR*, 1989, p. 1238). The sedation often caused by these medications, along with the risk of tardive dyskinesia, precludes the use of the major tranquilizers for most children with ADHD. However, these medications may have a role in helping to control impulsive and overactive behaviors in the rare situation when these behaviors present a danger to the child or others. Occasionally, the authors have seen these effectively used as a short-term addition to other treatments to help avoid hospitalization when overactivity or self-destructive behavior precipitates a crisis situation.

Clonidine

Clonidine (Catapres®) is an antihypertensive medication that has recently been used for treatment of attention-deficit symptoms. The mechanism of action is believed similar to that of the stimulant medications in that the catecholamine systems are affected. As clonidine has been studied less extensively than methylphenidate, the frequency of side effects is not as well documented. The place of clonidine in medical treatment of attention-deficit symptoms has yet to be determined with certainty. Since clonidine is also used for treatment of Tourette's syndrome, it may prove useful in children with attention deficit and tics or in those who develop tics on methylphenidate.

Clonidine has the potential advantage of administration by skin patch. Hunt (1987) studied 10 children who met DSM-III criteria for ADD and who scored more than 1.5 standard deviations above the mean on the parent and teacher

forms of the Conners questionnaire. These children were administered oral clonidine openly for eight weeks using the effective dosage determined in previous
study (5 micrograms/kg/day). Those with a favorable response to oral clonidine
were switched to transdermal clonidine administered via skin patch. They were
also treated with placebo, as well as low-dose (0.3 mg/kg) and high-dose (.06
mg/kg) methylphenidate for one week each in random sequence. Six children had
a preferential response to clonidine and continued on that medication. Three of the
nine children who received both the clonidine and methylphenidate had an overall better response to the methylphenidate and continued taking it after the study.
One of the most interesting features of this report is the skin patch application
of medication. The medication contained within the skin patch is slowly released
through the skin. No pills are required and the patches last in effectiveness for five
days. Many families liked the ease of administration, and the author concluded
that clonidine, especially with skin patch administration, may be the treatment of
choice for a group of children with the ADD syndrome.

Lithium

Lithium is a simple salt that has proven to be effective in the treatment of manic-
depressive disorders. The possibility that the overactivity of ADHD could be related
to manic symptoms has suggested trying lithium for treatment of ADHD. A good
response to lithium of an ADD patient was reported by Brown, Ingber and Tross
(1983). An 18-year-old patient with attention-deficit disorder by DSM-III criteria
initially showed improvement on pemoline in increasing doses up to 93.75 mg
per day over five weeks. Subsequently, lithium carbonate, 1200 mg per day, was
added. Once lithium levels reached 1.1 mEq/l, there was a marked decrease in
impulsivity, paranoid ideation and angry outbursts and ideas, as well as agitation
activity level. It was concluded that the lithium was most helpful for hot temper,
stress tolerance, impulsivity and affective lability. The question is raised as to
whether lithium may be an adjunct to pemoline. However, in this single case
report, crossover studies with other stimulants were not done to see if possibly
methylphenidate or amphetamine would be as effective or more effective than
pemoline in combination with lithium.

Studies of lithium by Greenhill, Rieder and Wender (1973) and Whitehead and
Clark (1970) were also reviewed by Brown et al. (1983). The first study employed
stimulant nonresponsive children as subjects. The second study had a small sample
size and lacked clear inclusion and response criteria. Brown et al. concluded that
the efficacy of lithium for hyperkinetic children or adults had not been determined.

Carbamazepine

The anticonvulsant carbamazepine (Tegretol®) has been suggested for treatment of
many childhood disorders. The structure of carbamazepine is pictured in Figure
9.9. One report by Pleak, Birmaher, Gavrilescu, Abichandini and Williams (1988)
found substantial adverse behavioral and neurological reactions in six boys, aged

l0 to l6 years, treated with carbamazepine for aggression in an inpatient setting. Negative reactions include mania, hypomania, increased irritability, impulsivity, hyperactivity, aggression, abnormal EEG and recurrence of absence seizures. Pleak et al. concluded that the frequency and severity of the adverse effects of carbamazepine were striking. They advised caution on the part of clinicians and researchers prescribing carbamazepine.

Other Medications

Many other chemical supplements have been used to treat ADHD symptoms. None has proven as effective as the stimulants or tricyclic antidepressants. Several examples are presented to represent the range of substances that have been administered to children in an effort to find effective treatments for ADHD symptoms.

D-phenylalanine is an essential amino acid. Zametkin, Karoum and Rapoport (1987) studied its effect on symptoms of inattention and hyperactivity. A group defined by parent and teacher behavioral ratings and cognitive measures was studied in a double-blind placebo comparison crossover study. Twenty mg/kg per day of d-phenylalanine was not associated with any improvement or deterioration in behavior.

The tetracyclic antidepressant mianserin was tested for effect on symptoms of attention deficit by Winsberg, Camp-Bruno, Vink, Timmer and Sverd (1987). No significant improvement was seen and side effects were encountered. Promethazine was studied by Zametkin, Reeves, Webster and Werry (1986). Eight children with ADD by DSM-III criteria were treated with promethazine in a double-blind study. The authors concluded that there was no improvement with promethazine. There was behavioral deterioration in four subjects that necessitated discontinuation of the drug in two cases.

Treatment of ADD children with essential fatty acids was studied by Aman, Mitchell and Turbott (1987) and found to have no effect on behavior. An antidepressant bupropion hydrochloride, was tested in a preliminary study by Casat, Pleasants and Van Wyck Fleet (1987). A group of 30 outpatient children, ages 6 to 12, was selected on the basis of DSM-III criteria and Conners hyperkinesis questionnaires. Improvement in clinical global impression and reduction in hyperactivity as reflected in the Conners Teacher Questionnaire were statistically significant. Minimal side effects were noted. Further studies are needed to determine if additional antidepressants may be helpful for attention deficit as well.

MEDICATION INTERVENTION AND THE BRAIN MODEL OF ADHD

In our discussion of the causes of ADHD (Chapter 2), we described a brain model for the attention system, and the concept of an attention center that projects to all areas of the brain and functions to modulate attention was presented. This attention center acts upon all areas of the brain to modulate a spectrum of attention from thoughtful and deliberate to quick and impulsive. On one end of the spectrum is highly focused behavior. The child is locked onto one target such as the teacher, book or even TV screen. Other factors, including extraneous noise, rattling of papers, speech or music emanating from a different source, are suppressed, as is the impulse to respond to these extraneous distractions. On the other end of the spectrum, the child is aware of many different surrounding activities, sounds and sights. The child is ready to respond to rustling of leaves or noises by running toward or away from the sounds. The ability to respond quickly to a sharp noise, rustling activity, or extraneous speech in some situations is more important than a thoughtful analysis. Impulsive activity based on quick response is sometimes needed; for example, in dangerous situations. Thoughtful, focused activity is more important in the classroom. Most normal children are able to change their behavior in many gradations along this spectrum. They can choose appropriate times for quick, impulsive actions and other times for deliberate, thoughtful responses.

Children with ADHD are not able to control their attentional skills. They may be intently concentrating when they should be aware of their surroundings, and they may be too easily distracted and ready to run off when they should be focused. Medication for ADHD works to enhance the functioning of the attentional system so that children can choose when to be sensitive to outside distractions and when to focus their attention. The attention center is stimulated by these medications with the result that the child has better control of himself or herself. The child's ability to interact in a purposeful way is greatly improved by medications (Whalen, 1987; Schachar et al., 1987; Pelham, 1987; and Barkley et al., 1984).

From this point of view, attention deficit is a result of the malfunction of the system that allows the brain to discriminate situations where focused, deliberate behavior is appropriate from situations where quick, impulsive actions are needed. This model allows us to differentiate ADHD from a learning disability. An ADHD child is unable to change as needed from focused concentration and deliberate action to impulsive action and sensitivity to his surroundings, whereas learning disability results from inappropriate processing and coordination of sensory input with memory and motor output. Medication intervention for ADHD improves the child's ability to control and focus attention, concentration and activity but usually has little if any direct effect on the ability to process and coordinate sensory imput, memory and motor output.

For example, a child with ADHD may have difficulty paying attention to the book being read but with medication intervention may improve the ability to concentrate on the printed words. A learning disability results from difficulty understanding or processing the words. A child with simple ADHD may appear to have difficulty reading because of a lack of concentration. If the distractibility and inattention are corrected, the child's reading will improve. If, however, the difficulty lay in understanding the written word and processing the information, improving the child's concentration will not improve the ability to obtain information from written words. In this case, appropriate attention to the book is a necessary, but not a sufficient, condition. Medication stimulates the attention center deep within the brain, but may have little effect on the cortical ability of the brain to process information. This model may aid in the understanding of the effect of medication intervention on ADHD symptoms and the lack of effect of ADHD on cerebral cortical dysfunction or learning disabilities.

Using this model also allows the practitioner to understand the nature of medication side effects. Stimulants adjust the functioning of chemical brain systems, including dopamine, noradrenalin, serotonin and possibly others. These chemical systems are involved in other functions of the brain in addition to attention and concentration. The other systems may also be stimulated by the medication and change their level of functioning.

For example, one can think of the child's appetite as a parallel system to the attentional system. Stimulating centers in a way that affects satiety may result in decreased interest in food. If the appetite system were more sensitive than the attention system, the result would be anorexia at a dose that would not affect attention. If one considers the attention system to be similar to the appetite system but in most children more sensitive to stimulate medications, one can understand why children will have some decreased appetite as they improve their ADHD symptoms. The sleep system can also be sensitive to stimulant medication. Increasing the dose of medication stimulates wakefulness and may interfere with sleep. When this occurs as an unwanted effect of medication, it is termed a side effect. Fortunately, in most children with ADHD the attention system is more sensitive to the effect of stimulant medication than other systems. In some children, however, the sleep or appetite systems appear to be more sensitive, and in other children the attentional system appears to be unresponsive to the effects of the stimulant medication.

ALTERNATIVES TO MEDICATION

Comparisons of medication risks and benefits with alternatives depend on understanding the alternatives to medication intervention. The alternatives include nonmedication intervention and nonintervention. There is very little evidence that medication intervention has a long-term effect on the child with ADHD symptoms, but it may have a very dramatic effect on the short-term outlook. Many of the beneficial effects of medication can be achieved in some settings with nonmedication-intervention programs. When medication is not employed, however, the results are less dramatic, do not generalize as well, and require more organization and effort on the part of the family and therapist. In addition, effective nonmedication-intervention programs may not be available to all children. Nonmedication-intervention programs are more costly than medication, both in terms of the financial resources required to support the therapy and also in terms of personal resources required by the family.

THE DECISION TO USE MEDICATION

Comparison of the risks of medication, benefits of medication and alternatives to medication is the recommended basis for making the decision concerning medication intervention. Baseline assessment and the expected benefits of intervention with medication are compared to the expected outcome without medication intervention. If children are at higher risk for medication side effects (such as those with tics, psychosis or a family unable to follow through with programs), this must be carefully weighed against the alternatives of nonintervention or nonmedication interventions.

The weighing of risks, benefits and alternatives to determine appropriate intervention is a common part of medical practice. Clinical judgment of the physician must be used. Involvement of the family can be important. The process of comparing risks, benefits and alternatives brings the decision-making process concerning medication intervention for treatment of ADHD closer to the decision-making process for other medical problems.

A PRACTICAL APPROACH TO ADMINISTRATION OF METHYLPHENIDATE

The best or optimal dose and schedule of medication might be considered to be the one that produces greatest benefits and least side effects. There are no studies that demonstrate the preferred means of determining the optimal dose or schedule of medication. This section will present some practical suggestions that may serve as a guide to the clinical use of methylphenidate when consideration of risks, benefits and alternatives leads to the conclusion that a trial of medication intervention is warranted. Many of these suggestions are applicable to other medications as well.

A multidisciplinary team is used for evaluation of ADHD and for supervising a treatment regimen. One member of the team functions as a case manager to coordinate the gathering of information concerning the effect of medication at differing dosages and/or time schedules. This information is then communicated to the physician in a way to allow appropriate medication adjustment.

Methylphenidate—How Often, How Much?

R. D., an eight-year-old boy with ADHD was started on Ritalin in the morning before school. His mother felt that, rather than helping, it seemed to aggravate the symptoms. His morning teachers, however, felt that he was dramatically better on the medication. His afternoon teacher didn't see much difference. How do these different observers reach such different conclusions? Methylphenidate reaches its greatest effect one to two hours after it is taken. The time it takes to lose one-half its maximum effect, or its half-life, is approximately four hours in most children. Medication taken at 7:00 A.M. will be most effective from 8:00 to 10:00 A. M. and then become less effective during the day. In this example, R. D.'s morning teacher observed him while the medication was fully effective and concluded that it was helping. His afternoon teacher observed him after the medication had lost much of its effect and saw little change. After school, his mother observed him during a period of rebound and felt that the medication was aggravating his symptoms. This example illustrates the importance of understanding the time course of medication effect. This section will present an approach to medication adjustment.

Medication begun at a very low dose (5 mg) and gradually increased, with information obtained about the child's performance at school and at home at each dosage change, allows maximum flexibility. In some children, the results are clear in only a few days. For others, it requires two weeks before the results of a medication change are clear. Initiating medication intervention with a very low dose often will allow children who are very sensitive to methylphenidate, either with a positive or negative response, to demonstrate this sensitivity. In these children, dosages that work well for other children may cause unacceptable side effects. For some children, a very low dose will produce the best response, and a higher or more frequent dose may produce fewer positive or more negative effects.

ADHD symptoms respond well to stimulant medication. However, symptoms of conduct disorder, oppositional behavior, specific learning disabilities, depression or other problems not the result of ADHD often are not improved with stimulant medication. Symptoms of attention deficit can be separated from other symptoms by careful evaluation. It is recommended that ADHD symptoms be clearly identified and that the dosage of methylphenidate be adjusted to a level that maximizes the effect on these symptoms. Feedback on a regular basis is necessary for this determination, and reevaluation of the target symptoms is needed. Techniques to obtain subjective and objective information from teachers and parents, as well as independent observation, are usually needed to determine the effect of medication and the optimal medication dosage.

As all children do not respond to the same dose or have the same time course of medication response, arbitrarily predetermining dosage amounts is not recommended. While it is simpler to place all medicated children on the same dose and schedule, arbitrary selection of amount and frequency of medication ingestion will result in too much or too little medication for some children. Medication adjustment, a single dose at a time, will produce more positive results and fewer side effects.

Once a single dose of medication is adjusted to optimal effect, one can determine whether a second dosage of medication is appropriate. Methylphenidate is most effective one to two hours after it has been administered. Evaluation two hours after it has been ingested will help determine if there is substantial improvement in attention-deficit symptoms. Evaluation at other times of the day is also needed. After four or five hours, the effect of medication may no longer be present. Six to twelve hours after the medication, the symptoms of attention deficit will often return to their premedication levels. For some children, the ADHD symptoms are actually worse in the period 6 to 12 hours after medication is administered than they were on days when no medication was administered. This is known as the rebound effect. If symptoms are troublesome at the six-hour time, whether this is caused by rebound or simply by the return to nonmedication functioning, a second dosage of methylphenidate may be helpful four hours after the initial dose.

Initiating a single morning dose of methylphenidate and following its progress through the day will allow one to separate side effects related to the presence of medication from side effects related to medication withdrawal or rebound. The second dose of medication, when required, may be administered at lunch time.

When the second dose is titrated independently of the initial morning dose, the amount of methylphenidate required may be less for the second dose than the first. Much of the clinical effect of the methylphenidate has dissipated after four hours. However, some medication effect is still present, and continuation of the medication effect with a much lower second dose may be possible. One-half to two-thirds of the morning dose may suffice for a noon dose.

By evening, the morning and most of the noon medication will have lost its effectiveness. Most children will function well in the evening possibly as a result of the effects of medication given earlier in the day. If rebound or return of ADHD symptoms is a problem in the evening, a third dose of medication may be helpful. Individual titration allows more flexibility in determining whether a third dose is helpful and what dosage is most effective. An after-school dose given between 4:00 and 6:00 P.M. may improve ADHD symptoms in the late afternoon and evening. This third dose may produce difficulty falling asleep at night and decrease appetite for dinner, however. If difficulty falling asleep or anorexia persists, it may preclude use of a late-afternoon dose of medication. If a third dose is required, a lower dosage than the morning and possibly even lower than the noon dose may be effective. Reevaluation of the ADHD symptoms can help determine the need for and value of the third dose of medication.

The determination of the optimal dose and administration time of medication requires careful monitoring. Some children with ADHD also have other disorders such as learning disabilities, oppositional behavior, depression, anxiety or social-skill deficits. The attention-deficit symptoms are likely to be the only problems responsive to stimulant medication. Use of non-attention-deficit symptoms to judge the effect of medication can result in overlooking medication effectiveness or can lead to dosage adjustments that are higher than optimal. When adjustment of medication results in dosages greater than 20 mg of methylphenidate, the target symptoms that were used to adjust medication should be reevaluated. Retitration of the medication may prove helpful.

For example, a ten-year-old fifth-grade boy taking 35 mg of Ritalin three times a day was seen because of persistence of ADHD symptoms as well as restlessness, sleeplessness and an increase in anxiety. A thorough evaluation revealed that the methylphenidate had been increased every time he had developed oppositional behavior under the mistaken belief that this was a symptom of attention deficit. When the episode of oppositional behavior subsided, it was thought to confirm the effect of the increased methylphenidate dosage, and subsequent episodes of oppositional behavior were further treated by increases in medication. Initially, the family was resistent to the idea of discontinuing the medication. After medication had been discontinued, an increase of attention deficit symptoms did occur, but a decrease in oppositional behavior, anxiety, restlessness and sleeplessness was also seen. When the Ritalin was retitrated to a dose of 15 mg in the morning and 10 mg after lunch, inattentive, distractible and impulsive behavior improved without the side effects of exaggeration of the restlessness, anxiety and sleeplessness. A single dose greater than 20 mg and a total daily dose of more than 60 mg should alert the practitioner that retitration may lead to better results at a lower dosage of methylphenidate.

Minimizing Anorexia and Insomnia

Anorexia is a common side effect of methylphenidate. In general, it is transient and self-limited. Many children will have decreased appetite and possibly even a pound or two of weight loss over the first few weeks. Appetite and weight will usually improve shortly thereafter. If the anorexia or weight loss is particularly troublesome, there are several techniques to alleviate this problem.

Administering the morning dose after breakfast may allow increased appetite for the morning meal. Increasing the caloric content of breakfast may increase the 24-hour caloric intake. A similar approach, with the noon dose administered after lunch, can sometimes be helpful in restoring a relatively normal appetite for lunch. If an afternoon dose of methylphenidate is administered, there may be some decrease in appetite at dinner. Giving the after-school dose of medication as early as possible and having dinner as late as possible may improve appetite for the evening meal. Some children will have a return of appetite near bedtime, and some families have found that a bedtime snack will increase the 24-hour caloric input. Many children have a dosage threshold for anorexia. A dosage of 10 mg may produce little anorexia, where 15 mg may produce significant anorexia. Titration of medication dosage to maximize therapeutic effects and minimize side effects may be useful in this situation.

Some children will have difficulty with sleeplessness after taking methylphenidate. There are at least two different reasons why this might occur. In one situation, the medication has a direct effect to stimulate wakefulness. This is often especially true if an afternoon or evening dose is used. This can be minimized by decreasing the afternoon or evening medication dosage. In some sensitive children, dosages that are so low as to barely affect the ADHD symptoms produce insomnia. Some tolerance to the sleep effects may occur, but sleeplessness may necessitate discontinuing methylphenidate and considering alternate medications.

A second explanation for sleeplessness is as a result of rebound. Increase in inattention and distractibility caused by rebound will prevent these children from concentrating on falling asleep. This rebound sleeplessness may appear similar to restlessness caused by direct effect of the methylphenidate. Observation of other symptoms during the day may give a clue to the occurrence of sleeplessness as a rebound symptom. Other symptoms of ADHD may also have rebounded. As the medication wears off, an increase in inattentive and distractible behavior may be seen. Children with rebound sleeplessness may actually fall asleep more easily with increased medication. For example, if a child receiving 15 mg of Ritalin once in the morning becomes restless in the afternoon and evening and has difficulty falling asleep, a second dose of 5 to 10 mg of methylphenidate either after lunch or immediately after school may improve the symptoms of restlessness at night. In these children, the medication may help them to settle down in order to fall asleep.

Noncompliance

Noncompliance is a possible explanation of medication failure. Sleator et al. (1982) found that many children in their study disliked the medication and tried to avoid taking it. They concluded that while the physician interview provides valuable information about noncompliance, other sources of information must be used to be certain medication is being taken as directed. Brown, Borden, Wynne, Spunt and Clingerman (1987) reported that in a study of 58 children with attention deficit involved in medication as well as nonmedication therapy, slightly more than one-half of these children completed a three-month treatment protocol. They concluded that it is often difficult to determine whether failure of medication intervention is the result of noncompliance. They found that some children become skilled at disguising their noncompliance. They reported that families may not be aware of the problem unless the prescription does not need to be renewed at the expected time or unless carelessly discarded medication is discovered in the sink or on the floor. The practitioner must keep in mind that various forms of noncompliance can be the cause of medication failure.

Generic Formulations

Generic formulations of medications are often less expensive than the brand-name medication and are usually as effective. Some questions have been raised in individual patients as to whether the generic methylphenidate is as effective as the Ritalin brand of methylphenidate. While it has been our experience that several children had a dramatic deterioration in effectiveness of medication when changed from brand-name Ritalin to generic methylphenidate, controlled studies have not been performed to test this question. Some pharmacies will change the manufacturer of their generic methylphenidate from time to time. A child who has one manufacturer's brand of generic methylphenidate one month may be on another manufacturer's methylphenidate the next month even though he receives his medication from the same pharmacy. The practitioner should be aware of this possibility. If a dramatic and sudden lack of response to methylphenidate occurs in a child who has previously been a medication responder, one possibility to consider is the switch from brand-name Ritalin to generic methylphenidate or from one manufacturer's generic methylphenidate to another's. In some children, changing back to brand-name Ritalin may reinstitute the effect that was lost by changing to generic.

Sustained-Release Methylphenidate

The four-hour half-life of methylphenidate often requires a second medication dosage while the child is in school. The advantages and the convenience of a single daily dose prompted the introduction of a sustained-release form of methylphenidate (Ritalin-SR®). One of the initial studies of sustained-release methylphenidate in 30 children (Whitehouse, Shah and Palmer 1980) indicated that standard methylphenidate had advantages over Ritalin-SR. However, the criterion for the diagnosis (minimal brain dysfunction) was not given and no placebo controls were used. Methods of evaluation included parent and teacher questionnaires (unspecified type) as well as the Bender Visual Motor Gestalt Test. For this study, the children selected were considered to be "doing well" on 10 mg of methylphenidate twice daily. Few behavioral differences were reported between the children given l0 mg of methylphenidate twice a day and those given 20 mg of Ritalin-SR once in the morning. However, the total score from parent and teacher questionnaires showed that standard methylphenidate was better than sustained-release. Despite significant improvement with regular methylphenidate in total score on both the parent and teacher questionnaires, the authors concluded that neither seemed clinically favorable.

The results of many other studies of sustained-release methylphenidate, however, have been disappointing. A comparison of the effect of standard methylphenidate and sustained-release was reported by Pelham et al. (1987). Thirteen boys with attention deficit as defined by Conners Questionnaires and clinical criteria were treated in a summer-treatment-program controlled environment. Although both medications were effective, standard methylphenidate was judged superior to the 20 mg sustained-release methylphenidate because most boys responded more positively to standard methylphenidate and because sustained-release methylphenidate had a slower onset of action as measured on a continuous performance task. The sustained-release did show some effect eight hours after ingestion, but that did not make up for its lesser initial effect.

A study of plasma levels reflects the clinical observations of the effect of regular and sustained-release methylphenidate (Greenhill, Cooper, Solomon, Fried & Cornblatt, 1987). These researchers reported that the average blood level from a single 20 mg sustained-release methylphenidate dose appears to be one-half that resulting from two doses of l0 mg methylphenidate, particularly in the afternoon.

Chewing the methylphenidate sustained-release tablets may be the reason for the lack of effectiveness in some children. This interesting hypothesis was suggested by Rosse and Licamele (1984) to account for some of the difficulties with sustained-release methylphenidate. Whether alternate means of ingestion of the tablets will improve the effectiveness of sustained-release methylphenidate has yet to be demonstrated.

Double-Blind Clinical Evaluation

Some authors have proposed determining medication effect by double-blind placebo trials in individual children (Ottinger, Halpin, Miller, Durmain & Hanneman, 1985). Citing results of a study of 118 children with attention-deficit disorder under double-blind conditions, Ullman and Sleator (1986) advocated use of a double-blind cross-over technique for all children given methylphenidate. Eighteen of the 118 children had nearly 50% improvement on the teacher rating scale for attention while taking placebo, and this was essentially the same response that they had to the best dose of methylphenidate. The authors concluded from this data that a significant group of children who appear to respond to methylphenidate may be responding to what they describe as nonspecific factors also present in the placebo trials. They urged all clinicians to use placebo trials and implied that this will allow children to have the benefit without the risks of medication.

Several questions are raised by placebo studies. These include: (1) What is the long-term effect of placebos? (2) Should children who respond be continued on placebo? and (3) Should children who respond to placebo simply be eliminated from consideration of medication intervention? The American Academy of Pediatrics (1987) has not recommended routine placebo trials as Ullmann and Sleator have advocated. It is not certain why double-blind trials have not become widespread in clinical practice. Possibly the difficulty in arranging for a placebo trial or understanding how to proceed if such a trial yields positive results has discouraged this practice. Nevertheless, some children seem to respond to medication at first, and then when the response wears off, they respond again to an increased dose. Possibly this group of children contains some who are placebo responders. It remains to be shown that double-blind trial administration of medication in clinical practice has a lower risk or greater benefit than other means of evaluation.

SUMMARY

How does one decide whether a child should be placed on medication for treatment of ADHD symptoms? We have suggested that the risks of medication and possible alternatives be compared with the benefits. Stimulant medication has a dramatic effect in improving a wide range of ADHD symptoms in 75% to 80% of ADHD children. Classroom behavior and interactions with peers improve. Even interactions between mothers and children change for the better. This effect appears to be the result of improved or "stimulated" functioning of the brain center, which determines whether concentration and deliberate action or quick response is appropriate. The mild degree of loss of appetite, difficulty falling asleep or irritability seen in many children as a result of stimulant medication can be viewed as the result of stimulation of other brain centers such as ones for sleep or appetite. These side effects usually resolve spontaneously and do not detract from the overall positive results.

Although it rarely occurs, some children develop severe depression or a toxic psychosis with delusion or hallucination, and 1% of treated children develop tics as a result of medication. While these symptoms usually disappear when medication is discontinued, reports of persistent tics and Tourette's syndrome raise the possibility of permanent injury from stimulant medication as a rare occurrence in some children. Other concerns, such as permanent growth suppression, however, have been dispelled by studies suggesting that children treated with stimulant medications will eventually reach projected height even if medication is continued through weekends and summer vacation. Concerns that medication treatment of ADHD might increase the likelihood of drug addiction, criminal behavior, suicide or other mental illness have also been proven, after study, not to be associated with stimulant treatment of ADHD in childhood.

Some factors increase the risk of side effects. Young children (below age six) and children with anxiety, depression, psychosis, tics or Tourette's syndrome are more likely to have side effects. Children with symptoms of disorders other than ADHD, such as learning disabilities, depression, anxiety, oppositional disorder or aggressive behavior, are less likely to improve with medication. A careful evaluation can increase the likelihood of benefit and decrease the likelihood of side effects. History and examination can be directed to separate ADHD symptoms from others and to search for conditions that increase risk of medication intervention. Multidisciplinary nonmedication behavioral intervention programs may increase the benefit of medication.

The practitioner must keep in mind that there are both medical and nonmedical alternatives to the use of methylphenidate. These include nonmedication (behavioral) interventions, as well as other medications. While other medications have been shown to be effective in treatment of ADHD symptoms, methylphenidate remains the choice of those prescribing for most ADHD children. Pemoline has the disadvantages of two-to-four week delayed onset of action and worrisome reports of liver function abnormalities in a few children. These may serve to outweigh such benefits of pemoline as effectiveness in single daily dose for many children and less restrictive government regulation. Amphetamines are associated with a higher incidence of anorexia and insomnia in some studies. Sadness is described in some children treated with dextroamphetamine.

Dextroamphetamine, which in the early 1970s was the most common medication used for treatment of ADHD symptoms, has been steadily declining as the medication preferred by prescribing physicians. Tricyclic antidepressants have the advantage of a single daily administration and non-controlled substance status. While they are often effective, some comparative studies suggest that tricyclics are not as effective as methylphenidate in treating ADHD symptoms in most children. They have the added disadvantage of slow onset of action (two to four weeks). However, for ADHD children with tics, depression, anxiety or unacceptable side effects from methylphenidate, imipramine may be the best choice. Other medication, including major tranquilizers, clonidine, anticonvulsants, antihistamines and others, may be helpful in some children but are not first-choice medications for most ADHD children.

By understanding the risks of medication and how to decrease them, the benefits of medication and how to increase them, and the alternatives to medication and how to use them, it is possible to make a reasoned and reasonable decision concerning medication intervention. In patients carefully selected so that the expected benefits outweigh the risks, medication intervention can be an effective addition to a nonmedication intervention program.

CHAPTER 10

Cognitive-Mediational Interventions

The cognitive-mediational strategies that are used with populations of developmentally impaired children, including those with attention deficit and learning disability, find their roots in the work of Luria (1959; 1961) and Vygotsky (1962). These Russian psychologists hypothesized that behavioral self-control is developed through a three-stage process. In the initial stage, children's behavior is controlled and mediated externally by others. In the second stage, children learn to control their own behavior but require self-generated external direction (talking to oneself) as a means of initiating and following through with tasks. By the third stage, children develop the ability to internalize mediational strategies and behavior is self-controlled through a covert, unobserved process. This theory appeared to best explain the self-control inadequacies that inattentive and impulsive children experienced and was attractive to a number of researchers. The 1960s and 1970s witnessed an increase in applied research attempting to develop strategies to assist inattentive children in developing skills and passing through these stages. As Keough and Barkett (1980) pointed out, cognitive-mediational training held the promise of reducing impulsive behavior and leading to more effective problem-solving strategies with good potential for generalization.

Early research studies were innovative and yielded positive, optimistic data (Palkes, Stewart & Kahana, 1968; Palkes, Stewart & Freedman, 1971). Eventually, this theoretical base was integrated with behavior modification technology. The resulting school of psychology has come to be known as "cognitive behavior modification" (Meichenbaum & Goodman, 1971; Meichenbaum, 1975; 1977). This school of psychology has gained widespread attention, and the techniques developed have been used with populations of developmentally impaired children, including those with learning impairments (Hallahan & Sapona, 1983), behavioral problems (Rhode, Morgan & Young, 1983), brain injury (Gajar, Schloss, Schloss & Thompson, 1984) and attention disorder (Christie, Hiss & Lozanoff, 1984). Positive effects for children with attention deficit have been observed in both special education settings (Hallahan, Marshall & Lloyd, 1981) and regular classrooms (Rooney, Hallahan & Lloyd, 1984).

The techniques initially developed by these researchers have been adapted and used to alter thinking skills in order to positively impact a variety of behaviors, including on-task performance (Harris, 1986), behavioral compliance (Christie et al., 1984), positive attribution (Licht, Kistner, Ozkaragoz, Shapiro & Clausen, 1985) and social skills (Kirby & Grimley, 1986). The basic premise for all of these strategies and techniques is that children's behavior can be altered by teaching them to think differently. Through different thinking, children gain self-control and the ability to modify their behavior as they interact with the environment.

Research in the area of cognitive strategies as a means of developing self-control has extended over the past 20 years and included techniques such as self-recording (Broden, Hall & Mitts, 1971), self-evaluation (Kanfer, 1970), self-reinforcement (Lovitt & Curtiss, 1969), self-punishment (Kaufman & O'Leary,

PROBLEM SOLVING SKILLS GROUP ASSESSMENT QUESTIONNAIRE

Child _____   Rater _____   Date _____

Directions: Listed below are a list of social skills which are important for social competence. Please read the description of each skill and circle the answer which best describes your opinion of this child's ability. Please use the space at the end of the questionnaire if you feel there are additional social related problems which this child exhibits.

This Child:

	is very poor at this skill.	exhibits this skill as well as others.		exhibits this skill better than others.
Recognizes problem situations	1	2	3	4	5
Accepts responsibility for problems	1	2	3	4	5
Projects the source of problems onto others	1	2	3	4	5
Able to solve problems independently	1	2	3	4	5
Able to solve problems with minimal support	1	2	3	4	5
Unable to solve problems independently without significant support	1	2	3	4	5
Able to generate alternative problem solving solutions independently	1	2	3	4	5
Frequently chooses inappropriate solutions to problems	1	2	3	4	5
(Please check) Frequently chooses: ____ aggressive solutions ____ assertive solutions ____ passive solutions					
Has a system for choosing the best problem solution	1	2	3	4	5

Figure 10.1 Problem Solving Skills Group Assessment Questionnaire. From S. Goldstein and E. Pollock, *Problem Solving Skills Training for Attention Deficit Children.* Copyright 1988 by Neurology, Learning and Behavior Center. Used with permission of the authors.

Is able to implement a problem solution	1	2	3	4	5
Appears able to understand the impact a particular problem solution may have in the future	1	2	3	4	5
Has a system to evaluate problem solving success	1	2	3	4	5
Listens during conversation					
Deals with own feelings appropriately	1	2	3	4	5
Deals with other's feelings appropriately	1	2	3	4	5
Accepts conseqences appropriately	1	2	3	4	5
Reacts to failure appropriately	1	2	3	4	5
Deals with peer pressure appropriately	1	2	3	4	5
Able to plan and reflect	1	2	3	4	5
Rewards self	1	2	3	4	5
Follows directions	1	2	3	4	5

Comments:

Figure 10.1 (continued)

1972), self-instruction (Meichenbaum, 1975), external cuing (Blick & Test, 1987) and attribution training (Reid & Borkowski, 1987). These techniques have been effective with inattentive children and hold promise of leading to positive changes in both home and school behavior. Although critics have argued that cognitive training may be beneficial for normal or learning-disabled children it is not efficacious in academically deficient ADHD children (Abikoff et al., 1988) and may not overall be clinically useful for inattentive children (Abikoff, 1985; 1987), even these critics acknowledge that within-group comparisons have demonstrated cognitive interventions effective in improving specific academic skills and teacher-reported behavior (Abikoff et al., 1988). As such, it has been increasingly recommended that these techniques be implemented with inattentive children at home and in school (Polirstok, 1987).

This chapter will define cognitive behavioral strategies, present a brief review of the literature in the use of these techniques with attention-deficient children, present ideas that the practitioner can use to teach these techniques and reference text and software materials that can also be used. An integrated cognitive-behavioral model based on the research literature will be presented to assist the practitioner to implement cognitive and behavioral change. The chapter will conclude by providing an overview of a six-session program to comprehensively teach problem-solving skills to ADHD children and adolescents (Goldstein & Pollock, 1988).

ASSESSMENT OF COGNITIVE SKILLS

Cognitive skills as they relate to problem solving, self-instruction and self-monitoring are not easy to evaluate in clinical or laboratory settings. Often the ADHD child's weakness with these skills is inferred from behavior reported by parents and teachers. Many of the commercially available cognitive-mediational training programs take all children through a series of steps designed to teach all of the basic skills and are not designed to identify each child's cognitive strengths and weaknesses through preassessment. It is the authors' experience that the majority of ADHD children rarely use any of these cognitive techniques as a means of problem solving. For those practitioners interested in preassessing each child, Goldstein and Pollock (1988) developed a preassessment questionnaire as part of a problem-solving skills group developed for ADHD children. (See Figure 10.1.)

SELF-CONTROL STRATEGIES

External Cuing

These strategies provide an external auditory or visual cue. Usually the cue is provided mechanically, independent of the teacher or parent; in some settings, however, teachers may directly provide a visual or auditory cue to the child. For example, students may be taught to check and see if they are on task every time a random beep sounds in the classroom.

Research

Cued self-recording was found significantly more effective in improving on-task behavior than non-cued self-recording in a study involving four inattentive, learning-disabled boys in a classroom setting (Heins, Lloyd & Hallahan, 1986). Although the difference between cued and non-cued self-recording conditions was not as significant for academic productivity, there was a dramatic positive difference in on-task performance. Barkley, Copeland and Sivage (1980) demonstrated improvements in attention to task and a reduction of misbehavior when children were signaled to self-record their behavior at random intervals in response to a prerecorded sound delivered through a tape recorder. Christie et al.(1984) used a teacher-signaled verbal or nonverbal gesture to cue the child in a classroom setting to record his behavior. In this study, students recorded a range of eight behaviors, including inattention, aggression, disruption and on-task performance. This form of signaled self-recording produced significant reductions in inattentive and inappropriate classroom behavior while increasing time on task. The procedures were used in a regular classroom, and children were provided with weekly feedback concerning their progress. The authors suggested that it was these two factors that increased the generalization of improvements to other areas of classroom performance and behavior.

Blick and Test (1987) successfully used a five-step cuing strategy to stimulate self-monitoring and self-recording with developmentally impaired adolescents. Students were trained to record their behavior in response to a verbal cue randomly presented through a tape recorder. Over the course of the intervention sessions, the cues were gradually faded until they were occurring 20 minutes apart. In the final step, the cue was faded completely, and the students were prompted to monitor their own behavior by watching a clock and marking a recording sheet containing preprinted clock times.

Strategies

AUDITORY CUES.   The most efficient way of delivering an external cue appears to be through the use of a tape recorder and a prepared, closed-loop audiotape. Although initially tedious to prepare, once completed, such tapes have an unlimited life expectancy. The cue can be a sound such as a beep or a single word. Published studies have not documented whether or not cuing without self-recording is successful in increasing on-task performance and attention. The authors have used a cuing strategy without self-recording successfully to improve children's task completion in the home. In all likelihood, cuing without self-recording in a classroom is also an effective intervention. Auditory cues can be used with both elementary and secondary students. This strategy works best during independent work periods. The initial tape should provide a cue at an interval ranging from approximately 10 to 90 seconds with a mean interval of 45 seconds. With older students who are involved in more complex tasks such as mathematics, the practitioner may wish to space the cues slightly farther apart.

VISUAL CUES.   Although teacher-directed cuing has been demonstrated to be effective, in the majority of classrooms it is impossible for the teacher to consistently provide visual cues to the student. A visual cue such as a digital or illuminated device that sits on a student's desk (Rapport, 1987) can be used but may be costly and somewhat cumbersome to manage and administer.

FADING CUES.   When external cues are efficiently faded, positive results obtained during cuing sessions are maintained. Fading is best administered by spacing out the cues and providing the student with a self-directed visual cue such as a clock to assist in determining self-recording times. The next step is to fade the self-recording procedure so that self-directed tracking continues without recording. The goal is that the student has developed the habit of self-monitoring her behavior on a regular basis and continues to do so even without the prompt of an external cue or the self-recording process.

Self-Recording

This strategy is usually paired with an external cue. The child is taught to make a mark in response to the cue, usually on some type of behavioral recording form. During self-recording, behavior is recorded without any attempt to judge the goodness or appropriateness of that behavior.

Research

Self-recording as a primary intervention has been found to be effective in producing behavioral change in places other than classrooms (Johnson & White, 1971; Kazdin, 1975) and classrooms (Heins et al., 1986; Blick & Test, 1987). Broden et al. (1971) found cued self-recording to be associated with a 48 percent increase in on-task behavior. Lovitt (1973) found that self-recording resulted in a significant decrease in inappropriate behavior. In conjunction, there was a dramatic improvement in appropriate behavior. The majority of studies that have been titled or referred to as studies in self-recording have involved some degree of evaluation. For this reason, these studies will be reviewed in the self-evaluation section. It has been suggested that self-recording does not have to be accurate to produce desirable changes in target behaviors. It has also been suggested that desirable effects associated with self-recording may require the addition of reinforcing contingencies in order to be maintained (Rosenbaum & Drabman, 1979).

Strategies

YOUNGER CHILDREN.   Although younger children can be taught a pencil-and-paper self-recording strategy, other tangible strategies may work better. Chips can be placed in a box on the child's desk and a cup placed next to the box. Each time a cue sounds the child must take the chip from the box and place it in the cup. Small circular stickers can also be used. When the cue sounds, the child takes the sticker and attaches it to a recording sheet. The process of developing the habit to self-record on cue is not difficult for younger children, especially since they are not being required in this process to evaluate their behavior.

OLDER CHILDREN AND ADOLESCENTS.   The simplest self-recording procedure would use a four-by-five-inch recording sheet divided into a grid of small boxes. The younger the child the more likely it is the boxes will need to be larger; thus, a larger sheet of paper may be required for recording. When the cue sounds, the child or adolescent is directed to place a mark, usually an X or a check, sequentially in the next available box. Recording usually follows horizontally from left to right.

OUTSIDE THE CLASSROOM.   Children can be taught to self-record to an auditory or visual cue in a variety of situations. Chip or paper and pencil recording systems can be used during clean-up time, at meals and even in the car. It is somewhat more difficult to implement self-recording techniques in situations where children do not have to remain seated, but patience and planning will prevail.

Self-Evaluation

Self-evaluation requires the child to record and to evaluate the accuracy, competence or appropriateness of his behavior.

Research

Self-evaluation has been used to improve on-task performance in the classroom (Blick & Test, 1987) and as a component in programs designed to teach self-control (Drabman, Spitalnik & O'Leary, 1973; Camp & Bash, 1981). It has long been suggested in the research literature that the effectiveness of self-evaluation is enhanced with the provision of externally provided criteria for self-evaluating performance (Kanfer, 1970). The criteria provided have varied. Blick and Test (1987) provided a fairly simple set of criteria and an evaluative system in which students were given examples of on-task behavior and graded themselves as a plus if they were engaged in the behavior when cued or a zero if they were not. Christie et al.(1984) provided a much more complex rating system that required the child to record one or more of eight different behaviors that she may have been engaged in when cued. Kirby and Grimley (1986) used self-evaluation as a process to reinforce the use of self-instructional techniques. After a self-instructional training program, children were provided during course work with a checklist containing six rows that listed the six problem-solving stages taught during their training program. When cued, the child was required to check the column that described the problem-solving stage she was engaged in at that moment. Kirby and Grimley hypothesize that it is not the child's accuracy that is important in recording but rather the use of the cue to remind the child to continue to use a systematic strategy during task work. Self-evaluation has consistently proven to be effective in implementing an increase in on-task behavior and work productivity (Kneedler & Hallahan, 1981).

The focus of many self-evaluation classroom studies has been on improving on-task behavior. However, limited research has suggested that increased time on task does not directly lead to improved academic performance (Klein, 1979). In response, some researchers have compared the benefits of having students self-evaluate productivity rather than attention to task, but at this point, it has not been demonstrated that having children evaluate one type of behavior instead of another is more beneficial (Harris, 1986).

Strategies

Mahoney (1977) provided a five-step model to teach cued self-evaluation to children. In the first step, the trainer explains and clearly defines what is appropriate or inappropriate behavior. Various examples are provided. It is essential that before proceeding to the next step the child understands each category of behavior. In the second step, children are taught to mark self-recording sheets when cued. In the third step, the facilitator models the entire procedure. In the fourth step, children are required to repeat out loud definitions of the behavioral categories they are to self-rate and the self-recording instructions. In the fifth step, children begin performing the procedure under the facilitator's direction. The facilitator then gradually fades direct supervision. Mahoney demonstrated success with this model using only a 15 minute training session. It is recommended that following holidays, illness or other periods away from the school the procedures for self-recording be briefly reviewed with the child. This holds true at home as well.

Self-Instruction

Self-instruction techniques are varied and have been limited only by the creativity of their developers. They range from single ideas to multistep interventions.

These techniques teach the child strategies for thinking differently and guiding his behavior just as if an external source, such as a parent or teacher, were there providing that guidance. This area comprises the majority of cognitive-mediational techniques presently used with ADHD children and adolescents. These techniques have also been used with adults (Dougherty & Redomski, 1987).

Research

From as early as 1968, outcome studies using self-instructional procedures in which children are taught to "talk to themselves" have been effective in modifying various cognitive skills (Palkes et al., 1968). Self-instructional strategies have been successful in reducing impulsive responding (Brown, 1980); increasing planning, concentration and reasoning (Meichenbaum, 1976); improving social skills (Shure, 1981); increasing the accuracy of academic work (Cameron & Robinson, 1980); and increasing generalization of skills to the regular classroom routine (Bornstein & Quevillon, 1976). These latter authors demonstrated that self-instructional training in an experimental setting appeared to generalize to the regular classroom in the form of increased on-task behavior.

Shure and Spivack (1978) described five distinct cognitive interpersonal problem solving skills that are essential for successful socialization. These included problem sensitivity, alternative thinking, means-ends thinking, consequential thinking and causal thinking. This model will be presented in Chapter 12 of this text.

The effectiveness of a comprehensive self-instructional training program has been repeatedly demonstrated in a variety of settings (Hinshaw et al., 1984; Konstantareas & Hermatidis, 1983). Kirby and Grimley (1986) describe verbal self-instruction training as an eight-step sequential process. Training begins by assisting the practitioner to identify and define the task, teaching a cognitive modeling strategy and eventually teaching the child to fade overt self-instruction and develop covert self-instructional skills. This model is easy to follow and to implement. It will be presented later in this chapter.

Copeland (1979) investigated the types of private speech produced by attention-deficit and normal boys. The hyperactive boys talked more than the normal boys when alone in the playroom. The hyperactive population engaged in a significantly greater degree of immature private speech, including exclamations and descriptions of self, while engaging to a lesser degree in more mature planning verbalizations. It is therefore logical to assume that immature speech is a reflection of the ADHD child's immature cognitive strategies. Gordon (1979) found that children with impulse control problems were also impaired relative to their same-age peers in establishing covert language skills. Such skills are necessary for effective self-instruction in problem situations.

It has been documented that modeling is an effective component in teaching attention-deficient children new behavior (Carter & Reynolds, 1976). Goodwin and Mahoney (1975) demonstrated that modeling as an initial procedure when combined with instruction, practice and reinforcement was successful in reducing physical aggression in attention-disordered boys. Modeling procedures are often initial steps in the process of self-instruction training (Camp & Bash, 1981).

Although some studies have failed to demonstrate significant positive effects from self-instruction training (Freidling & O'Leary, 1979; Douglas, Parry, Martin & Garson, 1976; Burns, 1972), Ross and Ross (1982) conclude that the disappointing results in some of these studies are a function of procedural deficits in the training programs. They conclude that many of these programs are "far too narrow in content and too situation-specific for generalization to occur" (p. 265). They suggest that a program which teaches the concept of self-control would have far more success. Based on their impressions, such a program should incorporate modeling, role play, games and the opportunity to successfully use self-regulation through the use of stories and imagery. Incorporating such techniques into self-instruction training has also been suggested by others to increase positive outcome (Schneider, 1978). Ross & Ross (1976) also report using these strategies successfully.

Kendall and Brasswell (1982) concluded that adding components of self-instructional training and cognitive modeling of problem resolution to behavioral interventions resulted in improved performance as measured by achievement tests and teacher reports of reduced impulsivity and increased self-control. Children receiving both behavioral treatment and cognitive intervention made more progress than those children receiving only the behavioral treatment. These researchers also reported improved self-concepts in those children who received the combination of cognitive and behavioral interventions. Data suggests increased positive attribution as a result of the cognitive training.

Strategies

A MODEL FOR VERBAL SELF-IINSTRUCTION TRAINING.   Kirby and Grimley (1986) have organized and synthesized the work of other authors into an eight-step verbal self-instruction training program. To use this model, the practitioner chooses a task for which successful performance requires a specific skill in which the ADHD child is deficient. Self-instructional training can be beneficial in increasing attention, reducing impulsive responding and modulating emotionality or arousal level. In a one-to-one setting, the practitioner models the task for the child and provides an overt verbal description while engaging in the task. The practitioner verbalizes the definition of the task, possible approaches for solving the task, a method for selecting a strategy and applying it, self-monitoring, self-evaluation, self-reward and selecting an alternative approach if the strategy proves unsuccessful. The practitioner guides the child through the task and then assists the child in developing verbal mediational strategies to guide himself. The practitioner then whispers self-instructions and teaches the child to do so. Eventually, the overt verbal instructions are faded, and the task is completed with covert self-instruction. Figure 10.2 presents an overview of this sequential training program with a specific task example.

PROGRAM FOR SUCCESS.   When teaching children self-instruction as a means of improving their performance, it is important to break tasks into component parts to ensure that the child very quickly achieves success as a result of using the self-

Step One: Task Selection

The clinician selects tasks that involve sustained focused attention and require the use of some type of systematic plan or strategy for successful completion. Information gained from the assessment procedures should be used to help the clinician select tasks with an appropriate level of difficulty for the child.

Example:
For the child who has performed poorly on the Matching Familiar Figures Test, the clinician could select a similar match-to-sample task.

Step Two: Cognitive Modeling

The clinician models the solution of the task. This modeling involves the clinician's talking himself or herself through the following six problem-solving stages:

Defining and Understanding the Nature of the Task
Example:
Clinician: "Let's see, I'm supposed to find the cowboy that looks just like the one below. The problem here is that all six cowboys up here look just alike. I could just pick any of them, but that would be guessing. I need some way to be sure I get the right one."

Generating Possible Ways of Approaching the Task
Example:
Clinician: "I could look carefully at each cowboy and then choose, but they might all still look the same. Maybe I could pick two or three that look the closest alike and then compare them with each other. Or maybe I could eliminate them one at a time until there is only one left.

Selecting a Strategy and Applying it
Example:
Clinician: "If I really want to do well at this, I'd better take my time and look at each one closely. I guess I'll try the elimination plan. OK, cowboy number one. Hat's the same, shirt's the same, buckle's the same—whoops! No, it isn't. Cross out cowboy number one. Cowboy two. Ah, the hat's smaller. I bet it's number three. Yeah, he looks good. I pick this one. But wait, my plan was to look at *each* one. Better keep going. Number three is a maybe. Now number four is out; his gun is missing. Number five. H'mmm, he looks the same as three. Number six is way out, his boots don't have heels. So, is it three or is it five? Let me compare each of them. Ah, I see it. Three has no buttons on his shirt. It's number five, and I'm sure of it. On to the next problem."

Self-Monitoring of Progress Toward Solution
Example:
At periodic intervals the clinician asks herself or himself, "How is this working out? My strategy was to use the elimination method, and it seems to work. I have to be careful not to start guessing though. This is hard work and kind of boring, but I've got to stick it out. Only three more problems."

Self Evaluation and Self-Reward
Example:
Clinician: "Done. Finally. Not bad; I think I got them all right. Except maybe the spaceship one. That was hard. I think I'll go back and check that one again. Let's see, it was four or six, and I picked six. Oh, Oh, the nose cone is too pointed. Let's look at four. That's it. Now I think I have them all right. Good for me. I usually do terribly on any problem that you have to be careful on, but if I settle down and talk myself through with a plan that I stick with, I can do as well as anybody. Maybe better. What a thinker I am. Class act."

Figure 10.2 Verbal self-instruction training. From E. A. Kirby and L. K. Grimley, *Understainding and Treating Attention Deficit Disorder*. Copyright 1986 by Pergamon Press. Used by permission of the authors and publisher.

Selecting an Alternative Approach when Unsuccessful
Example:
Clinician: "I'm working hard on this, but I keep making mistakes. I'd better check my strategy. I think I need a whole new approach here."

Step Three: Overt External Guidance

Next, the clinician has the child complete the task while the clinician verbally instructs him through it, following the same six problem-solving stages

Example:
The clinician says, "Now you solve the next one and I'll do your thinking for you. OK, you're looking at all the possible answers and thinking . . . what am I doing here now? I'm trying to find one that's exactly like the one below. What plan could I follow? I could pick this one, but wait, my plan was to look at *each* one carefully and eliminate them one at a time. Here I go."

Step Four: Overt Self-Guidance

Then, the clinician has the child complete the task again (or a similar one) while using the child's own self-statements to guide him toward a solution. This is a difficult step to teach because it requires the child's active involvement. Instead of considering steps three and four as separate procedures, the clinician should go back and forth (between this one and overt external guidance) by prompting the child's thoughts and then letting the child finish the thought.

Example:
Clinician: "Well, number three is eliminated, now I will. . . ."
Child: "Check number four."
Clinician: "Let's see, the hat is. . . ."
Child: "The same. The shirt is the same. The gun is—oh, oh, it's different."

During this step the clinician begins to capture the nature of the child's natural way of self-instructing and notes the kinds of self-statements used by the child. The clinician also notes the types of self-statements that would appear to help but are not being generated by the child. For example, the child might habitually avoid statements directing himself to consider the nature of a problem carefully and to pause to choose a deliberate strategy before beginning work on a task. He could also lack coping statements to deal with the frustration of being stuck. Modeling samples of each of these types of self-statements follow.

Task definition statements, for example, for a match-to-sample task such

as the MFF, a clinician could model like this: "What kind of problem is this? I need to figure out which one up here exactly matches the one below."

Coping self-statements to be modeled might include

"Wow, this is driving me nuts. I need to slow myself down and start over. I'll just go slow and easy. Boy this is hard. I can't do it. I'll just have to give up. Oh, no, I'm not supposed to say that. Now what do I do when I'm stuck? Oh yeah, let me see if there is another way of looking at this."

Figure 10.2 (continued)

277

Step Five: Modeling of Faded Overt Self-Guidance

The clinician models the whispering of the instructions to himself or herself while going through the task.

We have found that children are sometimes even more self-conscious about whispering than they are about talking to themselves. Rather than insisting that they actually whisper, we model and teach self-instructing in a low, barely audible tone. This step in the VSI training also demonstrates the disjointed, fragmented type of instructions that are more characteristic of the inner speech or thoughts we are attempting to develop. For example, a clinician might need to model

"Check two. Nope. Three. Hat. Buckle. Ah, ha, nope. Number four. Whew—boring. Stick it out. Careful. I think it's number five. Check six again. Yeah, it's five. Good. Not many more. Hang in there, hang in."

Step Six: Child Practice of Faded Overt Self-Guidance

The objective here is to help the child see the nature and usefulness of genuine self-instructions. The clinician listens carefully to the child and helps him generate his own thoughts and self-instructions rather than allowing him to copy the clinician.

Step Seven: Modeling of Covert Self-Instruction

In modeling this stage, the clinician moves his or her lips, looks pensive, pauses to check two alternatives by pointing at one and then the other, and so on. Also, the child is told before the task is modeled the kinds of things the clinician will be thinking about.

Step Eight: Child Practice of Covert Self-Instruction

This is the final step in Verbal Self-Instruction Training. The child now has to think his own way through the task at hand. Because this involves covert self-instruction, the clinician is unable to monitor directly the child's thinking. But observation of the child's behavior (e.g., did he evaluate two alternatives by pointing to one and then the other?) provides some clues to the clinician about how the child is approaching the task. To check how the child is providing self-instruction, the clinician might need to ask some clarifying questions such as

"What were you thinking just now?"
"Tell me the strategy you just used."

Figure 10.2 (continued)

instructional strategies. Tasks must also be presented sequentially, beginning with the simplest and working up to more complex tasks. It is also important for the practitioner to have an understanding of the child's overall intellect and abilities so that tasks chosen are not too far beyond the child's skill level. Children with language disabilities are at greatest risk for being unable to benefit from these interventions (Abikoff, 1985).

INCLUDE PARENTS AND TEACHERS.   Parents and teachers will have significantly more opportunities than others to help the child use and generalize self-instructional strategies. It is important for all adults involved on a daily basis with the child to understand the basis of the training program and its aims. It is recommended that the practitioner provide either a verbal or written summary of specific strategies the child is being taught. This will allow other adults to facilitate the use of these strategies in problem situations. Understanding on the part of parents and teachers will also help them to modify task demands and requirements as needed, increasing the likelihood that the child will succeed when a self-instructional strategy is used.

ENCOURAGE INDEPENDENCE.   Although the ADHD child begins by directly modeling self-instruction and problem-solving strategies presented by the practitioner, it is important to encourage and reinforce the child for modifying the practitioner's model and developing his own strategies. Kirby and Grimley (1986) point out that it may be helpful for the practitioner to consider each child's personality and determine the type and quality of self-instructional speech in which the child is most likely to engage. The practitioner can then gradually reinforce the child for doing so. Rote, uninvolved self-instruction is not likely to be very helpful or to generalize easily.

BUILD MOTIVATION.   Meichenbaum (1977) and others suggest that it is most important to make the inattentive child an active participant in learning self-instructional skills. The practitioner should be excited and responsive. Initially, games and art projects are better than school work for teaching the use of self-instructional strategies. Computer software can also be an effective teaching tool.

TEACH SIMPLE RULES.   Providing simple rules the ADHD child can use as a guide for applying self-instructional training can often be effective. For example, one such rule might be, "You must think of at least three alternative solutions to the problem you are facing before you decide what to do."

SUGGESTIONS FOR PRACTICING COGNITIVE SKILLS.   Mazes can be used to practice reflection and planning skills. Children with visual and perceptual strengths will enjoy perceptual tasks as a means of practicing reflection skills. Story problems can facilitate the use of self-instructional skills. Self-recording can be practiced using a number of techniques, including charts, tokens and even beads on an abacus. Playing a game such as checkers repeatedly, directing the child during the initial game not to use cognitive strategies and then to use a self-instructional strategy in subsequent games can help the child observe the difference in her performance. Provide self-evaluation cue cards, asking questions such as "Did I do my best?", "Did I understand what I have to do?", "Did I use self-instruction?", "Did I work independently?", and so forth. Planning strategies can be facilitated by helping the child learn to estimate simple things, such as how many blocks can be stacked in a minute or how many beads can be placed on a string. This helps the child work toward developing realistic appraisal and planning skills. Finally, the discussion of hypothetical situations, such as what the world would be like if we saw only in black and white, teaches critical and reflective thinking. This helps children identify the aspects of a stimulus that are most important to attend to. Simple stories and follow-up questions can be used. Such strategies teach ADHD children to consider all alternatives and can be facilitated by having a child generate lists of solutions to simple problems, such as ten ways to put out a fire or five things you could do if the heat in your house didn't work.

Self-Attribution

These techniques teach children to develop an internal locus of control by attributing success and failure to factors that potentially are within the child's ability to control. Two types of attribution have been described in the research literature. Antecedent attribution is considered to be a set of long-standing beliefs the child has about himself based on past successes and failures. These beliefs potentially can act as self-fulfilling prophecies when the child is faced with a new task. Program-generated attribution results from the child's experiences in an immediate situation. These are the thoughts or feelings the child develops based directly on what is occurring at the time. These thoughts or feelings then have an immediate impact on the child's behavior (Henker, Whalen & Hinshaw, 1980).

Research

The multiple failures experienced by ADHD children occur day in and day out over a long period of time and in a variety of settings. It is inevitable that repeated failure leads to the development of beliefs of helplessness, lack of ability to control one's environment in a positive way and lower self-concept (Weiner, 1979; Bandura, 1977). It is not surprising, then, that many ADD children develop an external locus of control (Linn & Hodge, 1982; Rosenbaum & Baker, 1984). They perceive themselves as controlled and manipulated by their environment. When they succeed, they believe it is the result of luck and external factors. When they fail, they perceive themselves as incompetent and inadequate. This is opposite from the positive self-attributions that we all need to succeed. Over time, the ADHD child is at increasing risk to build a large fund of antecedent attributions about lack of competence and skill. These attributions cannot help but have a negative impact each time the ADHD child faces a new challenge. It has been demonstrated that teaching alternate attributional ideas (i.e., that failure results from controllable as opposed to uncontrollable causes) to children with helpless attributions can successfully alter their thinking (Dweck, 1975), resulting in increased persistence and task performance (Licht et al., 1985).

Reid and Borkowski (1987) developed a training procedure to enhance both antecedent and program-generated self-attributions. Techniques taught to alter antecedent attribution included a discussion regarding the child's beliefs about causes of failure, an opportunity to reperform previously failed items in a successful manner and an effort to help children develop appropriate beliefs about the causes of success. Program-generated attributions were altered by providing consistent feedback to the child during task performance between the strategy the child was using and success. Short-term treatment effects demonstrated that children who received attribution training used more complex problem-solving strategies, were more willing to take responsibility for their behavior, expressed the belief that their effort affected their performance and displayed reduced impulsivity. At a ten-month follow-up, children who received both self-control and attribution training persisted in their use of new strategies and maintained their new attributions. These authors also reported that several severe ADHD children demonstrated decreased hyperactivity in the classroom and improved self-control as the result of the combined self-control and attributional training. They suggested that attribution training is essential for the continued use and generalization of improvements based on self-control or self-instructional training. Reid and Borkowski's program also demonstrated that the combination of attribution training, self-control instruction and strategy teaching had additive effects leading to improved performance. Bugental, Collins, Collins and Chaney (1978) in a much earlier study, reported that cognitive self-control training was effective in enhancing ADHD boys' perceived control over their academic achievement.

Reid and Borkowski (1987) also used a number of techniques to help children increase the saliency of attribution. They used each child's correct and incorrect responses as examples for teaching that child specific attributional ideas. Dweck (1975) had previously suggested that increasing motivation and desire to succeed is fostered best by teaching children to learn from their mistakes, using mistakes constructively as a means of modifying thinking and acting strategies.

Strategies

USE ANALOGIES.   At different ages, different types of analogies can be helpful in assisting children to understand the concept that they are in charge and in control of what happens to them. Combining humor with this model can also be effective. For example, the practitioner may point to his shirt and tell the child that if the child were to say she did not like the shirt, the practitioner would have a choice of never wearing it again or discounting what the child has said because the practitioner likes the shirt. The point is to help the child understand that it is not the events in the world that determine her behavior, but based on a rational-emotive model, it is the child's thoughts and feelings that affect her behavior. If she believes that effort can make a difference in outcome, she is more likely to try harder and increase the chances of succeeding.

USE REAL-LIFE MISTAKES.   As pointed out in the research literature, the process of teaching attribution can be facilitated by using real-life examples of the child's mistakes. It is important, however, to not allow such an interaction to be perceived by the child as a lecture or criticism. Instead, help the child in a benign way look at his own behavior and its consequences and learn alternate ways of thinking and behaving. Most children and adolescents will agree that if you approach a new situation believing that you are going to be unable to succeed, there is a greater likelihood you will, in fact, fail.

REVIEW UNCONTROLLABLE FACTORS.   ADHD children, based on the nature of their history, are often very quick to attribute their failures to external factors such as: (1) the teacher or parent does not like me; (2) I am unlucky; (3) I am not smart; and (4) the task was too difficult. It is important for the practitioner to work through these factors with the child and patiently help the child understand that in most situations it is not these uncontrollable factors that account for failure but a controllable factor such as the child's not using a particular self-instructional strategy when attempting to complete the task. It is important for the ADHD child to replace negative self-attributions with positive beliefs reflecting an internal locus of control.

AWARENESS.   It is important for the practitioner to provide the child with a tangible, internally based explanation as to why problems with attention span and arousal are causing difficulty. It is important to help the child recognize that problems in the world result from internal, as opposed to external, factors. This facilitates the process of getting the child to accept that by making internal changes things can go better. The ADHD child must be convinced that she can learn to pay attention, reflect, organize and plan more effectively. She must be convinced that if she learns to do these things, the demands placed upon her by the environment will be easier to meet.

Self-Reinforcement and Self-Punishment

These techniques are usually paired with a self-evaluative strategy. The child is required to determine a level of reward or punishment based on the data he has recorded about his behavior.

Research

SELF-REINFORCEMENT.   Chase and Clement (1985) demonstrated that when self-reinforcement was used as the sole intervention with a population of ADD children, academic performance was significantly improved. Similar results were obtained with children experiencing both hyperactivity and learning disability (Varni & Henker, 1979). Clement, Anderson, Arnold, Butman, Fantuzzo and Mays (1978) demonstrated similar positive findings in improving on-task performance for a population of children with behavioral disorders.

Chase and Clement (1985) also found that a combination of stimulant medication and self-reinforcement was more effective in improving academic performance than self-reinforcement alone. Surprisingly, they also discovered that self-reinforcement alone was substantially more effective for improving academic performance than stimulant medication alone. This finding is contradictory to earlier research that suggested stimulant medication was more consistent and reliable than self-control training in improving sustained attention (Anderson, Clement & Oettinger, 1981). Further research is needed to clarify this issue. Chase and Clement's findings also tend to support previous hypotheses by Wender (1971) and Barkley (1981), suspecting that stimulant medication results in children being more sensitive to reinforcement, with the result that combined treatments lead to more success.

SELF-PUNISHMENT.   Limited research has been conducted on the effects of self-punishment. In the majority of research studies, punishment is part of a response-cost system in which students earn positive reinforcements for appropriate behavior and then are externally penalized by losing those reinforcers for inappropriate behavior. Response-cost has repeatedly been found effective as a component of reinforcement programs. Meichenbaum (1977) hypothesized that self-instructional training will be more effective when paired with a procedure such as response-cost. In one of the few studies evaluating self-punishment, Kaufman and O'Leary (1972) demonstrated the maintenance of minimal disruptive behavior in a classroom setting when students were allowed to control the number of tokens they would lose for inappropriate behavior.

DEFINING BEHAVIOR

A critical initial step in successfully implementing self-control strategies is the practitioner's ability to choose and operationally define behaviors to be altered. The behaviors must be defined clearly, precisely and in a manner the ADHD child can understand. Many behaviors must be defined based on both overt and covert processes. For example, a child sitting and thinking about a response to an essay question before writing may not appear clearly on or off task to the external observer. The key to successful definition is to help the child understand from an internal perspective what constitutes a particular behavior. Clear, precise behavioral definitions of target behaviors is the essential first step. If behaviors are not clearly defined, interventions that follow will be compromised in their potential for success.

GENERALIZATION

The failure of some research studies to find generalization of self-instructional skills across situations in all likelihood results to a significant degree from a lack of opportunities for effective generalization. Self-instructional training, by its nature, is a strategy considered effective for promoting generalization of behavioral change (Stokes & Baer, 1977). Self-instructional training precipitates internal change. The skills learned by the child remain with the child and are, therefore, accessible in a variety of other situations. Although some studies have suggested that generalization can occur spontaneously (Bornstein & Quevillon, 1976), in all likelihood some structure or monitoring is essential to teach the ADHD child to use skills that he possesses and to promote generalization.

Rosenbaum and Drabman (1979) point out that the majority of studies evaluating generalization investigated time generalization. This refers to changes in behavior that occur in the therapeutic or experimental setting that endure in that setting over time when contingencies have been removed. However, it is usually setting generalization that is of greatest concern and interest to the practitioner. Setting generalization occurs when changes in target behavior obtained in the therapeutic or experimental setting transfer and are demonstrated in a different setting without program contingencies. A third type, response generalization, reflects changes in nontarget behaviors observed in the therapeutic or experimental setting during intervention. This form of generalization has also not been well investigated. The practitioner must consider these three types—time, setting and response—when planning for generalization.

EXTERNAL CONTINGENCIES

The majority of contingencies that parents and teachers are directed to provide are positive. Although most children will be motivated by external positive contingencies that they value, the practitioner must caution parents and teachers not to develop an extensive reinforcement system based on tangible rewards that then will be difficult to extinguish. It is important for the practitioner to help parents and teachers understand that reinforcement is idiosyncratic and the value of a reinforcer can easily be altered. For example, many clinical psychology students are told the story of the towel lady. This was a woman in an institutional setting who began hoarding everyone else's towels. Towels for this woman were positively reinforcing. They were such powerful reinforcers that no form of alternate positive reinforcer or punishment proved effective in extinguishing the hoarding behavior. The staff literally brought in a truckload of towels and filled this woman's room. She became overwhelmed and wanted the towels removed. The towels were then removed contingent on her not taking anyone else's towels and following the rules and limits of the institution over the coming week. The towels, which had initially been positively reinforcing desired items, now became aversive negative reinforcers with the woman working to get rid of them.

A reinforcement inventory in which children are asked to respond to their favorite games, foods, toys and activities can facilitate the process of identifying positive reinforcers that are idiosyncratic for each child. It is recommended that whenever possible, social reinforcers be used as opposed to primary or consumable reinforcers. Ideas for social reinforcement might include praise, physical affection and positive facial expression. Enjoyable activities might include renting videocassettes, taking trips or watching television. Secondary reinforcers could include tokens, points or other symbols that can be traded for primary or secondary reinforcers. Such a system might also give money in exchange for tokens or points.

It is also important for the practitioner to pair social reinforcement and an attributional statement with any secondary positive reinforcer. In this way, the child begins to develop the ability to work for praise and encouragement, as well as internalize the process of self-reinforcement. Clark (1985) states, "Encouragement, words of praise and a loving touch strengthen good behavior" (p. 23).

THE ROLE OF PSYCHOTHERAPY

In an insightful discussion of psychotherapy with attention-disordered children, Smith (1986) points out that the adjustment problems ADD children experience result not only from an interaction of physiological development and environmental demand but also from the child's ego-development. Smith suggests that the ADD child's cognitive impairments require the practitioner to modify traditional psychotherapeutic childhood techniques regardless of the therapist's therapeutic orientation. Treatment must also involve an integrated approach using other types of interventions in addition to psychotherapy. Individual psychotherapy has been found to be an effective intervention and component of a multitreatment plan for attention-deficient children (Satterfield, Cantwell & Satterfield, 1979).

The majority of ADHD children do not exhibit problems that require long-term psychotherapy. However, all ADHD children experience repeated failures, which places them at greater risk to develop an external locus of control, feelings of helplessness and an inability to understand why they have so much difficulty meeting the expectations of their environment. For these reasons, it is recommended that all ADHD children be placed in a short-term counseling program to assist them in developing an understanding of the manner in which they cope with their environment and the reasons for their difficulties. Counseling can afford them the opportunity to reduce feelings of helplessness, increase motivation and improve coping skills. Often these latter goals can be facilitated through individual or group, cognitive and behavioral intervention programs. Although the initial goals might also be accomplished in a small group-discussion setting, many ADHD children initially are not good candidates for such groups because of their difficulty sticking to a task, impulsive responding and hyperactivity.

It is also important for the practitioner during the counseling process to be sensitive to the fact that ADHD children frequently have issues, including feelings about themselves and family members, that can be dealt with during the counseling process. ADHD children experiencing significant problems with oppositional behavior, anxiety, depression, conduct disorder or adjustment difficulty probably require longer term psychotherapy from a well-trained psychologist, social worker or psychiatrist.

Explaining ADHD to the Child

Psychotherapy with ADHD children is briefly reviewed in this chapter because it, too, is a cognitive intervention. Regardless of the practitioner's psychotherapeutic orientation, we believe that there are a number of basic issues that must be covered with ADHD children of all ages. First, it is important for the child or adolescent to develop an understanding of the relationship of her attention, impulsive and overarousal problems to persistent failure to meet the environment's demands. It is important for the child to understand the common-sense definition of ADHD and be able to apply that definition as a means of understanding daily failure. This helps the child observe the manner in which temperamental difficulties impact her at home, at school, with friends and in the community. The goal is not for the child to use attention deficit as an excuse but rather as a benign, nonthreatening explanation for why she has experienced so much difficulty. The goal, as with self-recording, is to help the child become an active participant in the treatment process.

The authors concur with the recommendations of Ross and Ross (1982) that the practitioner should avoid the use of confusing terminology such as brain damage or minimal brain dysfunction. The authors disagree, however, with their recommendation that the practitioner make no attempt to provide a factual explanation to the child concerning attention deficit. It is important for the child to understand the concept of individual difference, the fact that these are problems that many children experience and that these problems vary based on the demands placed upon the child.

As previously noted, the authors have found that analogies can be immensely helpful in assisting children to understand the reasons for their difficulties. For example, the specific behavior of remaining on task, can be used to illustrate this point. An analogy can be made to the ripple effect when a stone is thrown into the center of a pond. The stone in this case is not remaining on task. The child is then directed to add the "ripples." The first ripple is that the child gains negative attention from the teacher. The second ripple is that other children in the class observe this process. The third ripple is that work is not completed and the child may not learn as much. The fourth ripple is that the teacher may become increasingly annoyed. The fifth ripple is that the children begin to realize that the ADHD child is causing frustration for the teacher. The sixth ripple is that the other children may then wish to avoid interacting with this child even during recess, because of their perception that by associating with this child they too may be disliked by the classroom teacher. The converse model of remaining on task and completing work is then presented, and the child can observe the significant impact that one specific behavior can have upon the entire school experience.

For the learning-disabled child, psychotherapy provides a good opportunity to discuss the fact that specific skill deficits will cause specific types of learning problems and that the children are neither bad nor stupid if they have difficulty learning. Again, analogies are an effective and very powerful way of helping children understand the importance that certain skills have in mediating success in given tasks.

Developing Internal Control

The second step in counseling is to help the child build motivation and develop a sense of internal control. Some therapy models at this point provide the child with specific activities during the week to facilitate the use of skills learned during the counseling process. Other therapeutic models may not provide or suggest homework. Many of these skills can effectively be taught in a small group setting. The rational-emotive model (Ellis & Harper, 1975) can be used effectively with the ADHD child. The practitioner must help the ADHD child understand that between the environment's act and the child's response come the child's thoughts and feelings. These thoughts influence his behavior. Many ADHD children do not realize that they have control over their behavior. If they are insulted, they can choose to become angry and aggressive, or they can choose to ignore and withdraw. The choice and locus of control is within the child. Many of the techniques used to teach positive attribution can be effectively used during the psychotherapy process.

The Role of Medication

Since many ADHD children receive stimulant medication, it is important to place medication within the perspective of this model. Once the groundwork is laid, this is a fairly simple process. It is important to help the ADHD child understand that "pills will not substitute for skills." Taking a pill will not make a child finish his math or listen to his mother. Again, analogies are helpful. Comparing the medication to a hammer helps the child understand that it is not the hammer that builds a good house but the manner in which the carpenter uses the hammer. It is essential that ADHD children take responsibility for and internalize the positive changes that may be evidenced as the result of medication treatment.

Even in a situation where the ADHD child may not receive short-term counseling, the practitioner must take time to help the child understand why medications are used, the role they play, the behaviors they may assist and the need for the child to be an active participant in order to take advantage of the assistance the medication may offer. Such discussion does not necessarily need to be provided by the physician but must be provided by someone whom the child trusts and to whom they will listen. With adolescents it is recommended that medication be used as a reinforcer rather than a punishment. Many adolescents, as they are beginning to increase their desire to control all aspects of their lives, resist the use of medication and perceive medication as another source of external control. In such settings, once the adolescent has been made an active participant in other nonmedication interventions, an explanation about the potential benefits of medication can be used as a reinforcer with the intent of having the adolescent request a trial of medication.

If medication is to be used, the child must be provided with a simple explanation as to what medication accomplishes, why it works and the fact that with or without medication the child is still responsible for, and can learn to be in control of, her behavior. The authors believe that this is an essential component of the medication counseling process. ADHD children frequently develop an external locus of control. As such, it is not surprising that a group of hyperactive children were found to view medication as solely responsible for successful experiences (Whalen & Henker, 1976). If a child believes and is reinforced for the concept that the medication is responsible for changing and controlling her behavior, she will not take responsibility for the changes she makes or internalize success. The common response that many practitioners have heard from such children is, "I didn't take my pill today; therefore, I cannot behave." When this mode of thinking develops, the practitioner is faced with another, secondary behaviorial problem, at times equally as difficult to deal with as other psychiatric problems of childhood such as anxiety, depression or oppositional disorder.

A Three-Level Program

Douglas (1980), using a three-level program to develop an internal locus of control, provides a good overview and description that lends itself to an individual counseling setting with attention-disordered children. Level 1 is designed to help children understand the nature of their deficits and the ways in which learning alternative means of behaving and thinking can help. During this stage, the child is provided with an explanation of the problem, ideas as to how the problem affects the child and the attributional concept that problems can be modified. In Level 2, the child's motivation and capacity to deal with problem solving is expanded. The child is taught specific activities, such as breaking tasks into component parts. Successful experiences are specifically arranged at home and at school. The child is taught the concept of self-monitoring and self-evaluation. During Level 3, specific problem-solving strategies are taught. These include teaching the child scanning and attention techniques, active listening, strategies to inhibit impulsivity and strategies to facilitate the generation of alternate solutions. The child also improves his ability to self-monitor emotional status, to rehearse responses and to develop strategies to successfully complete specific academic tasks.

More Stepwise Programs to Teach Self-Control

Barkley (1981) suggested a nine-step format for training children in self-control and problem-solving behaviors. The steps include: (1) teach self-recording; (2) teach children to recognize potential problem situations; (3) teach children to inhibit impulsivity; (4) teach children to analyze problem situations; (5) help children generate alternative solutions; (6) teach children self-evaluative procedures; (7) assist children in implementing solutions; (8) help children evaluate changes precipitated by implementation of solutions; (9) assist in the development of self-reward and self-punishment. Barkley points out that this process is very similar to the operational process of behavior modification, with the difference being that in this process the child acts as his own change agent.

Varni and Henker (1979) combined components of self-instruction, self-monitoring and self-reinforcement in both laboratory and classroom settings with the goal of improving reading and arithmetic performance. The combination of these interventions, especially the addition of the self-reinforcement component, increased academic performance and appeared to decrease hyperactive behavior.

AN INTEGRATED COGNITIVE-BEHAVIORAL MODEL

The authors agree with the conclusions drawn by Ross and Ross (1982) concerning the reasons many cognitively based interventions fail or do not demonstrate generalization. In all likelihood, similar reasons account for the failure of behavioral interventions to facilitate long-lasting change as well. In an effort to deal with these problems, the authors have expanded a stepwise model first suggested by Rosenbaum and Drabman (1979) to maximize the potential effectiveness of self-control training. Our present model also incorporates components of attribution training and opportunities for generalization. This model can be used both at home and in school. Figure 10.3 provides a sequential overview of the integrated cognitive-behavioral model to facilitate the development of self-control and behavioral change. The steps will be briefly explained and an example provided.

Define Behavior

Teach Self-Recording and Self-Evaluation

Provide Externally Administered Contingencies

Teach Self-Instruction and Attributional Techniques

Transfer Control of Contigencies to Child

Provide Opportunities for Generalization

Fade Contingencies

Intermittently Monitor and Provide
Maintenance Contingencies

Figure 10.3 An integrated cognitive-behavioral model.

1. *Define Behavior.*   The initial critical step requires the practitioner to operationally define the behavior to be modified. It is then essential for the ADHD child to demonstrate an accurate understanding of the definition of the behavior in question before beginning any type of self-evaluative procedure.

2. *Teach Self-Recording and Self-Evaluation.*   The initial goal of self-recording is to assist the ADHD child to become a better observer of her behavior. It is important for the ADHD child both to understand from a common-sense perspective the possible reasons for her behavior and to develop the ability to accurately observe and monitor her behavior. Suggestions for short-term counseling with ADHD children to facilitate this initial process have been made in this chapter.

Self-recording begins the critical process of helping the ADHD child to observe her behavior. The next step, self-evaluation, allows the child to begin making judgments about that behavior. During this phase it is important for the practitioner, parent or teacher also to monitor and evaluate the ADHD child's behavior. In a nonthreatening and nonblaming way, feedback is provided in an effort to increase the ADHD child's accuracy in self-evaluation and self-recording.

3. *Provide Externally Administered Contingencies.*   If the ADHD child's self-evaluative reports are inaccurate, it may be beneficial to initially provide reinforcement when the child's perceptions closely match the practitioner's observations. Once a criterion is met, externally administered contingencies can be provided based on positive behavioral change. It is suggested that positive reinforcement be the first choice of contingent intervention. Response-cost is probably a good second choice.

4. *Teach Self-Instruction and Attributional Techniques.*   As the ADHD child's behavior begins to change, it is important to begin providing the child with cognitive strategies to modify his behavior. Concomitantly, providing attributional training to reduce helplessness and develop an internal locus of control is also necessary.

5. *Transfer Control of Contingencies to Child.*   Once the child has demonstrated consistent change with externally provided contingencies, has developed cognitive strategies and has demonstrated the use of those strategies, she should be afforded the opportunity to judge, evaluate and reinforce her own behavior. Positive reinforcement is recommended as the initial intervention, although in some situations allowing the child to choose her own punishment for inappropriate behavior can also be beneficial.

6. *Provide Opportunities for Generalization.*   This is a critical and essential step in the process. It is important to provide supervised opportunities for the child to demonstrate and use skills. At times, planning for generalization can be frustrating but must be actively pursued before fading contingencies. Opportunities for time, setting and response generalization must be provided.

7. *Fade Contingencies.*   At this point, the child in all likelihood has begun to internally reinforce himself and will decreasingly require secondary reinforcers. Reinforcement can be faded gradually.

8. *Intermittently Monitor and Provide Maintenance Contingencies.*   It is recommended that at intervals beginning with one week and extending to one month, a brief refresher concerning appropriate behavior and the manner in which the child has made and maintained behavioral change be made. At that point, a positive reinforcer may be provided contingent upon the child's demonstration of continued behavioral change.

Each of the strategies suggested in this model have demonstrated the power to facilitate behavioral change. Some of these strategies have been combined and have experimentally demonstrated both additive and positive interactive effects. Although this model has not been extensively tested, the authors' experience has been that the organized and sequential application of these interventions maximizes the chance of precipitating positive behavioral change with long-lasting potential for generalization.

An example of on-task behavior in the classroom setting can be used to illustrate application of this model. Initially on-task behavior is defined as the child actively engaged in the activity in which the rest of the class is participating. In this case, it will be a mathematics work sheet. On-task behavior is defined as the child either thinking about or actively engaging in writing the answer to one of the problems. Thus, on-task behavior is both an overt and a covert process. The practitioner works with the ADHD child to help her clearly understand this definition through role playing and providing the child with multiple examples of both on- and off-task behavior. The child is then asked to self-record without making a judgment during math time whenever an audible beep sounds in the classroom. Once the child demonstrates the ability to self-record, she is afforded the opportunity to again demonstrate an understanding as to the definition of on- or off-task behavior and at that point is required to self-evaluate during math sessions. The classroom teacher also evaluates the child's behavior, and at the end of each math session brief feedback is provided to the child concerning her accuracy in recording and self-evaluating.

Once the child demonstrates accuracy, external contingencies, in this case points that can be redeemed for secondary reinforcers at the end of the week, are provided contingent on the percentage of on-task behavior. During a brief training time each morning, a verbal, self-instructional program is initiated, and the child is provided with suggestions and ideas to reinforce positive attribution and an internal locus of control. Once the child has demonstrated an understanding of the self-instructional techniques, they are briefly reviewed each time before a math session, and she is instructed to use these techniques to improve on-task behavior. As continued improvement is observed, the child is allowed to self-reinforce, and a number of other school situations are chosen for her where she can use similar techniques. Once generalization has been demonstrated, contingencies are faded, and the child's behavior is intermittently monitored during the remainder of the school year.

TEXT AND SOFTWARE MATERIALS TO TEACH SKILLS AND FACILITATE GENERALIZATION

Text Materials

There are a number of excellent texts that practitioners and teachers can use with children to teach them problem-solving and generalization skills.

Think Aloud (Bash & Camp, 1985)

This program builds very closely on both Meichenbaum and Goodman's original work in teaching verbal mediational strategies to impulsive children and Shure and Spivak's (1978) program to teach solution generalization, means-ends and consequential thinking. This program is designed for elementary school children. There are separate materials for different grades. Implementation is designed for use in a regular classroom with the entire class. The ideal group size seems to be ten children; however, the materials and procedures can be used separately and in a wide variety of settings, including one-to-one instruction.

The program first teaches children to think out loud through modeling a variety of problem behaviors. One lesson builds upon another, first teaching a basic problem-solving approach that asks the questions, *What is my problem? What is my plan? Am I using the best plan?* and *How did I do?* Subsequent lessons teach children to generate alternatives, interpret emotions, plan, take perspective, think logically, reason inductively and handle a variety of social situations.

The leader's manual provides a brief introduction, the specific skill objective to be taught, materials needed, suggestions for implementing the skill, role-playing activities and extension activities for the group leader. The manual also includes a rating scale for teachers to evaluate each child's progress as well as rating scales for trainers to evaluate the progress of others who are being taught to implement the program. Suggestions are made for dealing with problems that may occur during group settings, including behavioral difficulties and children who experience problems mastering the skills being taught.

Bash and Camp report that intellectually deficient or significantly emotionally disturbed children may not have the skills to benefit from this program. The program is based on research data suggesting that adequate development of verbal mediational skills coincides with the ability to use language to facilitate planning, problem solving, learning, and social interaction and the ability to use covert language to block impulsive responding.

Stop and Think Workbook (Kendall, 1988)

This 16-session program is designed for each child to have a workbook. A manual and notes for the trainer are also included. The program provides ideas and materials to teach cognitive strategies for psychoeducational tasks, games, social problems and dealing effectively with emotions. Kendall's program is easy to use with elementary school age children. This program can be used on an individual or small group basis. Unique to this program is Kendall's assertion that a component of affective education must be included in effective cognitive training programs. Many impulsive children are able to practice and learn cognitive strategies in a protected office or playroom setting. Unfortunately, many of these children reach their emotional boiling point before they review the best alternative in problem situations. This program provides an affective component in which children are taught to utilize strategies when they become overemotional. For the interested reader, Kendall and Brasswell (1985) have authored a text on cognitive-behavioral therapy for impulsive children. The text provides guidelines for assessment and treatment as well as ideas for working with parents and teachers. The appendix of the text also includes a manual for helping children to develop self-control.

Comprehension Capers: Main Ideas and Inferences (Ceaser, 1986)

This text, designed for grades one through six, is not a training program per se but provides over 200 reproducible masters that can be used to teach a variety of skills. The materials teach children to reason, classify, identify critical data and make constructive inferences. The materials lend themselves very well to group teaching situations.

Primarily Logic (Leimbach, 1986)

This brief workbook contains 42 lessons, one activity per lesson, to teach the ability to identify relationships, reason deductively, organize information and solve problems. Materials are reproducible and designed for elementary school children. These materials can be used in conjunction with other cognitive training programs. When used on its own, this text requires a significant degree of input by the practitioner.

Problem Solving, Planning and Organizational Tasks: Strategies for Retraining (Parker & TenBrooek, 1987)

This text was developed for use in rehabilitation programs for head-injured individuals. The materials lend themselves very well for use with adolescents. The text contains multiple activities to teach effective problem solving, including skills such as following directions and generating alternatives. The latter section is designed to follow Shure and Spivak's (1978) problem-solving model. The planning and organizing section includes skills such as cooperation, leadership and the application of problem-solving skills. Each section contains multiple activities outlined according to the primary goal, length of activity, strategies for teaching the skill and description of the task. The program is especially useful with adolescents as many of the activities relate to real-life adult-oriented situations, such as making a budget, finding an apartment, shopping or obtaining telephone service.

Blooming: Language Arts (Zachman, Husingh & Barrett, 1988)

This program is based upon Benjamin Bloom's (1956) taxonomy, a hierarchy of learning skills. The activities included are designed for elementary school children. The program includes activities to improve the child's ability to analyze and synthesize information, as well as to evaluate performance. Each activity is structured through Bloom's taxonomy and provides the practitioner with suggestions to facilitate knowledge, comprehension, application, analysis, synthesis and evaluation. These activities are not presented to be used as a comprehensive training program but as supportive activities to facilitate skill development.

Manual of Exercises for Expressive Reasoning (Zachman, Jorgensen, Barrett, Husingh & Snedden, 1982)

This text was developed to facilitate the development of logical thinking skills for children and adolescents. The text presents 15 thinking skill areas with exercises primarily consisting of questions ordered in a hierarchy of difficulty. Thinking skills covered in this text include classifying, comparing, deductive reasoning, sequencing, making inferences, identifying problems and determining solutions. This is a good text to use when a specific skill is to be taught on an individual basis. For example, when the goal is to facilitate consequential thinking, the text provides a list of 100 sample questions beginning with simple questions such as "The boy is riding his bicycle home, what will he do next?" to more complex questions such as "The stop light on the corner isn't working, what might happen?" It is the practitioner's job to facilitate discussion and conversation based on questions such as these. The only drawback is that the text provides minimal suggestions for facilitating the child's or adolescent's participation and interaction.

Cues and Signals Series (Wehrli, 1971)

Although this series was developed as a self-instructional program for improving visual accuracy, the nature of the task requires speed and proficiency in information processing and visual scanning for numerical information. The child or adolescent must reproduce a series of numbers from a sample in sequence based on randomly presented numbers on the stimulus page. The task can be modified in a number of ways, including scanning for a specific sum, difference or exact number.

Creating Line Designs (Womack, 1985)

This program includes four books for kindergarten through ninth graders. It is designed to promote growth in visual perception, tactile awareness and motor abilities. The task involves the child connecting various letters and numbers to form a preplanned design. This is an enjoyable activity and when instructions are followed, creates very interesting designs. Successful performance requires the ability to follow directions effectively and to think sequentially as well as logically.

125 Ways to Be a Better Student: A Program for Study Skill Success (DeBrueys, 1986)

This is an excellent foundational text to facilitate teaching basic study skills, problem solving as it relates to school survival and successful classroom skills. The activities facilitate organization and independence. There are numerous handouts and worksheets. Specific skills dealt with include organization, following directions, responsibility for behavior, test preparation and test taking. Many of the activities can be used independently in other programs, either for individuals or in a group setting.

Special Kid's Stuff (Farnett, Forte & Loss, 1976)

This large volume of activities for elementary school children is presented in an easy-to-follow format to facilitate independent work. Although many of the activities are primarily directed at improving reading and language skills, others are especially useful for ADHD children, including those that facilitate critical listening, finding contextual clues, thinking creatively, associating and developing study skills. The worksheets are reproducible and lend themselves very well to both individual and group work.

Odyssey: A Curriculum for Thinking

Foundations of Reasoning (Adams, Buschelia, DeSanchez & Swets, 1986)

Verbal Reasoning (Nickerson, 1986)

Problem Solving (Grignetti, 1986)

Decision Making (Feehrer & Adams, 1986)

Inventive Thinking (Perkins & Laserna, 1986)

This curriculum was developed as a Harvard University project by Jorge Dominguez and Richard Herrnstein and implemented in Venezuela. The goal of the program is to facilitate children's ability to perform a variety of intellectual tasks. These include reasoning, hypothesis generation, evaluation, problem solving and decision making. Therefore, many of the activities in the volumes referenced can be used effectively with ADHD children.

The program is built on a premise that a child's ability to deal successfully in the environment can be improved when additional ability, strategy, knowledge and positive attitude are engendered. Each manual is divided into several units with a number of lessons in each unit. The lessons are well organized and presented for introduction in a small group or classroom. Each lesson includes a rationale, the objective to be taught, the target behavior to be changed, materials needed and a method for implementing the skills within the classroom. The lessons and skills are presented in logical sequence. For example, the manual on problem solving contains a number of initial lessons designed to teach children to clearly define a problem before taking action. The program is meant to be used on a daily basis with elementary and secondary school students. The manuals can be used independently of each other. However, within each manual specific skills must be taught sequentially, and therefore these materials don't lend themselves to the teaching of an individual skill. The curriculum is a comprehensive compendium of skills and activities following a logical theoretical basis for cognitive development.

Problem Solving and Comprehension (Whimbey & Lochhead, 1986)

This text, designed for adolescents, provides both an outline of methods to increase effective problem solving and a wide range of exercises to facilitate generalization of problem-solving skills. Although the primary purpose of the text is to improve school performance, it is an effective tool for teaching ADHD adolescents more appropriate problem-solving skills. Problem-solving methods taught in the text include thinking out loud, cooperative effort and learning by observing others. Techniques, such as developing the ability to break a problem down into its parts and continuously checking for accuracy during problem solution, are also taught.

Willy the Wisher and Other Thinking Stories: An Open Court Thinking Storybook (Bereiter & Anderson, 1983)

This collection of 49 stories is designed to be read to elementary school children by an adult. At specific points in each story, children are asked questions that require them to analyze the information that has already been provided, evaluate what has happened up to that point, provide alternate solutions to the problems presented and anticipate what might happen at a future point in the story. These stories can be used effectively to improve listening skills and facilitate generalization of cognitive problem solving-skills, including identifying problems, generating alternative solutions and engaging in means-ends and consequential thinking (Spivack & Shure, 1974).

Logical Logic (Gregorich & Armstrong, 1985)

This is a workbook of reproducible worksheets to facilitate critical thinking skills in eight different areas, such as logical thinking and deductive reasoning. Each skill builds on the previous skills taught, and the workbook is best used in its entirety. The majority of the materials appear best suited for adolescents.

Adventures with Logic (Schoenfield & Rosenblatt, 1985)

This set of reproducible worksheets is designed for children in grades five through seven. The activities can be used independently and are designed to facilitate inference, deduction and creative thinking. The materials can be used with an entire class or with one child. The procedures outlined in this text can also to be used as generalization activities for problem-solving skills.

Software

Research in the use of computer technology to teach cognitive skills to attention-deficient children has been limited and has not yet demonstrated unequivocal positive success or the ability to facilitate transfer of skills learned to other situations. Nonetheless, computer technology holds great promise of someday being able to do so. A review of commercially available, general software is included in this chapter. (See Table 10.1.) Names and addresses of software manufacturers and distributors are provided in Appendix 4. Table 10.2 contains a shorter list of software that has been specifically designed to improve attentional skills. The majority of this software was developed for use with head-trauma patients. For example, Wang Neuropsychological Laboratory has developed an attention-training program offering five levels of attention training in the areas of selective, sustained, flexible and sequential attention.

Software is not presented because it can be used as a substitute for direct instruction of cognitive skills, because it teaches cognitive strategies without the direct supervision of an adult or because it teaches skills that are transferable to the real-life situation, but rather because software offers an alternative opportunity for children to practice and apply cognitive skills. When used as a component of a cognitive training program, with direct adult supervision to provide feedback, software offers the opportunity for repeated practice in an enjoyable and reinforcing situation. Most children enjoy computer games. The software may also serve as an intermediate step between instruction and real-life action.

A PROBLEM-SOLVING SKILLS GROUP

Goldstein and Pollock (1988a) developed a 21-skill program to teach effective problem-solving skills to ADHD children. The program is designed to be implemented in six $1\frac{1}{2}$-hour sessions over a six-week period. Although implementation of the program in terms of specific activities is different for children than for adolescents, the basic skills taught remain the same. The authors suggest that the implementation of this program is best in a small group setting, including from three to six children. Fewer than three children in a group does not allow for sufficient interaction or opportunity for role play. More children, especially those with attention and over-arousal problems, tends to be disruptive. A practitioner interested in implementing this program is referred to Goldstein and Pollock (1988a) for specific activities and suggestions both for dealing with problems during the session and for keeping everyone interested in group activities.

Goldstein and Pollock's program uses a reinforcement system titled Withitness, or WINS. WINS, in the form of token reinforcers, are provided frequently and consistently during group sessions. WINS are provided intermittently for appropriate behavior and group participation. The purpose of these reinforcers is to improve attention and participation during the group meeting and to build self-esteem. Depending on the age of group participants, WINS are exchanged for activities at the close of the session or for material reinforcers.

TABLE 10.1. Software to Facilitate Development of Attentional Skills

Name of Program	Source (Manufacturer)	Level (Age)	Reflection	Focus	Sustained Attention	Vigilance	Means-End Thinking	Selective Attention	Generating Alternatives
Choplifter	Broderbund Software, Inc.	7–Adult		X				X	X
Road Rally USA	Bantam Software	12–Adult	X						X
Pickadilly	Actioncraft	5–Adult	X	X			X		
Oregon Trail	MECC	11–15	X						X
David's Midnight Magic	Broderbund Software, Inc.	7–15			X	X			
Yahtzee by Gary A. Foote	Apple Computer Inc.	10–Adult		X			X		X
Frogger	On Line Systems	5–16					X		
Snack Attack by Dan Illowsky	Funtastic, Inc.	5–12						X	
Spies Demise by Alan Zeldin	Penguin Software	7–12			X	X			X
Sky Fox by Ray Tobey	Raymond E. Tobey, Inc.	12–Adult	X			X			
Gremlins	Atari Software. Warner Bros	8–12			X		X		
Ghostbusters	Activision	10–15			X		X		
Root Beer Tapper	Trademark - Bally Midway	5–12	X	X		X			
Conan	Datasoft, Inc.	7–16				X	X		
Wheel of Fortune	Sharedata, Inc.	12–Adult		X					X
Family Feud	Sharedata, Inc.	12–Adult	X						X
Kids on Keys	Spinnaker	7–12			X				X

TABLE 10.1. (Continued)

Name of Program	Source (Manufacturer)	Level (Age)	Reflection	Focus	Sustained Attention	Vigilance	Means-End Thinking	Selective Attention	Generating Alternatives
Typing Tutor I, II, III, IV	Image Producers, Inc.	9–Adult			X				
Winter Games Summer Games	EPYX	10–Adult		X	X	X	X	X	
Four In A Row	Problem Solving Public Domain	5–12	X					X	
Dazzle Draw by David Snider	Broderbund Software, Inc.	10–18					X		
Where in the USA is Carmen San Diego?	Broderbund Software, Inc.	12–18	X				X		X
Where in Europe is Carmen San Diego?	Broderbund Software, Inc.	12–18	X				X		X
Where in the World is Carmen San Diego?	Broderbund Software, Inc.	12–18	X				X		X
Cat 'N Mouse	Mindplay	7–12	X		X		X		
Facemaker	Spinnaker	5–8		X					
Stickybear Opposites	Weekly Reader	5–8			X				X
Stickybear Town Builder	Weekly Reader	5–8					X		
Gertrude's Secrets	The Learning Co.	5–10	X				X		
Think Quick	The Learning Co.	7–10	X						X

TABLE 10.1. (Continued)

Name of Program	Source (Manufacturer)	Level (Age)	Reflection	Focus	Sustained Attention	Vigilance	Means-End Thinking	Selective Attention	Generating Alternatives
Hide 'N Sequence	Sunburst Communications	8–12	X				X		
Word-A-Mation	Sunburst Communications	9–15	X				X		
Word Problems in Math 1,2,3	Scholastic Software	8–12	X	X			X		
Alien Addition by Jerry Chaffin & Bill Maxwell	D L M	6–8		X					X
Alligator Mix	D L M	6–8				X		X	
Dragon Mix	D L M	6–8				X		X	
Clock	Hartley	7–12				X			
Capitalization	Hartley	10–12	X		X				
States & Traits	Designware, Inc.	10–18	X	X	X				
Dyno Quest	Mindplay	10–14	X			X			
Operation Frog	Scholastic Software	10–18	X	X		X			
Mind Puzzlers	MECC	10–18		X					
Survival Math	Sunburst Communications	12–14			X				X
Bagels	MECC	8–12	X						X
Following Written Directions	Microcomputer Educational Programs	10–12					X		
Patterns & Sequence	Hartley	5–7	X		X				

TABLE 10.1. (Continued)

Name of Program	Source (Manufacturer)	Level (Age)	Reflection	Focus	Sustained Attention	Vigilance	Means-End Thinking	Selective Attention	Generating Alternatives
Word Families I	Hartley	6–8	X		X				
Word Families II	Hartley	6–8	X		X				
Pond	Sunburst Communications	7–14	X		X		X		
Mix & Match (Layer Cake)	Sesame Street by Applesoft Basic	7–12	X			X			
Peanuts Picture Puzzler	Random House	5–10	X	X					
Peanuts Maze Marathon	Random House	5–7			X				X
Logic Builders	Scholastic Software	8–12	X		X				
Moptown Hotel by Leslie M. Grimm	The Learning Co.	7–10					X		X
Moptown Parade by Leslie M. Grimm	The Learning Co.	7–10					X		X
Reader Rabbit	The Learning Co.	6–9	X				X		
Writer Rabbit	The Learning Co.	7–10	X				X		
Racetrack	Learning Well	10–14	X			X	X		
Rocky's Boots	The Learning Co.	10–14	X	X					

TABLE 10.1. (Continued)

Name of Program	Source (Manufacturer)	Level (Age)	Reflection	Focus	Sustained Attention	Vigilance	Means-End Thinking	Selective Attention	Generating Alternatives
Bake 'N Taste	Mindplay	7–10		X			X		
Time Capsule	Mindscape Software	8–12		X			X		
Missing Links	Sunburst Communications	8–16			X				
What's First? What's Next?	Hartley	7–10			X		X		
Pictures, Letters & Sounds	Hartley	7–10	X						X
Observation & Classification	Hartley	6–8			X		X		
Code Quest	Sunburst Communications	9–14	X						
Perplexing Puzzles	Hartley	9–14					X		
Facts & Fallacies	Hartley	9–14	X			X			
Odd One Out	Sunburst Communications	8–12							X
High Wire Logic	Sunburst Communications	10–12							
Cause & Effect	Hartley	9–12					X		X
Fact or Opinion	Hartley	9–12	X				X		
Analogies	Hartley	10–16							

TABLE 10.1. (Continued)

Name of Program	Source (Manufacturer)	Level (Age)	Reflection	Focus	Sustained Attention	Vigilance	Means-End Thinking	Selective Attention	Generating Alternatives
Adv. Analogies	Hartley	10–18				X			X
Sequencing	Hartley	8–12	X		X				
Associations	Hartley	10–14	X						
Speed Reader I	Davidson	8–16	X	X					
Speed Reader II	Davidson	8–16	X	X					
Spell It	Davidson	8–16						X	
Word Attack	Davidson	8–16						X	
Math Blaster	Davidson	8–16	X			X	X		
Grammar Gremlins	Davidson	8–16		X					
K.L.S Cognitive Educational Systems by Carl Lambert	Lambert Software Co. Portions Copyrighted by Microsoft Corp.	Wide Range	X	X	X	X	X	X	X

302

TABLE 10.2. Software Designed for Attention Training

Name of Program	Source (Manufacturer)
Computerized Progressive Attention Training (IBM Compatible Only)	Wang Neuropsychological Laboratory
Cognitive Rehabilitation Programs for Brain Injured & Stroke Patients by Odie L. Bracy, III, PhD Attention/Multiple Reasoning (Package of 10 Programs) Simultaneous Multiple Attention (Package of 10 Programs) Vigilance for Omissions (Package of 10 Programs) Vigilance (Respond to X) (Package of 10 Programs) Visual Tracking (Package of 10 Programs) Visual Reaction Stimuli (Package of 10 Programs) Individual Spatial Perception	Psychological Software Services, Inc.
Memory II: Visual Memory (Sequenced/Spatial) Visualspatial: Paddle Ball (Scanning) (Package of 10 Programs)	Psychological Software Services, Inc.
K.L.S. Cognitive Educational System by Carl Lambert	Lambert Software Co. Portions Copyrighted by Microsoft Corp.

Soft Tools
  '83 Simultaneous Multiple Attention (SMA)
  '83 Visual Search
  '83 Search
  '84 Sequential
  '84 City Map
  '84 Shooter
  '85 Visispan
  '85 Guess Which Design
	Cognitive Rehabilitation

Attention Scanning Reaction Time	Network Services
Computer Programs for Cognitive Rehabilitation (Volume 4—Attention)	Life Science Associates
Public Domain Cognitive Games (1987)	Saint Lawrence Rehabilitation Center

Each group session is divided into a number of parts. To begin, homework is reviewed, and skills taught the previous week are briefly demonstrated. During the next part, each new skill is taught and broken down into a step-by-step model for acquisition. For the interested practitioner, each of the skills will be defined and steps for implementation will be reviewed. Role play is then used to demonstrate and practice the skill. Homework is assigned for each skill. Role play and homework activities are not included in this chapter but are available.

It is suggested that the child's parents and teachers complete the Problem-Solving Skills Assessment Questionnaire. This allows the practitioner to identify specific deficiencies for each child and to make a point of emphasizing those skills for that child during the program. This in effect individualizes each child's program within the group setting.

Skills taught are divided into six sessions as follows:

Session I

Recognizing problems

Accepting responsibility for problems

Projecting responsibility for problems onto others

Session II

Solving problems independently

Solving problems with minimal support

Solving problems with significant support

Session III

Generating alternatives independently

Avoiding inappropriate solutions to problems

Choosing the best solution to a problem

Session IV

Implementing a problem solution

Understanding future impact of current solutions

Evaluating problem-solving success

Session V

Listening during a conversation

Following directions

Planning/reflecting

Rewarding self

Session VI

Dealing with own and other's feelings appropriately

Accepting consequences

Reacting to failure

Dealing with peer pressure

The following is an overview of each of these skills taught in the program and the steps suggested to facilitate teaching of the skills.

SKILL: Recognizing Problems

STEPS:

1. Stop!
2. State there is a problem.
3. List possible explanations of problem.
4. State the problem and explanation.

SKILL: Accepting Responsibility for Problems

STEPS:

1. State the problem.
2. List possible causes of the problem.
3. Decide which is the most likely cause.
4. Decide what parts you were involved in.
5. Think about ways to express your ideas.
6. Choose best way to express your involvement.
7. Exercise choice.

SKILL: Projecting Responsibility for Problems Onto Others

STEPS:

1. State the problem.
2. List possible causes of the problem.
3. Decide which is the most likely cause.
4. Decide what parts others were involved in.
5. Think about ways to express your ideas to others.
6. Express ideas.

SKILL: Solving Problems Independently

STEPS:

1. State the problem.
2. Think about steps involved in solving the problem.
3. Prioritize steps.
4. Choose when to work on problem.
5. Choose place to work on problem.
6. Perform steps one at a time.

SKILL: Solving Problems with Minimal Support

STEPS:

1. Identify the problem.
2. Think about steps involved in solving the problem.
3. List steps involved in solving the problem.
4. Listen to other person's ideas about solving the problem.
5. Compare solutions.
6. Choose steps to work on.
7. Work on steps one at a time.
8. Check steps with other person at conclusion of steps.

SKILL: Solving Problems with Significant Support

STEPS:

1. List possible problems.
2. Listen to trainer/person list problems accurately.
3. Identify problem.
4. Check out with trainer/person the problem.
5. Tell trainer/person you do not understand how to solve problem.
6. Trainer/person generates possible solutions.
7. Choose best solution.
8. Check out best solution with trainer.
9. Trainer cues first step.
10. Restate instructions.
11. Complete first step.
12. Repeat cuing and restating until all steps completed.

SKILL: Generating Alternatives Independently

STEPS:

1. List problems.
2. Identify problems from most important to least important.
3. Take action on most important problem; hold off on the less important.
4. List all alternatives for solving the problem.
5. Determine the consequences to each alternative.
6. Prioritize alternatives from most comfortable to least comfortable.
7. Verbalize strategies.

SKILL: Avoiding Inappropriate Solutions to Problem

STEPS:

1. Stop! (Count to 10.)
2. Think about your actions and verbalize them.
3. List solutions.
4. Think through steps of solutions.
5. Decide if solutions will get you into trouble or generate negative feelings.
6. List other ways to act.
7. Choose best way, best time and best place to act.
8. Communicate choice to others at appropriate time.

SKILL: Choosing the Best Solution to the Problem

STEPS:

1. Identify problem.
2. Gather information.
3. List possible solutions.
4. Evaluate each solution in relationship to present circumstances.
5. Think about steps involved in each solution.
6. Prioritize solutions.
7. Identify solution #1.

SKILL: Implementing a Problem Solution

STEPS:

1. Identify solution.
2. Gather additional information.

3. List additional solutions.
4. Consider consequences of additional solutions.
5. Pause—take additional time.
6. Reconsider original solution using new information.
7. Choose best solution.
8. Exercise choice one step at a time.
9. Evaluate.

SKILL: Understanding Future Impact of Current Problem Solving

STEPS:

1. STOP! THINK about solution (time, place, etc.).
2. Decide what you want to happen.
3. Decide if you control happenings.
4. Think about how you have done in the past.
5. Think about how your solution will affect you.
6. Think about how your solution will affect others.

SKILL: Evaluating Problem-Solving Successes

STEPS:

1. Identify problem.
2. Identify solution.
3. Think about how you completed tasks.
4. Decide if all steps were completed.
5. Reward yourself as soon as possible.

SKILL: Listening During a Conversation

STEPS:

1. Face person who is talking.
2. Attend to what is being said.
3. Wait your turn to talk.
4. Ask questions about topic.
5. Say what you think about the topic, clarify, etc.

SKILL: Following Directions

STEPS:

1. Listen.
2. Look at person who is talking.

3. Think about what is being said.

4. Wait your turn to talk.

SKILL: Planning/Reflecting

STEPS:

1. Define the goal/task.
2. Gather information.
3. List steps to complete task.
4. Think about each step in regard to previous experience.
5. Think about each step in regard to order, skills, resources, etc.
6. Ask for help, if needed.
7. Perform steps one at a time.
8. Think about each step as it is completed.
9. Complete all steps.
10. Think about how you did.

SKILL: Rewarding Self

STEPS:

1. Decide what you have done to deserve a reward.
2. List ways to reward yourself.
3. Choose the best way.
4. Say or do it as soon as possible following the task you are rewarding yourself for.

SKILL: Dealing with Own Feelings Appropriately

STEPS:

1. Think about how you feel.
2. Think about what you feel.
3. Determine what happened to make you feel this way.
4. List ways you could express feeling or ways you could act.
5. Choose best way.
6. Exercise choice.

SKILL: Dealing with Other's Feelings Appropriately

STEPS:

1. Observe other person.
2. Listen to what other person is saying.

3. List feelings you think other person may be having.
4. Identify a specific feeling you think other person is having.
5. Decide if you need to verify it with other person.
6. Think about ways you could show the other person you understand his/her feelings.

SKILL: Accepting Consequences Appropriately

STEPS:

1. Identify action you took or neglected to take.
2. Explain what your thinking was.
3. Ask other person what he/she thinks about the action.
4. List ways to react.
5. Select best ways to react.
6. Exercise best way.

SKILL: Reacting to Failure Appropriately

STEPS:

1. Decide if you have failed.
2. Think about what happened.
3. Determine why you failed.
4. Think about what you could do differently next time.
5. Ask questions; gather information.
6. Try again, using new information.

SKILL: Dealing with Peer Pressure Appropriately

STEPS:

1. Listen to what others want you to do.
2. Think about what could happen.
3. Think about what you want to do.
4. Think about what could happen.
5. Decide what is best for you.
6. Explain to others what *you* want to do (may include explanation of why you cannot go along with what others want you to do).
7. Suggest alternative plan.

SUMMARY

Cognitive-mediational interventions have repeatedly demonstrated the ability to facilitate behavioral change in ADHD children in a wide variety of situations and for a wide range of behaviors. These interventions hold great promise and are well accepted as essential components of a multitreatment program. This chapter attempted to categorize types of cognitive skills taught to children, review briefly the research literature for each skill and present specific recommendations to the practitioner for implementing these skills with ADHD children. Text and software materials that can be used to facilitate the teaching process were presented and reviewed. An integrated cognitive-behavioral model was suggested to provide the practitioner with a logical system to follow when attempting to use these skills to facilitate behavioral change. This chapter also reviewed a number of self-instructional training programs and presented a six-week training program used by the authors to teach problem solving to children and adolescents.

CHAPTER 11

Managing and Educating the ADHD Child at School

It is not surprising that the ADHD child has had increasing problems in our school system over the past 20 years. Successful performance is increasingly dependent on the ability to persist, maintain concentration for long periods of time, inhibit bodily movement, maintain an appropriate level of arousal and delay gratification until report cards are issued. Schools are demanding competence in these skills at earlier ages. It is essential for the practitioner to assist the ADHD child's teachers in understanding the mechanics of the educational system and the reasons why these particular children are at significant risk to be unable to meet the demands of the classroom. In school, ADHD children often develop a host of secondary behavioral and adjustment problems in response to frequent and repeated failure. The model presented in this chapter is not meant as a step-by-step, all-encompassing classroom management or educational system. Teachers are unique and very different in their styles. The guidelines and suggestions offered in this chapter are presented in a generic fashion. It is up to the practitioner to help teachers understand their particular interactional style and make use of specific interventions that may fit within that style. This chapter will also briefly review dimensions of teacher behavior in an effort to help practitioners identify teacher variables that may increase or decrease the ability to deal with an ADHD child in the classroom.

Effective management and education of the ADHD child in the classroom is a multistep process. The effective teacher must understand the ADHD child's behaviors from the perspective of developmental impairment. The teacher must be able to make the distinction between incompetent and noncompliant behavior. The teacher must understand, at least in a basic sense, the causes of these problems, the developmental course and the common symptomatic manifestations of ADHD in the classroom. The effects that specific behaviors such as punishment and negative reinforcement may have, secondarily, upon this population of children must also be understood. The second step involves helping the teacher identify and define problematic behavior in the classroom. Once identified, problems can be prioritized and interventions developed. Interventions will be situation-specific, implemented within the classroom or in a nonclassroom setting. Interventions are then stratified according to those that are designed to help the child manage himself versus those that alter the environment, thereby assisting the child to function more effectively.

ESSENTIAL BACKGROUND DATA FOR TEACHERS

The easiest and most economical way to educate teachers concerning definition, problems, cause and developmental course of attention disorders in childhood is to provide resource materials. Short texts and pamphlets written especially for teachers (Coleman, 1988; Goldstein and Goldstein, 1987; Friedman and Doyal, 1987; Silver, 1980b) are preferred. Interested teachers desiring more in-depth materials can be referred to Barkley (1981), Ross and Ross (1982), Loney (1987) or the opening chapters of this text. In the coming few years a number of training videotapes for teachers should also be available on this subject. It cannot be too strongly emphasized that the practitioner make certain the classroom teacher has a basic understanding of attention disorder before suggesting the implementation of classroom interventions that may require the teacher to make significant changes in style and routine. The teacher making change based on understanding will be an active, motivated participant. The teacher lacking in understanding and uncertain why these interventions may help will be a passive, frequently unsuccessful, change agent.

DEFINING PROBLEMATIC BEHAVIOR

It is essential for the practitioner to assist teachers both to define the child's behavioral difficulties and to specify the situations in which those difficulties are manifest. The assessment process often accomplishes this task, allowing the practitioner to provide the classroom teacher with a summary of the child's problems and their situational occurrences. It may also be beneficial for the practitioner to request teachers to prioritize behavioral problems of greatest concern and the situations in which they occur. Often it is impossible for the practitioner to address all of the ADHD child's behavioral and situational problems within the classroom simultaneously. By providing the classroom teacher with relief for the most problematic behaviors and situations, the practitioner immediately is seen as a valuable ally. The reduction of one or two severe problems often makes other behavioral difficulties much more bearable for the classroom teacher.

It is essential for the practitioner to help teachers operationally define behavioral problems and to take baseline data before initiating intervention. Data can be collected in a number of ways. Some behaviors lend themselves easily to one particular form of data collection rather than to another. Other behaviors can be scored and observed in a number of ways, depending specifically on the teacher's need.

An example of a classroom behavior, one which was briefly reviewed in Chapter 4, is the number of times a child leaves his seat. In a given period of time, the teacher may be concerned with the frequency of the behavioral occurrence. How many times does the child leave his seat during a half-hour lesson? A sample tally can record number of occurrences. In other situations, the absolute number of out-of-seat behaviors may not be as important as the amount of time spent out of seat. In this case, the teacher would record duration data and arrive at a time score for total number of minutes out of seat during the half-hour lesson. Finally, in some situations, neither frequency nor duration is as important as the pattern in which these behaviors occur. For example, a child may remain in his seat for the first 15 minutes but then be out of his seat 12 times in the last 15 minutes of the lesson. Recording either frequency or duration data for this child would not really help the practitioner and teacher understand the process of what is occurring in the classroom. In such a situation, interval recording is best. During a fixed interval such as 10 or 15 seconds, the observer either responds yes or no for the target behavior. It makes no difference whether the child is out of his seat once, twice or an infinite number of times during the interval. If the child is out of his seat even once, an affirmative score is given. The data is then observed on a continuum, and the intervals and the progression of the child's behavior during the half-hour lesson are noted. Interval data collection is also helpful since some classroom behavior problems are difficult to define in terms of a beginning and ending.

EDUCATIONAL PROGRAMMING

Teachers are often surprised to learn that all-encompassing, specifically developed classroom programs for attention problems are not available. A number of factors have contributed to this phenomenon, including the fact that for a long time problems with attention and overarousal were seen as transitional difficulties of 6- to 12-year-old children. There has also been a very strong emphasis on the use of medications as a means of helping children control themselves rather than on managing the child's differences through environmental manipulation. Finally, the emphasis on behavior modification and special education placement has resulted in teachers developing the attitude that children who are different in the classroom, regardless of their difference, must be educated outside of the classroom in a special education setting.

Numerous types of special classrooms and curricula have been suggested for attention-deficient children, but none has demonstrated magical properties. Some people have advocated an open classroom in order to allow children to choose whatever tasks and activities they would like to pursue. Open classrooms are often places where children have both considerable flexibility in scheduling and more individualized instruction. Research studies have not clearly demonstrated that the open classroom is beneficial for the attention-disordered child. The child may not create as many problems for the teacher in such a setting, but often very little else is accomplished.

In contrast to an open classroom, Strauss and Lehtinen (1947) hypothesized that on-task performance improves and activity level decreases when environmental stimulation is reduced. Minimally distracting environments continue to be advocated in special education classrooms through the use of individual cubicles. Again, research, at some points promising, has not clearly demonstrated that attention-deficit children significantly benefit from such an educational approach.

The practitioner, inside or outside the educational system, must understand reality within the special education system today. For whatever reasons, public education has chosen not to acknowledge problems with attention and overarousal as requiring special education assistance within the schools. Despite the fact that these are the most common problems of childhood, educators continue to provide programs based on available dollars and legislators' opinions, choosing to focus intervention almost exclusively on achievement. In reality, the majority of children with attention and arousal problems will spend most, if not all, of their time in a regular classroom setting. To the extent that the practitioner can assist teachers by providing practical, common sense interventions within the classroom, these children will benefit. Chapters 10 and 12 review problem-solving, cognitive attribution, self-control and socialization skills in depth. These skills are often provided in multisession programs presented over a number of weeks and offered to children in a small group setting. Although ADHD skill-deficient children appear to benefit most from a multiskill program, many of the ideas reviewed in these chapters can be extrapolated and given to teachers to use as interventions within the classroom.

The practitioner must also carefully listen in an effort to understand the teacher's style and which types of interventions might fit best with that style. At a later point in this chapter, teacher personality variables will be reviewed and a model of the effective teacher for an attention-deficit child will be presented. The classroom suggestions that follow are based on generalizations from a wide range of classroom research. They are divided between child-centered interventions designed to help the child with self-management and teacher-centered interventions that manipulate the environment and thereby make it easier for the child to function. It is important that the practitioner help teachers understand that teacher-centered interventions lead to immediate, effective management but may not facilitate long-term improvements in problems of incompetence when the interventions are no longer used. Child-centered interventions, on the other hand, are directed at helping the child develop skills to overcome a problem of incompetence, and success is measured in long-term, observable change following training.

Child-Centered Interventions

Directions

Compliance and task completion increase when teachers provide simple, single directions and seek feedback from the child. The ADHD child does not respond well to multiple instructions. Often, teachers are unaware of the complexity of instructions they provide in the classroom. It may be beneficial for the practitioner to help teachers focus on the manner in which they provide instructions in the classroom. For many ADHD children, the teacher's awareness of the complexity of instructions being given often results in a simplification of instructions and increased compliance by the ADHD child.

316 Managing and Educating the ADHD Child at School

REPEAT DIRECTIONS. Compliance within the classroom increases when the ADHD child is required to repeat directions. When group instructions are given, this intervention may be difficult to implement. It is suggested that once the group is given an instruction, the teacher then approach the ADHD child and request the child to repeat the instruction, even if the child has begun to comply. The teacher may approach with a reinforcer indicating that the child is doing a good job but nevertheless ask the child to restate the direction.

State Rules

Compliance with instructions and classroom procedure increases when the ADHD child is often required to state rules out loud. On an intermittent basis the teacher may ask the child to explain the rules of a specific situation. For example, before sending the ADHD child out to recess, the teacher may ask the child to quickly review the rules of the playground and the kind of behavior that is expected.

Produce Self-Directed Speech

In Chapter 10, strategies to increase cognitive self-monitoring and reduce impulsive behavior were presented. The core component of some of these strategies involves teaching the child to verbalize out loud. If the child produces self-directed speech audibly, he must stop, consider what he is going to do, listen to himself talk about the problem and consider potential solutions. Self-directed speech is a slowdown procedure that increases the likelihood that the child may consider other alternatives rather than making an impulsive, often inappropriate choice.

Teach Self-Pacing

ADHD children often function better if they can provide their own schedule and pacing for work completion rather than having an imposed timetable. In many classroom situations, this is not always possible. However, teaching the ADHD child to structure work and divide larger tasks into small parts that can then be approached and accomplished will increase task completion in the classroom. In some situations, self-pacing is facilitated by the teacher providing smaller portions of work, which increases the likelihood the child will successfully complete the task. Whalen and Henker (1985) demonstrated that during self-paced periods the intensity of the ADHD child's behavioral problems was lower than in situations in which the child's behavior was paced by others.

Provide Cues

Providing the ADHD child with external visual or auditory cues that do not directly involve teacher intervention can be beneficial in maintaining appropriate classroom behavior and fostering the completion of class work. External, self-monitored cues help the ADHD child to be an active participant in behavior change. An auditory or visual cue has been found to be as effective as direct teacher monitoring (Hayes and Nelson, 1983). Providing an auditory cue, such as running a tape on which an audible, variable stimulus reminds the child to check and make sure that she is working, has been demonstrated to result in increased on-task behavior and academic performance (Blick and Test, 1987).

The success of such a system requires the student to be motivated and cooperative. This intervention often works best with older students. The authors have successfully used a similar model in which an ADHD adolescent wore a portable cassette player and headphones so that the auditory cues did not disturb the rest of the classroom. In some situations with older students, it is also beneficial to have the student keep a record when the auditory cue sounds of whether or not she was on task. Studies have suggested that students who were more accurate in recording their behavior were on task more often than the less accurate recorders (Hallahan and Sapona, 1983). Self-management procedures such as this have also proven effective in stimulating generalization of skills (Stokes and Baer, 1977), a frequently encountered problem in teaching attention and reflection skills. The practitioner interested in expanding a repertoire of behavior analysis and recording skills in the classroom is referred to Tawney and Gast (1984).

Teacher-Centered Interventions

Transitions

ADHD children move easiest from formal to informal, focused to unfocused or structured to unstructured settings. If the teacher allows the ADHD child a few extra minutes in the morning to unwind and be off task, it makes it even more difficult to get the child settled down and focused on task requirements. The ADHD child is often the first to stop working even during small interruptions such as someone entering the classroom. She may be the last child to settle down and return to work after an informal break, such as recess. In team-teaching situations, she will have trouble moving from one classroom to another. She may be the last student to start working but the first to stop working. Keeping such informal transitions to a minimum, providing additional structure during transitional periods, providing positive reinforcement contingent on the child's ability to successfully complete the transition and helping the ADHD child settle into a formal setting again, can have a significant positive impact on the child's overall functioning in the classroom.

Teacher Pacing

Often, attempts to teach the ADHD child to pace himself prove difficult. In such situations, the teacher's ability to understand how much the child can successfully accomplish before difficulty with attention and distractibility becomes overwhelming can be very helpful. The teacher can then provide a small amount of work to ensure that the child will remain on task, provide reinforcement when the task is completed and very quickly provide another brief task. For the ADHD child, several shortened work periods will result in more work completion and fewer off-task behavioral problems than longer work sessions.

Consistent Routine

ADHD children function significantly better in a consistent setting. Varying the sequence of daily activities may be confusing, decrease attention to task and hamper work completion for the ADHD child. The impulsive, spontaneous teacher may match very well with the gifted, attentive child. The ADHD child, however, will experience problems in such a classroom.

KEEP THINGS CHANGING.   Within the routine, however, the ADHD child will function significantly better if provided with multiple, shortened work periods, variable tasks and intermittent, enjoyable reinforcers.

Allow Movement

We are now well aware that it is the inattentive, disorganized, impulsive style of the ADHD child that primarily interferes with successful classroom performance, not the child's activity level. It is important for the practitioner to help teachers focus and prioritize their goals for the ADHD child in the classroom. Most teachers will designate organization and work completion as priorities. It is important to help teachers understand that the ADHD child, even when functioning successfully in the classroom, may exhibit more restless, overactive behavior than other children. This pattern of behavior need not be a detriment if teachers are flexible and the child is completing work and being positively reinforced.

Feedback

Teachers frequently observe that there appears to be a direct relationship between the amount of one-to-one instruction ADHD children receive and their compliance and task completion. It is obvious that attention-deficient children function significantly better if they can be provided with immediate feedback and increased teacher attention. In some situations, moving a child's desk closer to the teacher's facilitates positive interaction. In other situations, teachers should have the opportunity to employ adult aides or even children from upper grades as peer tutors during independent work periods. It is also important for teachers to understand the role of both positive and negative reinforcement. Often, the social feedback ADHD children receive from teachers is negative and contributes to the child's view of the world as a place where she does not often succeed and where she complies with requests to avoid aversive consequences. Some teachers must be coached to provide numerous positive instructions, reinforcers and social feedback to the ADHD child.

POSITIVE REINFORCEMENT.   White (1975) found that in the early elementary school grades, teachers exhibit a significant degree of positive reinforcement for desirable behavior. By middle elementary school and through secondary school, however, teachers begin paying increasingly greater attention to undesirable behavior and less attention to appropriate behavior. This naturally occurring pattern places the ADHD child at a greater disadvantage since in the first few grades when teachers appear to be making a conscious effort to positively reinforce their students, the ADHD child often does not receive his share. In the later grades, as teachers exhibit less positive reinforcement, perhaps because they feel it is not needed, the ADHD child is at even greater risk as an increasing pattern of negative reinforcement develops between this child and the teacher. The practitioner must help teachers understand that the appropriate application of positive reinforcement has repeatedly been demonstrated to increase both on-task behavior and work completion (Kirby and Shields, 1972).

If teachers are going to structure special positive reinforcement programs in the classroom, it is important that such programs begin at a level at which the ADHD child can succeed and be positively reinforced. All too often, teachers set up wonderful behavioral programs but set criteria too high initially, and the ADHD child never tastes success. The practitioner must assist teachers to define the problematic behavior in an operational sense and obtain a level of baseline occurrence. It is suggested that at first reinforcement be provided when the child is at or slightly better than baseline. For example, if a child is out of his seat ten times during a work period, reinforcement can be provided initially if the child is out of his seat no more than eight times. As the child succeeds, the necessary criteria for reinforcement can be gradually tightened, requiring fewer out-of-seat behaviors during a given period of time.

Bushell (1973) cautions that some consequences teachers provide for children are irrelevant and neither strengthen nor weaken the behavior that they follow. Although the teacher may feel that placing stars on a chart or providing a toy are consequences that all children will work for, this may not be the case. Although some children may be motivated by these consequences, others may not be. Therefore, the fact that certain consequences follow a child's behavior may neither strengthen nor weaken the chances for that particular behavior to reoccur. Bushell refers to consequences that are irrelevant as "noise." These are neutral consequences that have no effect on the behavior they follow. The practitioner must make certain that consequences chosen in the classroom are reinforcing and not "noise." A reinforcement inventory completed by the ADHD child often facilitates this process.

NEGATIVE REINFORCEMENT.   The most powerful event in the classroom for the ADHD student appears to be the pattern of negative reinforcement that develops between student and teacher. Clark and Elliott (1988) found that negative reinforcement was rated by teachers as the most frequently used classroom intervention. It is important to help teachers understand the role they play in providing the ADHD child with a negative reinforcer to begin tasks but not to complete them. Within the classroom setting, ADHD students frequently return to the task at hand in an effort to avoid an aversive consequence, usually the teacher's attention to the fact the child is off task. Once the teacher's attention is removed, the child has been negatively reinforced and stops working. Thus, ADHD children in the classroom are both victims of their temperament, which makes it difficult for them to complete tasks, and their learning history, which reinforces them for beginning but frequently not for finishing.

There are a number of simple ways to help teachers deal with this problem. If the teacher is going to use negative reinforcement, it is important to pay attention to the ADHD student until the assignment is completed. This, too, is a negative reinforcer, but it teaches the child that the only way to get rid of the aversive consequence, teacher attention, is not just to start but to complete the task at hand.

A second alternative involves the use of differential attention or ignoring. The term differential attention applies when ignoring is used as the negative consequence for exhibiting the undesirable behavior and attention is used as the positive consequence for exhibiting the competing, desirable behavior. This is an active process in which the teacher ignores the child engaged in an off-task activity, but pays attention immediately when the child begins working. Many teachers avoid interaction with the ADHD child while she is on task for fear of interrupting the child's train of thought. It is important, however, to reinforce the child when she is working so that a pattern of working to earn positive reinforcement rather than working to avoid negative reinforcement is developed.

Differential attention is a very powerful intervention when used appropriately. Teachers must also understand that once they begin ignoring inappropriate behavior, they must continue to ignore that behavior despite escalation, or run the risk of intermittently reinforcing the negative behavior, thereby strengthening its occurrence. For example, if a teacher decides to use differential attention for a child's out-of-seat behavior, but becomes sufficiently frustrated after the child is out of her seat for ten minutes that she then pays attention to the child, this will reinforce rather than extinguish out-of-seat behavior.

DIFFERENTIAL REINFORCEMENT.   When consequences are provided for two competing behaviors, this is referred to as differential reinforcement of other behavior (Sulzer-Azaroff and Mayer, 1977). It is important for the practitioner to help teachers understand that this can be a very powerful intervention. The target behavior that is to be decreased can be provided with a negative consequence, such as ignoring or punishment, when it occurs, while the competing positive behavior can be praised and reinforced when it occurs. Competing behaviors might include teasing or playing cooperatively, aggression or negotiation and emotional outbursts or self-control when frustrated. Differential attention is a differential reinforcement procedure.

Incompetence Versus Noncompliance

As outlined for parents in Chapter 13, it is equally important for teachers to understand the distinction between behavior resulting from incompetence, which must be dealt with through education, and behavior resulting from noncompliance, which must be dealt with through appropriate consequences. The practitioner may find it helpful to use many of the techniques in Chapter 13 with teachers as well. Often the teacher-student relationship is very similar to the parent-child relationship.

BE POSITIVE.   It is important for teachers to understand the need to tell ADHD students what they want to have happen rather than what they do not want to have happen. This appears to be a very simple concept but it is the essence of being positive. If a student is exhibiting a behavior that the teacher does not like, instead of pointing out that behavior, the teacher can tell the ADHD student what she wants to see happen instead. The emphasis on what is to be done as opposed to what is to be stopped will help the ADHD child understand the task demands and teacher's needs. This also avoids the frequent dilemma of the child following the teacher's direction to stop a particular behavior but then engaging in an alternate nonproductive behavior. By counseling teachers to tell the ADHD student specifically what they want to have happen, the stage is set, if the student doesn't follow through, to punish noncompliance.

Multiple Reinforcers

It is important for the practitioner to help teachers develop a hierarchy of the behaviors that they would like to see the ADHD child exhibit in the classroom. For example, in response to out-of-seat behavior, many teachers may initiate a reinforcement system to increase in-seat behavior. Although the child may earn multiple reinforcers for remaining in his seat, this does not guarantee that he will engage in constructive or appropriate behavior while remaining seated. Often multiple levels of reinforcement must be initiated. For example, the child can be provided with a reinforcer for sitting and a second reinforcer for working while sitting.

FAVORITE REINFORCERS.   Paine, Ridicchi, Rosellini, Deutchman and Darch (1983) found that additional recess, free time in class, material reinforcers, field trips and games in class were the five most frequent reinforcement ideas suggested by elementary school students. Intermediate grade students more frequently favored activities that involved interaction with teachers, including acting as an assistant in grading papers, carrying on a discussion or playing a game on a one-to-one basis.

Response Cost

Most teachers understand response cost as a system in which students lose positive reinforcers they have earned for appropriate behavior when they exhibit inappropriate behavior. A slightly altered form of response cost has been found effective with hyperactive children (Rapport, Murphy and Bailey, 1982). Under this system, the child is initially provided with the maximum number of points or tokens that can be earned during a school day and must work throughout the school day to keep those tokens. Possibly because ADHD children have a long history of not working well for positive reinforcement, a system in which they are provided with all of their reinforcement initially and must work to keep it may appear more motivating. A response cost system can be as simple as chips in a cup or marks on a chart placed on the student's desk or pinned to the student's shirt, or as complex as the Attention Training System (Rapport, 1987). The Attention Training System is a remote-controlled counter that sits on the student's desk. This device provides the student with a digital read-out showing the number of points he has earned. Using a remote-control device, the classroom teacher can add or remove a point from anywhere in the classroom contingent upon the child's on- or off-task behavior.

Use Cognitive Interventions

Although referred to by a variety of labels, such as cognitive behavior modification, self-control procedures, problem solving or attributional training, these interventions share a basic foundation in that they attempt to teach children to think differently and through different thinking to modify their behavior. Such strategies, when combined with stimulant medication and behavior modification, have led to significant improvements in classroom functioning for the inattentive child (Horn and Ialongo, 1988; Pelham et al., 1980). Although allegations have been made that cognitive self-control training alone or in combination with other interventions is neither particularly helpful nor as helpful as the use of stimulant medication (Abikoff, 1985; Abikoff and Gittelman, 1985), other researchers in the field have suggested that such strategies may be particularly effective in reducing impulsive behavior (Horn and Ialongo, 1988).

Build Success

It is most important that interactions with ADHD students end successfully. Because of the pattern of negative reinforcement that ADHD students frequently elicit from teachers and the multiple failures they frequently experience, they often end up being punished without being given the opportunity to succeed. Teachers must be counseled that they need to be certain that the ADHD student has an opportunity to try again, succeed and be praised. Teachers must be helped to understand that many ADHD children develop a view of the world as a place where they are unable to succeed and over time develop feelings of helplessness and poor motivation. It is important for the practitioner to help teachers develop a system to provide frequent positive reinforcement for the ADHD student's successes, no matter how minor they may be.

Prepare for Changes

Unexpected or unexplained changes often precipitate significant behavioral problems in ADHD children because of their tendency to become overaroused easily and their difficulty in moving from one setting to another. Teachers may be counseled to help the ADHD child prepare for changes by mentioning the amount of time remaining in a work period and by taking the child aside to explain any change in routine that might occur later in the day. This will help the ADHD child anticipate changes and respond more appropriately.

Adjust Expectations

The practitioner must help teachers understand that successful performance of the ADHD child in the classroom is as much the result of changes in the teacher's expectation as it is of the provision of additional educational, behavioral or medical interventions. Some teachers develop extensive reinforcement systems that do not take into account the ADHD child's developmental impairments. As noted earlier, the very child that a specific classroom intervention may have been designed for may not have the competence to succeed, thus creating increased frustration for everyone involved. It is helpful for teachers to understand that in some settings, the best immediate solution for a child with a short attention span is to structure the environment so that the child is not required to concentrate for long periods of time. Cognitive and behavioral interventions can then be developed to slowly increase the child's concentrational skills.

Preventive Strategies

The practitioner must help teachers anticipate potential problems and develop preventive, as opposed to reactionary, strategies. A thorough understanding of the ADHD child's skills and abilities facilitates preventive intervention. Some teachers may benefit from considering the task demands placed upon the ADHD child during a typical day and planning specific strategies for situations where problems are anticipated. In a preventive model, teachers can be taught to intervene by modifying the environment, such as altering the demands placed upon the ADHD child, or by modifying the child through the use of educational opportunities to increase competence. Although preventive strategies may not totally avoid problems, they certainly will help to minimize the severity of problems and retard the development of secondary adjustment problems resulting from repeated failure.

BEGINNING THE SCHOOL YEAR.   One of the best preventive strategies is to educate a new teacher about the ADHD child's history and abilities. Parents often hesitate to inform teachers about the child's previous academic and behavioral problems in an effort to avoid teacher bias. Although this approach is valid, more often than not, it leads to increased problems because during the first few weeks of school, the teacher places pressure on the ADHD child to conform without understanding that the child cannot do so. It is important for the practitioner to understand, and help parents to understand, that the teacher is a professional and part of the child's treatment team. It is beneficial for parents to meet with the ADHD child's teacher before the beginning of the school year. It may also be beneficial for parents to allow the practitioner working with the ADHD child to speak with the teacher. The first few weeks of school are critical in determining consistent classroom routine, normative behavior and the teacher-child relationship. The informed teacher can closely monitor the ADHD child during the first few weeks of school, identify and understand potential problems and begin preventive intervention strategies.

Further Suggestions

Some teachers may request detailed programs or models to implement in the classroom either because there are a number of ADHD or behaviorally difficult children in that classroom or because the teacher simply wishes to develop alternative skills. Teachers can be referred to texts by Paine et al. (1983), Sulzer-Azaroff and Mayer (1977), Bushell (1973), or Buckley and Walker (1970). These texts provide very specific suggestions for structuring and modifying classroom routine.

THE PRACTITIONER AS CLASSROOM CONSULTANT

It is important for the practitioner to be sensitive to the teacher's ability and the demands of the classroom. Some teachers are unable to make significant changes in their teaching style or may not have the time to implement more extensive interventions. It is important that the practitioner not encourage a power struggle between the child's family and the school in an effort to obtain interventions within the classroom. In some situations, changing the child to another teacher or providing out-of-school interventions is in the long-term best interest of the child.

Teachers often feel alienated and misunderstood by professionals outside of the classroom or educational system. Community-based professionals often make recom-
mendations and provide reports directly to parents concerning what should happen in the classroom, without ever communicating with the teacher or understanding that teacher's personal style. This creates secondary problems rather than contributing to successful intervention and effective management of the ADHD child's problems within the classroom. As a practitioner outside of the school system, it is important for you to communicate with teachers. Communication can be encouraged by sending a brief accompanying letter with the teacher questionnaires during the evaluative process. It may be beneficial to ask the teacher to provide input concerning specific areas of problems, their current concerns and questions they would like to see addressed in an evaluation. Once permission is obtained from the parents, providing the educational team with a copy of the written evaluation or making a follow-up phone call to the classroom teacher also helps to establish a professional link between yourself and the school, setting the groundwork for future communication. For physicians, teacher's feedback and observations of the child's behavioral change in the classroom in response to medication is essential. If teachers perceive that they are respected and their input is valued, they become an important and valuable component in the child's treatment program.

For psychologists, both in and outside of the school system, it is important to communicate with teachers and understand their personality styles and classroom systems. Suggestions for behavior management and change must be made within the context of the existing system. As described later in this chapter, some teaching styles and personalities will simply not adapt well to certain behavioral recommendations. Making those recommendations rigidly without understanding the teacher's style and personality will result in increased problems and, in all likelihood, increased resistance from the teacher. Teachers must also be encouraged to communicate with the practitioner whenever concerns are raised or help is needed. The message from the practitioner to the classroom teacher must be clear: *You are an essential part of the ADHD child's treatment team.* This is true both for special education and regular education teachers. Frequently, special education teachers can act as a liaison, providing additional assistance and ideas to the regular classroom teacher.

Dealing with Noncompliant Parents

One of the most frustrating aspects of attempting to evaluate and treat ADHD children is dealing with parents who experience the very same cluster of temperamental problems as their child. This often precipitates an inability to follow through with recommendations. Even more frustrating are parents who, for whatever reasons,

either deny or choose to ignore the child's problems and are unwilling to participate to help their child. This situation tends to create significant problems for
the practitioner within the school setting. Some parents are unresponsive to the
educational team's request for increased parental support at home and in extreme
situations deny the school system the right to provide special education services.
In such situations, it may be beneficial for the classroom teacher to refer such
parents to an outside practitioner or family physician to discuss the child's current
behavioral and possible medical problems. It is important for teachers not to engage
in a power struggle with parents in which the basic issue becomes the school's
advocacy for the child to be placed on medication for behavioral problems. This
is an inappropriate position for the school to be in and frequently results in more
anger and resentment from parents than compliance.

Managing Medication

Chapter 9 contains an overview of methods for collecting essential data that
the physician requires to effectively manage medication. It is important for the
practitioner to help teachers understand that the use of psychoactive medications
with children is scientifically sound and that treatment decisions are based on
changes observed in the child on an ongoing, rather than on a one-time evaluative
process. The practitioner must provide classroom teachers with a realistic overview
of medication and the areas of problems that can be addressed through medication
intervention. Teachers, like the rest of the population, can form very distorted
opinions about medications, ranging from ideas that they may cause all kinds of
additional problems and are unwarranted to viewing medications as a "miracle
cure."

TEACHING STYLES

There is no support for the notion that a generic set of teaching skills is effective
for most students in most situations. Few, if any, specific teacher behaviors are
appropriate in all contexts. Several patterns of behavior appear to be consistently
related to learning gains for all students. Effective teachers focus on academic
goals; carefully select instructional goals and materials; structure and plan learning
activities; involve students in the learning process; closely monitor student progress;
and provide frequent feedback concerning progress and accomplishments.

Effective teachers develop the ability to organize and maintain the classroom
learning environment in order to maximize time spent engaged in productive
activities and minimize time lost during transition periods or for disruptions that
require disciplinary action. The ADHD child's tendency to disrupt classroom
functioning can stress even the most effective teacher. Kounin (1970) used the
term "withitness" to describe the successful classroom teacher. "Withit" teachers
are organized and manage time well. They do not tolerate negative behavior, allow
interruptions during class activity, socialize extensively during academic times or
engage in nonteaching behaviors to a significant degree during class time.

ugg suggestedm studentslassroom discipline with in studentsley (1986) suggested that effective teachers develop a workable set of rules in the classroom;
respond consistently and quickly to inappropriate behavior; structure classroom
activities in an effort to minimize disruption; and respond to, but do not become
angry or insult, the disruptive student. Students in classrooms where these four
goals were successfully implemented demonstrated greater improvements in behavior and academic work than students with similar attentional problems in other
classrooms. The effective classroom teacher for the ADHD student must also be
well organized, an efficient time manager, flexible and able to handle multiple
task demands. That teacher must set realistic goals for the ADHD student and find
ways of helping the student achieve those goals. The effective teacher must be able
to quickly discriminate between the ADHD child's incompetent or noncompliant
behavior. Interventions must be applied efficiently and consistently. The effective
teacher for an ADHD student must be able to maintain an ongoing awareness of
the entire classroom's activities, even when focusing one-on-one with the ADHD
student. The effective classroom teacher is able to carefully time interactions for
maximum effect. Such a teacher is democratic, responsive and understanding. The
kindly, optimistic, friendly teacher will be better able to accept and meet the needs
of the ADHD student.

The autocratic teacher, who may be intolerant and rigid in providing directions,
will experience difficulty with the ADHD child's frequent inability to follow
those directions. The aloof, distant, condescending teacher, stiff or formal in
relationships with students or unable to view students as children, will experience
difficulty with the ADHD child's differences. The restricted, rigid teacher, able to
recognize only the need for academic accomplishments, focusing only on the very
good or very bad and impatient with students who do not fit expectations, will
have difficulty with the ADHD child. The hypercritical, fault-finding, threatening
teacher will be frustrated by the ADHD child's inability to change quickly. The
hopeless, pessimistic, unhappy teacher with a tendency to categorically view all
misbehavior and unfinished work as the result of willful disregard will not develop
a good relationship with the ADHD child. Finally, impulsive, short-tempered,
disorganized teachers will also experience difficulty caused by the similarity in
their behavior with that of the typical ADHD child.

To the extent that the practitioner is aware of these dimensions of teacher style
and behavior, he or she is in a better position to determine which types of classroom
interventions may be most successful. For example, the rigid, autocratic teacher
must be educated about, and willing to accept, the ADHD child's incompetencies
if that child is to succeed in class. The disorganized teacher must be helped to
structure and organize if the ADHD child is to be expected to complete tasks, and
so on.

It is not difficult to informally assess teacher style through parental reports
concerning the teacher's past behavior and interaction with parents, written data
provided by the teacher to parents, review of the teacher's written comments on
the ADHD child's work, the effort the teacher exerts in providing the practitioner
with needed assessment data, telephone conversations with the teacher and finally,
the ADHD child's self-report concerning the teacher.

It is also important for the practitioner to remember that standards set by teachers often act as self-fulfilling prophecies for students. When expectations are high, students achieve at higher levels, exhibiting fewer conduct problems. However, just as with parents, the ADHD child's off-task, inappropriate behavior has a coercive effect in shaping the teacher's behavior. It is not uncommon that over time, poorly performing students are praised less and criticized more.

SUMMARY

Teachers play a critical role in the successful school experience of the ADHD child. This chapter provided the practitioner with suggestions for educating teachers regarding specific child- and teacher-centered interventions that may be beneficial. It is important for the practitioner to be available and to be of support to the classroom teacher. Initially, the practitioner must educate teachers concerning basic background and developmental aspects of attention disorders. The practitioner must understand each teacher's style and capabilities before recommending classroom interventions. The interventions suggested in this chapter were designed to be applied in any form of classroom structure or routine. It is important for the practitioner to be sensitive to the multiple daily demands placed on teachers and the increased pressure teachers experience when faced with educating one or more ADHD children. As with interaction with parents, the practitioner must be supportive and available to the ADHD child's teachers.

CHAPTER 12

Social Skill Training for ADHD Children

A child's ability to develop and maintain appropriate peer relationships is considered to be an important predictor of positive adult adjustment and behavior (Cowen, Pederson, Babigan, Izzo and Trost, 1973). It is well recognized that ADHD children are at significant risk to experience difficulty developing appropriate social and peer interaction skills as the result of their inattentive, impulsive, easily overaroused style. Although DSM–III-R (APA, 1987) introduced some ADHD diagnostic, descriptive behaviors related to social problems (i.e., often interrupts or intrudes on others), social problems are often overlooked or excluded when considering the diagnosis of ADHD. Based on the SNAP checklist, Pelham and Bender (1982) found that problems with peer interaction were as efficient in distinguishing ADHD from normal children as were problems with attention span, impulsivity and hyperactivity. This chapter will provide a review of the research literature as it relates to socialization problems ADHD children experience. Definitions and methods of assessment for social skills and social competence will be discussed. A model for teaching a single social skill independently from a group training program will be presented. A number of commercially available social skills programs will be discussed, and a six-session group training program developed by Goldstein and Pollock (1988b) will be presented.

RECENT RESEARCH INTO SOCIAL PROBLEMS

The past ten years has seen a dramatic increase in research in the area of social competence and social skill development. Entire texts have been devoted to the subject (Strain, Guralnick and Walker, 1986; L'Abate and Milan, 1985). Teacher observations of ADD children's social interaction frequently note problems with fighting, interrupting and being more disliked (Pelham and Bender, 1982). Campbell and Paulauskas (1979) reported that mothers of hyperactive children observed similar social problems. Barkley (1981b) found that 80 percent of parents of hyperactive children provided ratings that suggested that their children were having serious problems playing with other children. In this study only 7 percent of the non-hyperactive control group children were reported as having such problems. In fact, hyperactive adolescents and adults with histories of hyperactivity also recognized the problems they experienced in developing and maintaining friendships (Hoy,

Weiss, Minde and Cohen, 1978; Weiss, Hechtman and Perlman, 1978). It has also been suggested that the social problems of many ADHD children may increase with age (Waddell, 1984).

Peer Relations

Children of all ages also very quickly become aware of the hyperactive child's socialization difficulty and perceive her negatively (Milich, Landau, Kilby and Whitten, 1982; Klein and Young 1979). It has been suggested that rejection by peers is an important predictor of psychopathology (Milich and Landau, 1981). It is therefore of considerable significance that ADHD children are disliked by their peers. Pelham and Bender (1982) found that of 49 hyperactive children, only 2 were not nominated as disliked more often than nonreferred peers. In an excellent review, Pelham and Milich (1984) suggested that ADD children differ from other children and experience "behavioral excesses leading to rejection and social skill deficits leading to low acceptance"(p. 560).

Classroom observation studies have consistently found hyperactive children to exhibit greater negative verbalizations and physical aggression in comparison to their peers (Whalen, Henker, Collins, Finck and Dotemoto, 1979; Abikoff et al., 1977). Pelham and Bender (1982) found that in group play situations, hyperactive children exhibited ten times as many negative verbalizations directed at others and three times as many acts of physical aggression. It is not surprising that this pattern of behavior very quickly results in the ADHD child being less accepted and more rejected in social situations. Unfortunately, this is the child that is least able to cope with the frustration of peer rejection. Often a vicious spiral develops. In response to rejection, the ADHD child attempts to exert control over the other children or to express unhappiness or anger toward the other childeren. This results in more inappropriate behavior and increased rejection. Research has also suggested that these problems occur in both structured and unstructured settings, affecting the ADHD child in all areas of his interaction with the environment. The practitioner must be cautioned, however, that the total number of social interactions or the frequency of positive interactions does not appear to distinguish hyperactive from normal children (Pelham and Bender, 1982; Riddle and Rapoport, 1976).

Ross and Ross (1982) point out that since children frequently judge their own self-worth in terms of the opinions of others, peer rejection for the ADD child results in diminished self-esteem. This then leads to an inappropriate effort to gain acceptance in the peer group and further rejection by that group. This further limits the ADHD child's potential for normal social interaction by restricting his opportunities to develop and practice more appropriate skills.

Specific Skill Deficits

Studies attempting to define the specific skill deficits that account for the ADHD child's peer problems have suggested that the ADHD child experiences a wide range of problems including difficulty with off-task behaviors, disruptive behaviors, impulsivity, immature or aggressive responding and difficulty with basic communication. It has also been suggested that hyperactive children have difficulty adapting their behavior to different situational demands (Whalen, Henker, Collins, McAuliffe and Vaux, 1979). Hechtman, Weiss and Perlman (1980) demonstrated that when hyperactive young adults were presented with hypothetical vignettes requiring social judgments along with multiple-choice responses, they performed as well as a normal group of young adults. However, in a parallel free-response procedure in which no answers were suggested, the hyperactive group had significant difficulty generating appropriate social responses. Although it hasn't been replicated, this pattern is probably true of ADHD children as well. While researchers have repeatedly attempted to identify behavioral precursors of peer problems (Coie and Kuperschmidt, 1983), it is not surprising that a specific pattern of difficulty has not been identified for ADHD children because of the heterogeneity of problems they experience.

Aggression appears to be a very stable trait that does not diminish with age (Loeber and Dishion, 1983; Olweus, 1979). It is now recognized that aggression is a frequent component of the behavior problems ADHD children experience. It is also a negative predictor for positive treatment outcome (Loney and Milich, 1981). It appears that nonaggressive and normal children experience lower levels of peer rejection as they get older while their ADD and conduct–disordered counterparts with aggressive problems continue to be rejected (Ross and Ross, 1982). Additionally, ADD children experiencing a greater degree of hyperactivity were found to receive higher teacher ratings of aggression and disruption than their less hyperactive ADD peers (Edelbrock et al., 1984).

Pelham and Bender (1982) have suggested that impulsivity is more highly correlated with peer problems than hyperactivity. Further, ADD females are more similar to normal females on peer ratings than ADD males are to normal males. It has been suggested the ADHD females have fewer problems with aggression but more problems with mood and emotion than their ADHD male counterparts. Finally, although some researchers suggest that the onset of antisocial behavior among ADHD adolescents results from frustration with school and peer rejection, others have offered the alternative explanation that it is an early pattern of aggressive behavior that best predicts later adolescent antisocial problems (Kramer, 1987).

Cognitive-Mediational Deficits

It has been observed and well documented by research that the cognitive-mediational deficits hyperactive children experience have a negative impact on their ability to develop and maintain appropriate social relationships (Asher and Gottman, 1981). However, studies evaluating specific factors such as social perspective-taking, emotional labeling and attribution as they relate to the socialization process have been inconsistent in suggesting that these play a significant negative role in the ADHD child's ability to socialize (Pelham and Milich, 1984). These authors pointed out that "the question remains whether these social, cognitive processing deficits lead to or result from disturbed social relations, or perhaps instead represent a common, underlying mechanism (e.g., inattention, impulsiveness)" (p. 563).

Given the reported problems with generalization of newly learned cognitive skills that ADHD children experience, social skill programs standing the best chance of success must: (1) build in generalization opportunities for demonstration of skills in the child's daily environment; (2) provide external and then internally controlled consequences; and (3) follow the child for a long period of time. It would also appear that a combination of treatment interventions will best facilitate both target and nontarget behavioral generalization. Hinshaw, Henker and Whalen (1984b) demonstrated that with a combination of reward, self-instruction training and stimulant medication, ADHD children displayed almost normal levels of both inappropriate and appropriate social behavior. Other studies have found that stimulant medication alone improves positive social interaction for ADHD children. It has been suggested, however, that the beneficial effects of stimulant drugs on social competence may be limited to certain children, such as those who are highly aggressive or significantly overactive (Pelham and Bender, 1982).

Social Competence Versus Social Skills

Bailey and Simeonsson (1985) make a distinction between social competence and social skills. Social competence requires an evaluative judgment regarding the efficiency of a child's behavior within a specific context. It is the behavior, not the child that is judged. In contrast, social skills are specific strategies used to successfully perform social tasks in order to be judged as socially competent (Gresham, 1986). The teaching process requires the operational identification of social-skill deficits and the introduction of strategies to teach new social skills with the goal of improving social competence.

Walker, Todis, Holmes and Horton (1988) define two types of social competencies required for successful adjustment. The first are those that facilitate compliance with rules and the demands of the environment, such as listening, following directions and displaying appropriate work habits. The majority of these skills are taught in self-instructional progams for ADHD children. A second group of skills facilitates positive social interaction. Such skills include understanding how to begin and maintain conversation, compliment others and resolve conflict. It is these skills that are often the focus of most social skill programs.

In this text, the authors have chosen to distinguish between problem-solving training and social skill building. The assumption is that before social skills can be taught, the ADHD child must master the basics of self-instruction. Many of the newer social skills programs actually combine social and other skills with communication training (Walker, et al., 1988); or self-instruction, effective communication, dealing with stress and coping with excessive emotion (McGinnis, Goldstein, Sprafkin and Gershaw, 1984; Goldstein, Sprafkin, Gershaw and Klein, 1980). A number of these programs will be reviewed at a later point in this chapter.

Other researchers have pointed out that children with a wide range of developmental impairments commonly experience social competence problems, including helplessness, peer rejection, lack of acceptance by peers and poor self-esteem resulting from a combination of repeated social, behavioral and academic failures (McConnell and Odom, 1986; Gresham and Elliott, 1984).

Although many previously developed social skill programs have relied on intuition and theory to identify and define the range of social skills required for social competence, newer programs are using experimental research and statistical analysis (Walker et al. 1988). In an excellent review, Schloss, Schloss, Wood and Kiehl (1986) point out that approximately half of all social skills studies from 1980 through 1986 do not report a rationale for the selection of social skill goals. Goals for the majority of such programs are determined by social comparison (observation of normally functioning individuals) and subjective evaluation (input from other observers) (Kazdin and Matson, 1981). The result of this body of research has suggested that the perspective of the rater is also a factor in determining which types of skills are considered important. In the past, most evaluation of social skills was made by a third party such as a parent or teacher. Increasingly, children themselves are being asked to rate and evaluate their own and other's behavior. Parents and teachers tend to focus primarily on social skills that facilitate behavioral compliance and self-control while children and adolescents are more interested in the quality of their relationships with others. The former would appear to be more reliant on the development of appropriate cognitive-mediational skills, while the latter is primarily dependent on social competence.

Cox and Gunn (1980) suggest that children may lack social competence because they do not possess a repertoire of appropriate behavior, because they possess the behavior but have not had enough opportunity to practice and develop competence or because they experience emotional problems that interfere with effective problem solving and social interaction. It would appear that for the majority of socially incompetent ADHD children, the first two explanations are most salient. Many ADHD children have not developed an effective repertoire of social skills. Others possess the skills and are able to demonstrate their knowledge during a discussion or role-playing experience, but they are often inefficient in using these skills in the environment because of a lack of opportunity to practice or generalize due to their impulsive, inattentive, easily overaroused style. It is also important for the practitioner to recognize that appropriate social response varies with age. Researchers have demonstrated the importance of being sensitive to the child's age when identifying a lack of social competence and the specific social skills in need of remediation (Kelly and Drabman, 1977).

Definition of Social Skills

There has been increasing emphasis on concisely and operationally defining specific social skills that are necessary for children to exhibit social competence. In doing so, researchers have identified a number of classes of social skills, including physical factors such as eye contact and posture (Tofte-Tipps, Mendonca and Peach, 1982); social responsivity, such as sharing (Bryant and Budd, 1984); and interactional skills such as initiating and maintaining conversation (Whitehill, Hersen and Bellack, 1980). The attempt has been made to define these behaviors in such a way that they can be validly and reliably measured. In a broader perspective, the situations in which these behaviors must be successfully exhibited have also been reviewed and identified.

All-encompassing social skill and communication training programs have varied in the number of specific behaviors they operationally define and evaluate and for which training components are provided. Walker et al., (1988) defined 31 behaviors relating to peer, adult and self-relation skills. Peer skills include interactive abilities, such as complimenting and offering assistance, as well as coping skills such as negotiating and expressing anger. Adult-related skills include disagreeing appropriately with an adult and working independently. Self-related skills include developing self-control and accepting consequences for one's actions. Walker et al.'s program, titled ACCESS, is designed for adolescents.

Goldstein et al. (1980), in another program designed for adolescents, defined 50 skills in the areas of beginning and advanced socialization, skills for dealing with emotions, alternatives to aggression, dealing with stress and planning ability. In a program designed for elementary school children, McGinnis et al. (1984) defined 60 behaviors covering classroom survival, friendship making, dealing with feelings, alternatives to aggression and dealing with stress. These three programs are characteristic of the range of skills taught in a variety of other skill-building programs.

Dodge, McCluskey and Feldman (1985) collected and factor analyzed teacher-generated suggestions for social problems children experienced at school. Their factor analysis yielded five clusters of problems, including difficulty entering and joining the peer group, dealing with provocation by others, responding appropriately to failure, meeting social expectations and meeting teacher expectations.

As part of a social skills training program developed for ADHD children, Goldstein and Pollock (1988b) identified 23 critical behaviors in which many ADHD children frequently lack competence. Each of these skills is defined in the outline of the program that appears at the end of this chapter. These skills incude basic interactional ability such as beginning, listening during and ending conversations; joining others engaged in activity; working cooperatively; and resolving conflict.

ASSESSMENT

Assessment for children deficient in social skills is a two-step process initially involving identification of those children who are socially incompetent and lacking skills, and then specifically defining each individual's skill deficits. In classroom situations in which a practitioner is going to offer a social skills training group, this type of assessment is a critical component. In such a situation, it is easiest to ask teachers to nominate students who lack social competence. In many other situations, especially those involving an ADHD child receiving a comprehensive evaluation, assessment of social competence and skill is an integral part of the evaluative process. In this case, teachers are not asked to nominate students with problems but to define the types of problems a specific child experiences. The Teacher and Parent Social Skills Assessment forms reviewed in earlier chapters offer a fairly quick opportunity to obtain an overview of the ADHD child's aggressive or withdrawn socialization problems, as well as a brief observation concerning the child's ability to participate in group settings. Although these questionnaires are useful in identifying and beginning the evaluative process for ADHD children with socialization difficulty, they are not specific enough to use as a prescreening device before initiating a social skills group.

A number of social skills questionnaires are designed to specifically define social skill deficits. These questionnaires were developed as prescreening devices for the social skills programs they accompany. McGinnis et al. (1984) developed a 60-item teacher rating scale for elementary school children. Goldstein et al., (1980) developed a similar 50 item questionnaire for adolescents. Neither of these questionnaires is norm-referenced, and the data they generate is used qualitatively to identify specific goals for each child in the social skills group. Walker et al. (1988) offers the only adolescent norm-referenced social skills questionnaire that lends itself as a device for social skill group screening. The ACCESS Placement Test is a 30-item questionnaire designed to screen critical social skills. All three of these questionnaires can be used as in-depth evaluative devices before initiating any social skills training program. Goldstein and Pollock (1988) developed a 23-item questionnaire as a pre- and postassessment instrument for the social skills taught in the Social Skills Training for Attention Deficit Children program. The questionnaire appears in Figure 12.1.

Self-report inventories and student interviews offer the practitioner the opportunity to obtain feedback about the ADHD child's or adolescent's perception of her problems. Not only can this information provide insight in terms of the accuracy of the child's report, but this data can be effective in developing a hierarchy of skills and goals which are most important for each child to achieve from the child's point of view. Both of the Skill Streaming programs offer self-report questionnaires that parallel the observer behavior rating scales in these programs (Goldstein et al., 1980; McGinnis et al., 1984). For the interested practitioner, Cartledge and Milburn (1980) provide an outline of topics to be discussed in a social skills child interview. Topics include obtaining the child's perceptions of his ability to solve problems, join ongoing activities, receive and accept compliments and express a contrary opinion.

Another method that may be helpful in identifying socially deficient children is the use of peer ratings or sociometrics. Sociometrics, when used in an appropriate manner, offer the classroom teacher and practitioner the opportunity to obtain the perceptions children have about their peers. Additionally, the correlation between teacher observations and peer ratings has consistently been found to be at least moderate (Landau, Milich, and Whitten, 1984). Sociometric information is often helpful in identifying the shy or withdrawn child who may frequently not come to the attention of the classroom teacher. Sociometric techniques include asking each child in the class to respond to questions such as whom they would most like to sit next to, work with on a project or are best friends with.

Based on sociometric data, Mainville and Friedman (1976) found that hyper-

SOCIAL SKILLS GROUP ASSESSMENT QUESTIONNAIRE

Child _____ Rater _____ Date _____

Directions: Listed below are a list of social skills which are important for social competence. Please read the description of each skill and circle the answer which best describes your opinion of this child's ability. Please use the space at the end of the questionnaire if you feel there are additional social related problems which this child exhibits.

This Child:

	is very poor at this skill.	exhibits this skill as well as others.	exhibits this skill better than others.	
Meeting new people.	1	2	3	4	5
Beginning a conversation.	1	2	3	4	5
Listening during a conversation.	1	2	3	4	5
Ending a conversation.	1	2	3	4	5
Joining an ongoing activity with others	1	2	3	4	5
Asking questions appropriately.	1	2	3	4	5
Asking for a favor appropriately.	1	2	3	4	5
Seeking help from peers appropriately.	1	2	3	4	5
Seeking help from adults appropriately.	1	2	3	4	5
Sharing.	1	2	3	4	5
Interpreting body language.	1	2	3	4	5
Playing a game successfully.	1	2	3	4	5
Suggesting an activity to others.	1	2	3	4	5
Working cooperatively.	1	2	3	4	5
Offering help to others.	1	2	3	4	5
Saying thank you.	1	2	3	4	5
Giving a compliment.	1	2	3	4	5
Accepting a compliment.	1	2	3	4	5
Apologizing.	1	2	3	4	5
Understanding the impact his or her behavior has upon others.	1	2	3	4	5
Demonstrating the ability to understand other's behavior.	1	2	3	4	5
Rewards self	1	2	3	4	5
Follows directions	1	2	3	4	5

Comments:
_____
_____

Figure 12.1 Social Skills Group Assessment Questionnaire. From S. Goldstein and E. Pollock. *Problem Solving Skills Training for Attention Deficit Children.* Copyright 1988 by Neurology, Learning and Behavior Center. Used by permission of the authors.

active students were not rated as highly as others by their peers and were more likely to be rejected than accepted. Whalen and Henker (1985) found that normal children are often reluctant to select the ADD child for activities that potentially could have direct personal or social consequences (i.e., loaning money). These authors also found that normal children, when given a choice, preferred interaction with depressed, as opposed to ADD, children on a consistent basis. Carlson, Lahey, Frame and Walker (1987) found that attention-disordered 6- to 13-year-old children with and without hyperactivity, when compared to normal children, received significantly fewer most-liked nominations and more least-liked nominations. Identical patterns were found for both the children experiencing attention disorder with and without hyperactivity; however, those with hyperactivity were nominated significantly more as the child who fights most.

Although observation in a playroom or natural setting is also an excellent way of obtaining clear and precise data concerning a child's social skills, such opportunities are not frequently afforded the practitioner. When possible, observation of the ADHD child, especially on the playground, is recommended. This data may greatly increase the practitioner's insight concerning the ADHD child's problems. Often, school personnel, such as a psychologist or special education teacher, can be of assistance in obtaining observational data from the playground.

The coercive effect that the ADHD child has upon adults has also been demonstrated with peers. Observational research has been novel in mixing pairs of normal and ADHD children together and requiring cooperation in either a laboratory, home or analogue school setting. A wide variety of research in this area has consistently demonstrated the ADD child's interactional problems (Mash and Johnston, 1983). Whalen and Henker (1985) refer to ADD children as *negative social catalysts* because of their ability to elicit inappropriate behaviors from those around them.

Most recently, Clark, Cheyne, Cunningham and Siegel (1988) observed an ADHD and normal boy pairing in comparison to pairs of normal boys in a number of settings. The dyads with the ADHD child demonstrated a greater frequency of aggression and less cooperative activity than the control dyads. In a study observing social communication patterns of ADHD and normal elementary school boys during social role playing, Landau and Milich (1988) found that the ADHD children failed to modulate their social communication behavior as task demands shifted. Normal children did not demonstrate this problem. This pattern of behavior on the part of the ADHD child caused the normal child with whom the ADHD child was interacting to alter his response patterns even more in an attempt to meet task demands. The results of this study suggest that in many situations the social behavior of ADHD children may result from skill deficit and be independent of environmental demands.

TEACHING A SINGLE SOCIAL SKILL

In some situations, the practitioner may wish to pick a specific skill or problem to work through and develop alternatives with the ADHD child. Kirby and Grimley

(1986) pointed out that many ADHD children, because of their impulsivity and inattention, possess only limited awareness of their socialization difficulty and so frequently deny or project the source of their problems onto others. They may not be open to participating in a social skills group. Often, however, even the most impulsive, denying child will accept responsibility for some aspect of a specific problem. In some situations, it is best to start with that problem rather than placing the child in a group with a list of skill deficits that have been observed by others but that the child is unwilling to acknowledge.

A five-step cognitive, problem-solving skills model can be used effectively to teach a single social skill (Shure, 1981; Spivack and Shure, 1974). In a series of works, these authors suggested that cognitive mediation plays a strong role in the development of appropriate interpersonal problem-solving skills in children. This model is easy to implement to teach a specific social or interpersonal problem-solving skill to an ADHD child.

The first step involves helping the child to develop sensitivity for the problem at hand. Although this step may appear obvious to the practitioner, it is frequently taken for granted by adults that in a problem situation both they and the child see the problem in a similar fashion. Especially with ADHD children, this is frequently not the case. If this step is not satisfactorily met, the following steps will not meet with success. Often the ADHD child's definition of the problem may be very different from the adult's. The child may project the source of the problem onto others. He may even deny that there is a problem. The practitioner must work patiently with the child to reach some resolution and point of agreement concerning the problem. For example, in the case of the child who is not prepared and ready to go when the rest of the family is ready to leave the home, the child's explanation of the problem may be, "I didn't have enough time," while the parent's explanation may be, "You did not make good use of your time." The practitioner must work to help the child compromise and accept a definition of the problem for which he is able or willing to take some responsibility.

The second step involves having the child generate alternative solutions for the problem. Many children are unable to generate alternative solutions on their own. However, the practitioner must avoid lecturing the child and providing all of the possible solutions. A novel approach to this situation is to make a written list, either on a piece of paper or blackboard, of all the potential solutions to the problem. The practitioner may even suggest humorous solutions in an effort to encourage the child to participate. In the case of the child's being unable to dress in time to leave with the family, humorous suggestions made by the practitioner could include, "You could go out in your pajamas," or "You could never leave the house again." Humor is a valuable tool in helping the child feel comfortable and not on the hot seat during this process. Before proceeding to the third step, a comprehensive list of possible alternative solutions must be generated.

The third and often critical step, *means-ends thinking*, involves taking the child step by step through the process of the determined solution to the problem. In the case of the child being dressed on time, eventually a list of alternative solutions is generated, and together the child and the practitioner pick what appears to be the most attractive or best solution. Often, this is a process that requires the fourth step, teaching the child to think consequentially and consider the impact this particular solution is going to have upon himself and on others.

In some situations, the child may insist on a solution that the practitioner does not perceive as the best. In such a situation, it is best not to debate with the child concerning her choice of solution but to use means-ends and consequential thinking in an effort to help the child determine whether, in fact, this is the best solution. In some situations, the practitioner may wish to pick a second solution as the best choice and together with the child work through both solutions. Once a solution or solutions are agreed upon, the practitioner then helps the child break the solution down into specific steps that must be implemented. In the case of the child being ready, the solution may be for the parent and child to make a list of exactly how much time each task the child must complete will take and have the parent provide external cues to the child based on that timetable.

Finally, an attempt is made to link this particular problem and event with other past events and potential future behavior or problems. Once the timetable solution for being ready to leave on time is implemented, the practitioner can help the child look at how this particular solution may apply to other problems in the child's life, as well as the impact this solution is going to have on the child's relationship with others in the future. This helps the inattentive child develop a sense of causality that her behavior is not a series of isolated, unrelated events (Kirby and Grimley, 1986). Children deficient in these five problem-solving steps, in all likelihood, are going to experience problems with social competence. By using a number of specific, parent-generated examples, this model also can easily be taught to teachers and parents of ADHD children.

Judging Success

Success of a social skills training program may be difficult to assess. Postprogram questionnaires or playground observation can be used to measure change. Skills learned, however, may not be immediately demonstrated or generalized in the environment. From a common-sense perspective it is fair to assume that if a child's deficiency in a number of basic social skills results in social incompetence, teaching the child those skills increases the likelihood the child will be more socially competent.

It is clear that simply teaching a specific response in a specific situation is not the goal of social skills training. Children must not only learn the skill but learn to be flexible and organized in applying the skill. It is for this reason that cognitive training is essential for ADHD children before being taught social skills. In clinical practice, it has been the author's experience that socially incompetent children do benefit from social skills training. Some learn the skills and use them very well. Others learn the skills but continue to require prompts or additional intervention. It is rare that the time spent in social skills training does not reap some return benefits.

REVIEW OF COMMERCIALLY AVAILABLE SOCIAL SKILLS TRAINING PROGRAMS

Adolescent Curriculum for Communication and Effective Social Skills (ACCESS) (Walker, Todis, Holmes and Horton, 1988)

This program builds upon Walker's years of research on social competence and teaching social skills to children and adolescents. The program consists of 31 sessions and is designed to be implemented in a small group setting. A student study guide is available for each participant. Each skill lesson is composed of ten steps, including a review of the previously taught skill, the introduction of the new skill, an opportunity to practice and develop an understanding of this skill through discussion and role play and a contract in which each participant makes a commitment to when and with whom the new skill will be practiced for the coming week. The ACCESS program is very well organized and with some practice, not very difficult for a teacher or practitioner to administer. Unique to this program is the Triple A Strategy, a technique taught to adolescents in the program to facilitate appropriate problem solving and social interaction. Triple A stands for Assess, Amend and Act. The strategy is used throughout the skill building lessons.

Asset: A Social Skills Program for Adolescents (Hazel, Bragg Schumaker, Sherman, and Sheldon-Wildgen, 1981)

Asset is a video program designed to teach social skills to both typical adolescents and those who are having significant interactional problems. The program contains eight videocassettes dealing with social skills, including giving feedback, peer pressure, problem solving, negotiation, following instructions and conversation. Vignettes are provided focusing on each of these skills. The video format can be used effectively with adolescents to stimulate discussion. In addition to the videocassettes, the program includes all participant materials and a leader's guide.

Skill-Streaming the Elementary School Child (McGinnis, Goldstein, Sprafkin and Gershaw, 1984)

Building on an earlier work for adolescents, the skill-streaming series is primarily designed for instruction in a small group setting but can be used in a large classroom. The authors suggest that the groups be held three to five times per week for approximately 20 minutes for students in lower grades and as long as 40 minutes for students in upper elementary grades. The program requires the teaching of 60 skills and conceivably could last an entire school year. The outline is not as detailed as the one for the ACCESS program, but skill-streaming offers a number of suggestions for implementing the program and maintaining children's interest. The text also contains a section to assist in managing behavior problems during group sessions. That section includes suggestions for avoiding problems as well as dealing with problems after they occur. Numerous examples are provided to assist the practitioner to develop an understanding of the specific techniques suggested.

Skill-Streaming the Adolescent (Goldstein, Sprafkin, Gershaw and Klein, 1980)

This text is very similar in format, structure and content to the *Skill-Streaming the Elementary School Child* text. The program contains 50 behaviors that are to be taught in a small group or classroom setting. The steps necessary to implement the teaching of each skill, suggestions for role playing and suggestions for the practitioner or group leader in teaching the skill are provided. The text also contains an annotated bibliography of studies examining the effectiveness of structured learning, which is the basis for the skill-streaming program. Goldstein and McGinnis (1988) have recently released a video program illustrating the structured learning concepts and training procedures. The video can be used to facilitate understanding and effective use of the skill-streaming programs.

Think Aloud: Increasing Social and Cognitive Skills, A Problem-Solving Program for Children (Bash and Camp, 1985)

This program was reviewed in Chapter 10 since the bulk of the training uses verbal mediational activities to improve cognitive skills and problem solving. The program was originally developed as an intervention for aggressive children. In this program designed for elementary school children 7 of 30 lessons are directed at helping children improve social skills. Many of the intervention suggestions are quite useful.

Getting Along with Others: Teaching Social Effectiveness to Children (Jackson and Monroe, 1983)

This program combines a direct intervention approach with systematic instructional methods. Numerous teaching strategies and techniques are offered for teaching 17 "core social skills" and coping with 18 common behavioral problems. The utility of this program is its application in the real-life setting as problems are occurring.

The Prepare Curriculum: Teaching Prosocial Competencies (Goldstein, 1988)

This program is designed for both children and adolescents, especially those experiencing significant aggressive or social withdrawal problems. The curriculum covers ten interventions dealing with areas such as problem solving, interpersonal skills, controlling anger, managing stress, being cooperative and dealing effectively in groups. As with Goldstein's other publications, the text provides detailed suggestions and methods, using games, role playing and group discussions to facilitate group participation and motivation.

AWARE: Activities for Social Development (Elardo and Cooper, 1977)

This program was developed for use by both parents and professionals to help children develop appropriate social skills. Specifically, the program is designed to help children understand thoughts and feelings of self and others, improve their ability to accept individual difference,solve interpersonal problems and increase respect and concern for others. The program itself consists of four units designed to implement these goals. Each unit contains numerous discussion activities presented in a format consisting of three major sections, including a brief objective stating the skill to be taught, an overview explaining the process of teaching the skill and activity and discussion ideas for implementation. The text is easy to follow and use. Because each of the objectives is well defined, the text can also be used as a resource to deal with a specific problem (i.e., dealing with jealousy). The program is designed to be implemented in a small group setting but can also be used on an individual basis.

A SAMPLE SOCIAL SKILLS TRAINING PROGRAM FOR ADHD CHILDREN

As an extension of their cognitive training program, Goldstein and Pollock (1988b) developed a 23-skill program to improve social competence in ADHD children. The program is designed to be implemented in six 1 1/2-hour sessions over a six-week period. The authors suggest that implementation of this program is best in a small group setting, including from three to six children. Fewer than three children in a group does not allow for sufficient interaction or opportunity for role play. More children, especially those with attention and overarousal problems, tends to be too disruptive. For the practitioner interested in reviewing a comprehensive set of social skills and steps for teaching, the remainder of this chapter will present an overview of the program. The skills presented are defined generically, although it is clear that they vary in specific definition based on the age of the child or adolescent. As with other programs reviewed earlier in this chapter, many practitioners will require assistance with suggestions for implementation, dealing with problems during the group, keeping children interested and tips for facilitating generalization. For the practitioner seriously interested in providing social skill training in a group setting, a review of the chapters in the skill-streaming texts for dealing with these problems is recommended.

Goldstein and Pollock's program uses a reinforcement system titled With-it-ness, or WINS. WINS in the form of token reinforcers are provided frequently and consistently during group sessions. WINS are provided intermittently for everything ranging from sitting and working with the group to demonstrating social behaviors such as providing appropriate feedback to others and demonstrating skills being taught. The purpose of these reinforcers is to improve attention, participation during the group and self-esteem. Depending on the age of participants in the group, WINS can be exchanged for activities at the close of the group or for material reinforcers.

Each group session is divided into a number of parts. During the first part of the session, homework is reviewed and skills taught the previous week are briefly demonstrated. During the next part, each new skill is taught and broken down into a step-by-step model for acquiring the skill. Role play is then used to demonstrate and practice the skill. Homework is assigned for each skill. The overview of this program will present a session-by-session breakdown of skills taught, followed by an outline of each skill and the steps suggested to learn that skill. Role play and homework activities will not be presented but are available. The interested practitioner is referred to Goldstein and Pollock (1988b).

It is suggested that the child's parents and teachers complete the Social Skills Group Assessment Questionnaire. This will allow the practitioner to identify specific deficiencies for each child and make a point of specifically emphasizing those skills during the program. This, in effect, individualizes each child's program within the group setting.

Skills taught are divided into six sessions as follows:

Session I

Listening

Meeting people—introducing self, introducing others

Beginning a conversation

Listening during a conversation

Ending a conversation

Joining an ongoing activity

Session II

Asking questions appropriately

Asking favors appropriately

Seeking help from peers

Seeking help from adults

Following directions

Session III

Sharing

Interpreting body language

Playing a game successfully

Session IV

Suggesting an activity to others

Working cooperatively

Offering to help

Session V

Saying thank you

Giving a compliment

Accepting a compliment

Rewarding self

Session VI

Apologizing

Understanding the impact your behavior has on others

Understanding others' behavior

The following is an overview of the skills taught in this program and the steps suggested to facilitate teaching of these skills.

SKILL: Listening

Attend to speaker and acknowledge what is said.

STEPS:

1. Face person who is talking—"eye contact."
2. Sit quietly.
3. Attend to what is being said.
4. Wait your turn to talk.

SKILL: Meeting New People

Introduce self

STEPS:

1. Look at and acknowledge other person.
2. Decide if you want to meet other person.
3. Choose correct time to meet other person.
4. Walk up to other person.
5. Say your name.
6. Wait for person to tell you his/her name. Ask person's name if he/she doesn't tell you.
7. Tell other person something about yourself.

SKILL: Introducing Others

STEPS:

1. Look at and acknowledge other people.
2. State name of one person and tell him/her name of other person.
3. State name of second person and tell him/her name of first person.
4. Say something that both people have in common or that might interest both of them.

SKILL: Conversations

Know how and when to converse with another person/persons

STEPS

1. Choose whom to talk with.
2. Show interest.
3. Choose when to talk.
4. Start talking in friendly way.
5. Stay on the topic.
6. Listen to what other person says.
7. Ask questions.

SKILL: Ending a Conversation

STEPS:

1. Decide why to end a conversation.
2. Decide when to end a conversation.
3. Choose what to say.
4. Wait until other person stops talking.
5. State what you have to say to end the conversation in a friendly way.

SKILL: Rewarding Self

STEPS:

1. Decide if you deserve a reward.
2. List the ways you could reward yourself.
3. Select best way you could reward yourself.
4. Reward yourself as soon as possible.

SKILLS: Asking a Question; Asking for Help; Asking a Favor

STEPS:

1. Decide what to ask.
2. Decide who to ask.
3. Plan how to ask at appropriate time.
4. Choose appropriate time.
5. Get person's attention.
6. Tell person what you need in a friendly way.
7. Thank person.

SKILL: Asking for Help with a Problem

STEPS:

1. Decide what the problem is and if you need help.
2. Decide who you could ask for help.
3. Select the person you want to ask to help you with your problem.
4. Tell that person your problem and ask for help.

SKILL: Following Instructions

STEPS:

1. Listen to what is being said.
2. Ask questions about topic until you clearly understand.
3. Repeat the instructions to yourself.
4. Complete task one step at a time in order given.

SKILL: Sharing

STEPS:

1. Decide if you have something to share.
2. Decide with whom to share.
3. Choose best time to share.
4. Offer in an honest way.

SKILL: Interpreting Body Language

Pay attention to facial expressions and body movements.

STEPS:

1. Face person and watch.
2. Look at facial features of subject.
3. Identify feeling of subject.
4. Look at body stance of subject/positioning.
5. Identify what subject is feeling.
6. If unsure, check out verbally.

SKILL: Playing a Game

STEPS:

1. Review the rules of the game.
2. Understand the rules of the game.

3. Decide who starts, takes second turn, etc.
4. Wait for your turn.
5. Think about how you played.
6. When game is over, say something positive about the game.

SKILL: Suggesting an Activity

STEPS:

1. Decide on an activity you want to do.
2. Decide with whom you could do the activity.
3. Select someone with whom you want to do the activity.
4. Decide what to say.
5. Decide when to say it.
6. Say it in a friendly way.
7. If answer is "no," ask, "What would you like to do?"

SKILL: Working Cooperatively

STEPS:

1. Decide what you want to do.
2. Decide how you want to work.
3. State your position.
4. Be a good listener while others state their positions.
5. Read other person's body language.
6. Act thoughtfully.

SKILL: Offering to Help

STEPS:

1. Decide if someone needs help.
2. Decide if someone wants help.
3. Think of what you could do to help.
4. Decide how to ask if you can help.
5. Choose best time to help.
6. Offer help.
7. Help person.

SKILL: Saying Thank You

STEPS:

1. Decide if someone did something you want to thank her for.
2. Decide ways to thank.

3. Choose best way to thank person.
4. Choose best time to thank person.
5. Thank in a friendly way.
6. Tell person why you are thanking her.

SKILL: Giving a Compliment

STEPS:

1. Decide what you want to tell someone.
2. Decide how you want to say it.
3. Choose a good time to say it.
4. Choose a good place to say it.
5. Give the compliment in a friendly way.

SKILL: Accepting a Compliment

STEPS:

1. Decide if you were given a compliment.
2. Acknowledge compliment.
3. Say, "Thank You."

SKILL: Apologizing

STEPS:

1. Decide if you need to apologize for something.
2. List various ways to apologize.
3. Choose best way to apologize.
4. Choose best time to apologize.
5. Choose best place to apologize.
6. Apologize in honest way.

SKILL: Understanding the Impact Your Behavior Has on Others

STEPS:

1. Decide which behaviors are important to you.
2. Stay in control of those behaviors.
3. State your position.
4. Think about how others feel.
5. Think about what others might say.
6. Help others follow rules.

SKILL: Demonstrating the Ability to Understand Behavior of Others

STEPS:

1. Listen to what person is saying.
2. Watch what the other person is doing.
3. List reasons why person is saying and feeling what he is.
4. Choose best reason.
5. Decide if you need to say or do anything, e.g., suggest another activity, change subject, etc.
6. Follow through.

SUMMARY

Research suggests that the majority of ADHD children experience either social incompetence or aggression, or a combination of both problems. Although medications have been effective in reducing aggressive problems, a component of social skills training is essential for the ADHD child experiencing problems with social skills and competence. This chapter reviewed the research literature concerning ADHD and socialization problems and provided definitions and methods of assessment for these skills. A model for teaching a single social skill independent of a group training program was presented. Commercially available social skills programs were reviewed, and a comprehensive program developed by Goldstein and Pollock (1988b) was presented.

CHAPTER 13

Teaching Parents to Cope with and Manage ADHD Children

The model presented in this chapter is designed to facilitate the practitioner's success in modifying the manner in which parents interact with their ADHD children. The philosophy, approach and techniques described have been developed specifically for ADHD children but will be effective with all children. The model presented is not a comprehensive parent program but can be used in conjunction with a wide range of group or individual parent training programs.

INCREASING PARENTAL COMPETENCE

Understanding the Cause of ADHD

The first step in increasing parental competence is assisting parents to understand the primary cause of the ADHD child's behavior. Many of the published materials or clinical services available to parents stress the use of techniques at the expense of understanding. By following the model in this chapter, the practitioner will help parents to move beyond dependence on a handful of techniques or on a parent training manual. Because the philosophy and model presented in this chapter can be used with a wide range of programs, the conclusion of this chapter will include a review of several excellent programs, ranging from those designed for children who are significantly noncompliant to those structured for more normally functioning individuals. Many of these programs are helpful for parents of ADHD children; however, success may be intermittent and short-lived unless parents develop an understanding of the ADHD child's behavior, their interaction with the child and the effect problems with attention and arousal level are going to have upon the child on a long-term basis.

Seeing the world through the eyes of the ADHD child is also important for parents. This assists them in coping when the demands day in and day out become stressful. Simply providing parents with a number of basic behavioral techniques will not, over time, lead to long-lasting change. As a result of the nature of their temperament, ADHD children present an unending collection and variety of problems. For example, parents must be helped to understand that punishment will be successful when it is applied appropriately for problems of noncompliance but will not succeed when it is chosen as the intervention for incompetent behavior.

Pamphlets (Goldstein & Goldstein, 1989; Silver, 1980a), short texts (Parker, 1988; Coleman, 1988; Friedman & Doyal, 1987; Wender, 1987), and videotapes (Goldstein, 1989b; Friedman, 1988) can facilitate the educational process.

The most efficient way of teaching parents this parenting model is to meet on an individual basis over one or two sessions, separated by approximately two or three weeks. Many parents need individual time to interact with the practitioner and ask questions. This affords the practitioner the opportunity to make certain the parents understand why the ADHD child experiences so much difficulty meeting the demands of his environment. These parents are then better prepared to participate in a parent training program with greater confidence and ultimately greater success.

It is also recommended that the practitioner take into account parental style and temperament when suggestions are made for more effective management within the home. The earlier discussion of teacher style is also applicable to parental style. Often, data generated during a parenting style interview can help the practitioner develop a better understanding, not only of the parents' awareness, skills, and abilities, but of their temperament as well. For example, impulsive, easily overaroused parents must be first taught to master their own temperament before teaching them strategies to master their children's temperament. Such strategies will not be used effectively if parents are not able to control their own emotional level in the face of problems.

Distinguish between Noncompliance and Incompetence

The second step in the process of increasing parental coping and management skills is to assist parents to make a distinction between behavior that results from incompetence and that which results from noncompliance. The former must be dealt with through education and skill building, while the latter is dealt with through punishment. The majority of parents will agree that a large percentage of their ADHD child's behavior problems results from incompetence rather than purposeful noncompliance. The ADHD child's difficulty settling into a task, lack of persistence, tendency to become overaroused and easily frustrated, impulsive behavior and restlessness often result in a wide variety of nonpurposeful behaviors that are clearly disturbing to others. Parents must be helped to understand that, over time, these behaviors result in a significant number of "quit it, stop it, cut it out, don't do that" responses as a steady diet from all areas of the environment. Parents must also be helped to understand that, over time, ADHD children are at significant risk to perceive their social environment as restrictively controlling and dissatisfied with their performance, which then results in the child becoming increasingly oppositional. By successfully distinguishing between incompetent and noncompliant behavior, parents can reduce negative feedback, increase compliance and success, and stem the tide of the development of oppositional behavioral patterns.

Before proceeding further, it is essential that the practitioner make certain parents understand the distinction between incompetence and noncompliance.

Numerous examples tied specifically to the child in question may prove helpful. It is important for parents to understand that if they punish a child for impulsivity, there is a strong likelihood that the child will be remorseful and promise to behave better. Unfortunately, the next time the child is in that situation the impulsive need for gratification will outweigh any capacity to stop, think and plan, resulting in a reoccurrence of the problem. Developing an understanding of this critical issue not only helps parents relabel the majority of their ADHD child's behavior, but acts as a motivator in changing the way in which they deal with the majority of problems. Again, simple analogies may be helpful. A parent would not punish a five-year-old child unable to read and expect that punishment would increase the child's reading capacity. Instead, the child would be educated and helped to develop a basic foundation of reading skills. Parents of ADHD children must be helped to understand that punishing inattentive, impersistent, restless, overaroused or impulsive behavior holds little chance of changing that behavior.

Teach Positive Direction

Once parents understand this distinction and can begin to differentiate their ADHD child's behavior, the third step is to teach positive direction. By offering positive directions, parents can make the distinction between behavior resulting from non-compliance and that resulting from incompetence. This assists parents in determining whether punishment or skill building is the most appropriate intervention.

Human nature appears to direct all of us to point out that which we don't like. When a child exhibits an aversive behavior, most parents respond by directing the child to stop doing it. The focus on what is to be stopped as opposed to what is to be started may not be an issue for most children since they spend the majority of their time meeting parental expectations. The ADHD child, however, frequently does not meet expectations and may then receive a steady diet of negative directions. This does not help the child understand what is to be done.

The best example might be the case of a child with his feet on the wall. The parent directs the child by saying, "Take your feet off the wall." This sounds like a positive direction, but in fact, the child is being told to stop doing something rather than being told what to do instead. This leaves the range of all other behavioral possibilities open to the child. He may then take his feet off the wall and place them on the coffee table. The child has complied with the parental request but is now doing something else that is aversive and may increase parental anger. The problem escalates. The parent then directs the child to take his feet off the coffee table only to have the child place his feet on the bookcase.

Another example, from the CBTU Parent Training Program (Jensen, 1982), portrays a child receiving a spanking and protesting, "But Mom, I said ship!" In a previous interaction the child was directed to not say the word *shit*. This was an intelligent child. In an effort to meet the social demands of his friends, he found a word that sounded similar, *ship*. His plan was to say the word ship, which would allow him to fit into his social group but also follow his mother's direction. His mother, who may have experienced some difficulty with auditory discrimination, unfortunately cannot make the distinction. The problem is the mother's because the child was directed what not to say, as opposed to what to say, when he became angry or frustrated.

It is recommended that the practitioner direct parents to practice telling their children what they want instead of what they don't want for at least a week before beginning any other intervention. This sounds like an easy task. Most parents, however, will report that old habits are difficult to change. Many parents find themselves focusing on what is to be stopped without considering the nature of their actions. Again, the purpose of this model is to assist parents to think about what they do and how they interact with their children rather than passively applying behavioral techniques. In some cases, parents will frustratingly report that it is easy to see what they don't want the child to do but much more difficult in that instant to decide what they want the child to do instead. A good rule is to remind parents to ask themselves, "What do I want to see the child doing instead of what he is doing right now?" At the very least, the child can be directed to go to her room. Parents with histories of a large percentage of negative direction often report increased compliance and fewer problems when they begin telling the child what they would like to see happen.

Positive direction can be used to help parents make the distinction between incompetence and noncompliance. If the child is directed to place his feet on the floor (assuming the parent has his attention) and he does not comply within 15 seconds, this has nothing to do with attention deficit-hyperactivity disorder but clearly reflects noncompliance. It is at that point that a punishment will prove beneficial in the long run and increase compliance when parental directions are given. It is important to help parents understand that once they make a request, they must remain to see what happens. If a parent asks a child to place her feet on the floor, walks out of the room and comes back ten minutes later and the child's feet are on the wall, that parent cannot be certain whether the child's feet on the wall now is the result of incompetence or noncompliance. The parent has no idea whether the child complied for a few minutes and then was distracted by whatever she was doing and again her feet climbed up the wall.

Parents of ADHD children are also instructed that part of this model involves being a control system for the child and that following this model will greatly reduce negative confrontations. An example of an ADHD child playing in the house with a friend illustrates this process. The ADHD child becomes overly loud because he does not track the volume of his voice, just as he does not track many other variables when he is distracted. The parent then makes a positive direction for the child to speak in an inside voice. The child complies for a few minutes, but ten minutes later his voice is loud again. For most parents this results in an escalation of parental intervention and by the third offense is a major failure with the child being sent to his room and the friend being sent home.

Parents of ADHD children, however, are counseled to make the distinction between incompetence and noncompliance. If the child is asked to lower his voice and he complies for a period of time but his voice gradually becomes louder again, this is not the result of noncompliance but rather of incompetence. The parent then makes another positive direction requesting the child to speak in an inside voice. The parent acts as the control system for the child. During a one-hour play session, the parent may have to remind the child a number of times to speak in an inside voice. The question the parent must ask himself is what happens after the request is made. If the child complies, then he is making an attempt to meet parental demands. If over time the child has a problem again, it is most likely the result of incompetence and, therefore, the child is entitled to another positive direction. In this situation, the results are a number of small successes rather than one large failure.

Parents can be counseled to reflect the process they observe by telling the child it would be great if he could remember to follow the direction for more than a few minutes. However, the parent is aware that the child is not engaging in this behavior purposefully and will repeatedly remind the child so long as the child is compliant when the reminder is made. Approaching the problem this way then allows the parent to work with the child in an effort to create interventions that may increase the child's competence to monitor his own voice. A number of suggestions for such strategies will be presented later in this chapter.

End Interactions Successfully

In the fourth and final step of this model, parents are also directed to make certain that they end interactions successfully. ADHD children have long histories of failure. Typically, the child creates a problem and is punished, perhaps being sent to her room for an indeterminate period of time, with no effort made for the child to return to the situation and comply with the parental request. Assuming the child's behavior resulted from noncompliance, it is essential that the child be returned to the situation and comply. The message must be very clear to the child that regardless of the time involved she will eventually comply with parental requests. For this reason, parents are directed to use short punishment periods designed to clearly give the message that the parent is dissatisfied and to quickly return the child to the problem situation, allowing an additional try at compliance.

One of the major goals of this model is to assist parents in seeing the world through the eyes of their ADHD child. It is also important for parents to understand that in many ways the ADHD child's ability to change over time may be limited. A child provided with negative consequences for inappropriate behavior and positive consequences for more appropriate behavior will eventually improve his behavior and even when the consequences are withdrawn, will in all likelihood maintain that behavior as the result of internal change. Because ADHD children frequently lack the ability to successfully internalize and be responsible for their own behavior, they may perform well under a structured reinforcement system but be unable to maintain those changes without such a system. Again, helping parents to make the distinction between incompetence and noncompliance frequently allows them to accept the fact that they may need to continue providing a significant degree of structure for their ADHD child to maintain positive behavioral changes.

STYLES OF PARENTAL INTERVENTION

Effective discipline and behavior management for ADHD children does not sim-ply involve providing parents with a "how to" manual and training them in a set of specific techniques. Children with ADHD are at significant risk to experience persistent frustration in response to the environment. Effective parenting for the ADHD child is a multistep process. Parents must be helped to develop an under-standing of how and why the ADHD child behaves the way she does. Parents must also be helped to develop an understanding of the role they play in interact-ing with their child. This parental role is comprised of dimensions of behavioral interaction. These behaviors comprise a "menu" from which parents choose their responses to their children. Parents frequently attempt to reduce or eliminate a child's problematic behavior in either preventive ways (before problem occurs) or reactionary ways (after problem occurs). Using either of these methods, parents can act to change either the child or the environment. The combination results in four alternative levels for parental action. These are illustrated in Figure 13.1. Parents can act preventively either by anticipating a problem and teaching the child more competent skill or by manipulating the environment. They can act in a reactionary manner after a problem has occurred by attempting to change the child through punishment and skill building or by manipulating the environment to reduce the chance that the problem will reoccur.

Often parents respond in a reactionary fashion with punishment designed to change the child's behavior. Since the majority of children exhibit neither sig-nificant nor frequent behavioral problems, this level of intervention is usually successful. For ADHD children with skill deficiencies, a reactionary, punishing intervention designed to alter their behavior is usually ineffective and improves neither competence nor the chance of succeeding the next time. With an ADHD child, parents must be helped to understand that repeated and increasingly reac-tionary measures often lead to increasing behavioral problems. It is important for parents to understand the level at which they respond to their ADHD child. If a reactionary, punishing intervention is ineffective, parents of ADHD children must be willing to consider that the problem may result from incompetence and be willing to attempt an intervention at a different level.

The younger the child, the more successful parents will be if their interventions are directed at manipulating the environment in a preventive manner. With older children, interventions that either teach skills or punish inappropriate, noncompliant behavior and that are directed at the child rather than the environment are often more effective. Parents must be helped to understand that with older children, it is more difficult to effectively direct the environment. Two-year-olds are much easier to control than six-year-olds. Additionally with younger children, parents' ability to anticipate problems and act preventively by manipulating the environment is essential, along with building the child's skill and competence. Such interventions allow parents to avoid escalation of problem behavior and the frustrating pattern of repeatedly reacting to similar behavioral problems.

It is important for the practitioner to help parents of ADHD children think

WHAT CAN PARENTS DO?

Points of Parental Response

The problem: Child getting into kitchen cabinets

PREVENTIVE LEVELS

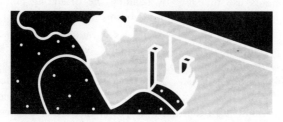

Modifying the Environment	Modifying the Child
"The locks on the cabinets will keep you out of trouble."	*"You've done a good job learning which cabinets not to open. I have a reward for you."*

REACTIVE LEVELS

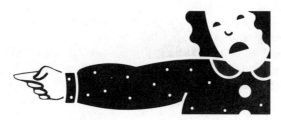

Modifying the Environment	Modifying the Child
"I am sick and tired of you making a mess in the cabinets. Get out of the kitchen."	*"I am going to punish you for getting into the kitchen cabinets again. Maybe time-out in your room will help you remember to stay out of the cabinets."*

Figure 13.1 Alternative levels for parental action. From S. Goldstein and P. Hinerman, *Language and Behavior Problems in Children*. Copyright 1988 by Neurology, Learning and Behavior Center. Used with permission of the authors and publisher.

creatively and understand the levels at which they interact with their children. Parents must be made aware of the alternatives that are always available. If they respond with a reactionary intervention designed to change the child and success is not experienced, persisting with interventions at that level will create frustration for both the parent and the ADHD child. This will, in all likelihood, lead to the development of further problems.

Management Techniques

Time Out

Time out is an effective intervention for children between the ages of 4 and 12 years. Many parents use time out by sending the offending child to his room where he may watch TV or play with toys. In this model, time out serves as both a punishment to let the child know his parents are dissatisfied with his actions and an instructional opportunity to quickly bring the child back to the situation to comply. Time out is used for noncompliance and not as an intervention for incompetence.

When the child is noncompliant, as in the case of being requested to place his feet on the floor and responding that he will not do so, he is immediately sent to time out. It is recommended that the time-out chair be in the same room as the offense, preferably facing a wall or corner. The only requirement is that the child's bottom remain on the chair. The child may cry or talk to himself, but may not play with toys or be talked to by others. The time-out period is one minute. This is such a short amount of time that even the most hyperactive ADHD child can easily comply and control himself if he chooses to do so. This brief time out also allows the child to almost immediately return to the problem situation and again attempt compliance.

The purpose of time out is not to make the child feel bad or make the parent feel better. The purpose is to consistently let the child know when she is being noncompliant and allow her to return to the situation quickly to make a second attempt at compliance. When the child has returned to the situation, the reason for time out is briefly stated by the parent and the direction is again stated. In this case, the child is directed to place his feet on the floor. If the child's feet remain on the floor for the next 10 to 15 seconds, the interaction is ended with a verbal, positive reinforcement by the parent. If 15 minutes later the child's feet are on the wall, most parents escalate in their annoyance and anger. For the ADHD child a second positive direction is given to place his feet on the floor. The distinction must be made between noncompliance and incompetence. If the child responds appropriately, a verbal reinforcer is offered. If the child again refuses, time out is initiated. The child starts at the same level of time out, one minute.

If the child is seeking to pick a fight and exercise opposition and control with his parents, he may come out of the time out and immediately respond negatively to the repeated direction by engaging in the behavior a second time. It is easy for the parent at that point to make the distinction that this is behavior that is purposeful and therefore must be punished. There is no need for a positive statement. The child is sent back to time out and one additional minute is added. In this way, even in repeated situations, time out does not turn into an all-afternoon affair. Once the child returns from time out, again the positive instruction is given and the parent waits for compliance. If the child does not comply, the interaction continues and another minute of time out is added. This is a battle the child cannot win. Eventually the child will comply and be reinforced. Once that happens, parents may then wish to provide a cognitive explanation, indicating that the child's choice of actions is his, but sooner or later he will comply and it is certainly easier for everyone when he complies sooner. He may be told that time spent working towards compliance could be spent doing something else much more enjoyable.

The issue of noncompliance with the direction to go to time out or stay in time out must be dealt with. In the case of the child either refusing to go to time out or attempting to change the subject by throwing a tantrum, parents are directed to use differential attention. This example will be described further in the next section. If the child gets out of the chair before the minute is over, she is asked to return to the chair and instructed that if she leaves the chair a second time, the clock will be started over and she will be given one spank. For younger children, a clap of the hands is often an effective accompaniment with the word *spank*. Some parents are unwilling to use a single spank, and this component is not essential. However, if they are unwilling to follow through, a spank should not be used as a threat. Researchers have found that hyperactive children respond well to mild forms of corporal punishment (Hanf, 1978). If the parent wishes to use the spank, it is recommended that this be the only situation in which spanking is used so that it maintains its effectiveness as a significant intervention. Each subsequent time the child leaves the chair, one spank is given and time is started over again. Regardless of the number of times the child leaves the chair, only one spank is given each time and no penalty time other than starting the clock over is added to the time-out period.

Some parent trainers advocate restraining noncompliant children or physically dragging them to time out. This is not recommended for the ADHD population of children. One of the reasons our prisons do not rehabilitate is that the majority of individuals in prison perceive themselves there because they were unfortunate enough to be caught, convicted and placed behind locked doors. If a child is physically restrained in a punishment, her perception of the reason for being engaged in that activity is focused on the parent being inappropriate and unfair rather than on the fact that she has made a mistake and should accept the negative consequence as penalty. If the child is voluntarily sitting in the time-out chair, she must resolve the cognitive dissonance for being in that situation by telling herself that she has done something wrong and this is her punishment. This greatly increases the likelihood that punishment will be effective in reducing noncompliant behavior.

Differential attention can be used effectively to deal with both the child refusing to go to time out and the one refusing to remain in time out. The practitioner must be cautioned, however, that there are some children who refuse to buy into any level of intervention. Some children will continuously escalate in their opposition until they have a major tantrum and are out of control. Such children may require a safe, padded, illuminated, ventilated time-out booth. Occasionally, if needed, parents will construct such a booth and use it as a final or last intervention if less restrictive forms of time out are not accepted by the child. In most cases, the child tests the parent's intention to use the time-out booth once or twice and then no longer escalates to the point where the booth is necessary. There are some children, however, who do not benefit from this level of intervention either. Frequently, these children are severely disturbed, and their problems are much greater than just ADHD. Often these children may require psychiatric hospitalization.

Differential Attention (Ignoring)

Many parents ignore. They ignore the good, the bad and just about everything else their children do. Parents must be helped to understand that ignoring is an active process requiring them not to pay attention to behavior they don't like but immediately to pay attention in a positive way when the child begins to exhibit more acceptable behavior. Parents must also be helped to understand that in the majority of situations, once they make a direct request of the child and the child is noncompliant, ignoring her at that point will be an ineffective intervenition. The only time ignoring is recommended following a direct request for the child to follow through with punishment and the child engages in an additional aversive behavior in an attempt to manipulate, control or alter the situation. At that point, ignoring the child provides a clear message that parents will not deal with the child when he is being inappropriate or noncompliant. When the child once again gains self-control, the parent can return to the situation, reinforce the child for being in control and again direct the child to follow through with the punishment, usually time out. This process is again a "battle" the child cannot win. Some children may repeatedly test such a situation. Parents are instructed that by the third time they return and the child is not compliant, it is beneficial for them to add an additional aversive consequence, such as earlier bedtime or restriction from television if on the next request the child does not comply. It is rare that a child will continue to be noncompliant when a second aversive consequence is introduced.

Overcorrection (Positive Practice)

In some situations, the child engages in a behavior such as slamming a door, and the parent may then reply that "doors need to be shut quietly. " The child is not going through another door, and so there is no opportunity to assess the issue of compliance versus incompetence. Most parents in such situations will have the child return and attempt to go through the door in an appropriate manner. When this process is repeated a number of times, it is referred to as overcorrection. Overcorrection is a good intervention for both incompetent and noncompliant behavior. Although overcorrection of a nonrelated behavior (i.e., having an autistic child stand up and sit down when he self-stimulates) is used as a punishment, practicing an appropriate behavior uses overcorrection as an intervention for incompetence. It is helpful for the practitioner to assist parents to develop an attitude in which they approach the child in such situations with a smile and give a very clear message that this is not punishment. If we do not read well, we practice. If we do not kick a soccer ball well, we practice. If we do not close doors well, we also practice. Research suggests that behavior in which we engage repeatedly, in a similar fashion, becomes automatic. Having the child practice ten times consecutively walking through the door in an appropriate way will increase the likelihood that the next time the child goes through a door she will act appropriately.

Parents are directed to further explain to the child that if there is a problem the next time, it simply means there was not enough practice and the number of practice sessions is doubled. The practicing of appropriate behavior is an excellent intervention, working well with a wide range of behaviors, including forgetting to flush the toilet, to hang up a coat or to wash hands before dinner.

Interventions with Young Children

Because of the wide variation of what is considered normal attentional and related skills in young children, it is especially important for the practitioner to make certain that the child's parents have realistic expectations for their child, even if the child is attention-disordered. The overly rigid parent with inappropriate expectations will very quickly reinforce a pattern of problematic behavior in the child, much of which will not stem from a physiological basis but from the child's inability to meet excessive demands. With younger children, it is also extremely important to rule out the possible contribution to the child's behavioral problems of other developmental impairments, especially language disability.

Pediatricians are becoming increasingly responsive in identifying and providing support to parents with difficult infants. With difficult infants and toddlers it is essential to increase parental competence by: (1) providing education concerning the nature and pattern of the child's behavior; (2) helping parents understand the role they may play in reinforcing that behavior; and (3) teaching behavior management skills. Effective daily management of the difficult infant and toddler is a crucial determinant of long-term outcome. Parents approaching a difficult offspring with skills, patience and tolerance will diffuse power struggles and prevent the development of further problems. Parents approaching a similar child with anger, irritation, anxiety and ultimately emotional withdrawal will certainly enhance the development of secondary problems. As parents learn management skills, the practitioner must be supportive and available to help when problems arise.

One of the most frequent complaints about difficult infants are problems with sleep. Parents must be helped to explore numerous alternatives in an effort to find some specific routine or pattern that will enhance sleep. The range of possibilities includes rocking, a monotonous noise such as a metronome, playing of a lullaby or use of a pacifier. Some parents report that the only way they get their infant to sleep is to put the child in the car and drive around the block. Recently a product has been marketed that can be attached to the child's crib and provides a vibration simulating a moving automobile, along with a monotonous car-like sound. Parents have reported that this induces sleep as effectively as driving the child around the block.

Parents also complain about problems with restlessness during waking hours. Frequently, visual, auditory or tactile stimulation can be effective in reducing restless behavior. Many parents have found that a pacifier reduces irritability. Although some parents feel guilty about using a pacifier, parents of difficult infants and toddlers should be supported by the practitioner in using, within reason, any intervention that works. It is recommended, however, that the use of a pacifier must be slowly eliminated as the child reaches two years of age. Extinction of pacifier use in older toddlers is an extremely difficult and stressful process.

Parents of difficult infants must be counseled to be prepared for activities such as bathing and changing. It is essential that both parents play an active role in the care of the child and have enough breathing space so that they do not feel overwhelmed by the child's demands. A monthly group for parents of difficult infants in which ideas are shared and a brief presentation is made by a community-based professional is often an effective and valued support.

Interventions for Adolescents

By age 12, interventions that are effective with younger children very quickly lose their potency. Time out and overcorrection are often reacted to with resistance by the adolescent. Differential attention is an effective technique regardless of a child's or adolescent's age. With adolescents, it is often helpful to get the family together and teach negotiation and contracting skills (Robin, 1979; Robin and Foster, 1989). Robin's program will be briefly reviewed at the close of this chapter. Adolescents who refuse to participate in parental interventions or who are passively resisting participants cannot be forced. It is, therefore, most important for the adolescent to feel as if his opinion is important and his input will be considered in the rule- and decision-making process. Adolescents with long histories of ADHD problems have well-developed, often dysfunctional, patterns of behavior that are habitual and often resistant to intervention. Helping the adolescent feel comfortable and in control of the treatment process may facilitate change.

It is recommended that at least a brief period of psychotherapy be considered for all ADHD adolescents to help them understand their history and current problems as well as to make them active participants in the treatment process.

It is also recommended that the use of medications with the ADHD adolescent be used as a reinforcer rather than a punishment, and not immediatly offered. For the passive or mariginally involved adolescent, the medication will provide another issue and further opportunity to rebel. On the other hand, if medication is presented as an intervention that may help, but the adolescent will not be provided with medication until she demonstrates more effort in therapy, at school and socially, there is a likelihood of greater treatment progress and compliance once medication use is initiated.

Strategies That Help

Response-Cost

Most parents understand the use of positive reinforcers as a means of motivating children. Few, however, understand the use of response-cost. Response-cost is a form of punishment. By nature of their repeated problems, ADHD children do not earn as many reinforcers and may find it difficult to be motivated to earn a reinforcer that they may perceive they can never obtain. Response-cost turns the tables. The child is provided with the entire reinforcer going into the situation and must then work to keep the reinforcer. Instead of giving the child a $2.00

allowance at the end of the week when she behaves appropriately, parents may place $2.00 in nickels in a jar on a shelf that is visible to the child. So long as she behaves appropriately, the $2.00 belongs to her. Every time there is an infraction that has been clearly defined and agreed upon between parents and child, a nickel is removed from the jar. Many ADHD children, because of their reinforcement histories, perform much better when they are working to keep what they already have rather than to earn something they do not have.

Negative Reinforcement

Earlier in the text, negative reinforcement was explained at some length. It is important for the practitioner to make certain parents understand the powerful effect negative reinforcement has on ADHD children. Over time these children develop a view of the world in which they are repeatedly working to get rid of aversive stimulation rather than to earn positive stimulation. Some parents find it difficult to break this cycle. In such situations, it may be beneficial for the practitioner to teach parents to modify their use of negative reinforcement so that it is used in a constructive manner. In a situation in which the child is sent off to complete an activity, parents are instructed to repeatedly check on the child after short periods, increasing the likelihood that when they approach the child he will be engaged in the target task and can be positively reinforced. In the event the child is not on task, parents are then instructed to remain with the child until the task is completed. The child may work to get rid of the aversive consequence, parental attention, but learns that the only way to do this is to complete the task.

Cognitive Self-Monitoring

As discussed earlier in the text, ADHD children function very well if parents can identify behavior that results from incompetence and provide external structure and support in response to that incompetence. Cognitive self-monitoring is a technique that provides external cues to assist children in monitoring themselves. For example, during a play period instead of the parent coming in and directing a child to speak in an inside voice, a timer can be set to ring every ten minutes. The child is instructed that when the timer rings she is to make certain that her voice level is appropriate and she is following all of the rules. She is then to reset the timer and return to play. Cognitive self-monitoring has also been used effectively by the authors to assist children with morning routines. Cooperatively, the parent and child structure a schedule of required activities and the time allotted to complete those activities. An audiotape is then made by the child in which he directs himself concerning what he is supposed to be doing at that moment and then may also include a favorite song on the tape. Each morning the parent comes in and starts the tape. The tape then acts as an external cognitive cue, assisting the child to complete all necessary morning activities.

The Size of Punishment

Frequently, partial loss of a privilege or possession is a more aversive punishment than complete loss. Again, ADHD children have a long history of not obtaining positive reinforcement and losing many privileges. The loss of an additional privilege may have very little long-term impact. Structuring punishment so that all is not lost as the result of one infraction provides continued opportunity for the ADHD child to at least receive partial positive reinforcement. For example, the child is ten minutes late coming home for dinner. Rather than restrict the child from going out the next day, the loss of an equivalent amount of time or double amount of time in coming home earlier the following day is a better intervention. Instead of taking the child's entire allowance, taking half or two-thirds leaves the child with enough money that she has something to spend but not enough to purchase all that she may want. The mind set is important. Rather than the child approaching the situation saying that she has nothing and simply forgetting about it, the child has something but not enough to get what she wants. This may stimulate more reflection and increase the likelihood that the child will benefit from this punishment experience.

Suggestions to Facilitate Home Behavior of ADHD Children

Schedules

Changes in schedule and routine can be disturbing to all children but especially seem to bother ADHD children. A consistent schedule within the home, including specific time periods and routines for morning and evening activities, chores, homework, play time, television time and dinner are helpful. Parents can also be directed to explain changes in routine ahead of time so that the ADHD child can understand what is to come and anticipate change.

Rules

Clear and concise rules of behavior for the ADHD child are essential. The practitioner may wish to suggest that rules as well as consequences for breaking them or for appropriate behavior be written down and posted in a prominent place. Consistent management is essential. If a rule is broken and a determination is made that this resulted from noncompliant behavior, a negative consequence should follow every time.

Instructions

ADHD children should be provided with simple, clear instructions, frequently with physical demonstration if possible. Instructions should then be repeated back by the ADHD child. Reinforcement should be provided if the child understands and follows directions at the first request. Parents are advised not to give more than one or two instructions at a time. If a task is difficult, the practitioner may assist parents to develop the skill of breaking a task into smaller parts and sequentially directing the child.

Control Stimulation

Although a minimally distracting environment will not guarantee increased time on task, such an arrangement certainly can be beneficial. It is suggested that a specific, minimally distracting location be chosen for homework. For the easily overaroused ADHD child, it is suggested that play sessions be limited to one or two children at a time and that parents take an active role in choosing appropriate playmates.

The Practitioner as Parenting Consultant

It is important for the practitioner to understand that the behavior and management problems most ADHD children present for their parents are chronic and often repetitive. Parents of ADHD children are often frustrated when they successfully deal with one set of problems only to discover that a new problem arises. Often many of these problems result from incompetence, which is not as frustrating for parents to deal with once they can make that distinction and understand the basis for the child's behavior. Providing a parent training program or a few individual parent support sessions over a period of a few weeks will usually prove beneficial, but may not have a lasting effect if parents are then turned loose and do not have the opportunity to seek additional assistance as new problems arise. Given the chronic nature of these problems, it is important for the practitioner to be available on a long-term, as-needed basis to assist parents.

REVIEW OF COMMERCIALLY AVAILABLE PARENTING PROGRAMS

In *Defiant Children: A Clinician's Manual for Parent Training* (1987), Russell Barkley provides a parent training program with a strong behaviorally based foundation. The original basis and philosophy of this program Dr. Barkley credits to Constance Hanf, Professor Emeritus at the University of Oregon Health Science Center. In this program, parents are first taught to attend to and interact appropriately with their children and then are instructed on the management of noncompliant behavior. *Defiant Children* expands on that model, including a system of secondary reinforcement (chips) and techniques to assist impulsive children in planning and developing self-control. In the introductory chapter, Dr. Barkley states that his program is designed for children between 2 and 11 years of age, primarily those with noncompliant, acting-out problems. Dr. Barkley states that "Where children are problematic in listening to parental commands or requests, or in adhering to household or neighborhood rules, this program will prove quite effective" (p. 2). Dr. Barkley notes that the goals of the program are to improve parental management skills, increase parental knowledge of the causes of childhood misbehavior and improve child compliance to parental commands. The manual is well written, and information is presented in a cohesive, easily understood format. Parents can be taken through the program in eight to ten weeks. Handouts and additional materials are also included in a separate accompanying workbook.

Fleischman, Horne and Arthur (1983) have developed and researched a parenting program for families with children experiencing significant aggressive and out-of-control behavior. The Troubled Families Treatment Program is designed to be implemented on an individual basis. The program assists the practitioner through all steps, including initially meeting with the family, teaching basic communication and behavioral skills and dealing with special problems and difficult families. The program can also be implemented in a group setting. Reproducible record-keeping and handout materials are also provided. This can be a very helpful program when dealing with a family in a family therapy setting.

In the *Children's Behavior Therapy Unit Parenting Program* (1982), William Jensen has organized a structured, behaviorally based, eight-week parent training program for parents of ADD children. The program is described as a "step-by-step at-home approach to changing children's behavior" (p. 1). Parents are provided with an 80 page handout that very closely parallels each week's presentation. Information concerning the physical and behavioral effects of stimulant medications is incorporated into the program to help parents understand the interaction of behavior management and medication in bringing about behavioral change. The Parenting Packet is well organized, and complex behavioral techniques are presented in a straightforward, easily understandable fashion.

Wade Horn of the Children's Hospital National Medical Center has developed a 12 week, behaviorally oriented parent training program for parents of attention disordered children. Dr. Horn (personal communication, 1988) notes that much of the material in his parenting program is broadly based on the prior work of Gerald Patterson, Rex Forehand and Russell Barkley. Each parent session is 90 minutes. The manual is well organized. Weekly sessions begin by introducing basic behavioral principles, teaching charting and paying attention to desirable behavior. Specific sessions are devoted to time out, compliance training, behavioral contracting and management of school-based behavioral problems. Dr. Horn augments the program by including Becker's text *Parents Are Teachers* (1971) and Patterson's text *Living with Children: New Methods for Parents and Teachers* (1976) for parents to read.

Breena Satterfield (1988) presents a fairly basic behaviorally oriented parent training course for parents of ADHD children. The program structure and content are very similar to the previous programs reviewed. Of greater interest to the practitioner is an additional, open-ended conjoint child-parent group that Ms. Satterfield has pioneered. The group continues to run from week to week as children complete treatment and others enter treatment. The goals of the group are to improve peer relations, social skills, child and adult communication and to provide additional training for parents. The unique aspect of this group is the fact that it is made up of dyads consisting of a child and a parent. During the group time, each parent is assigned someone else's child as his or her responsibility. This affords parents the opportunity to watch another adult attempt to manage their child as well as to use their parenting skill with someone else's child. Ms. Satterfield (1988) reports that she has found this particular intervention of significant benefit, both to the children and their parents.

Michael Pokin, in *Active Parenting* (1986), has developed a six-session parenting program that can be presented in a group setting or through a series of videocassettes. The program is less oriented toward specific behavioral techniques and more directed at teaching parents to cope with their feelings, encourage their children, communicate effectively, develop mutual respect, and provide natural and logical consequences. Components of this program interface nicely with other more behaviorally oriented parenting programs. Active parenting, when used alone as a general program for more impaired, noncompliant or attention-disordered children, may be too oriented toward feelings and emotions at the expense of teaching behavioral management.

Systematic Training for Effective Parenting (1982) by Don Dinkmeyer and Gary McKay is a parent training program based on the teachings of Rudolph Dreikurs. As Dinkmeyer and McKay note, systematic training for effective parenting (STEP) provides a democratic philosophy of child training. The parent's handbook is easy to read and contains numerous charts and tables summarizing key points. The program is applicable to all children and works best with children who do not experience significant behavioral problems. The basis of the program implies that children have active control over their behavior and the goals of their misbehavior include gaining attention, power or revenge, or displaying inadequacy. The program teaches communication, natural and logical consequences, and methods to build children's confidence and feelings of worth.

Robin (1979) and Robin and Foster (1989) described a problem-solving communication training program for treating parent-adolescent conflict. Robin notes that the program is designed to teach family members methods of effective communication, approaches to resolve conflicts and disputes, ways of restructuring inappropriate attitudes and effective skills to help family members relate in an adult-to-adult manner rather than an adult-to-child manner. The program teaches problem solving, communication training, cognitive restructuring, and approaches for generalization. Robin's program is designed to take place in 7 to 12 sessions with the intent that the skills taught to family members can be used without the assistance of the practitioner. The program has a wide applicability and can be used effectively with families of ADHD adolescents.

In *SOS: Help for Parents* (1986), Lynn Clark has written a very practical, well-organized and comprehensive guide for helping parents deal with behavior problems in children. Dr. Clark has also developed a professional trainer's kit to assist the practitioner to teach parenting skills in a group setting using the *SOS* text as a reference and resource guide. Dr. Clark's text includes sections on fundamentals of behavior, effective discipline, basic behavioral skills, dealing with noncompliance, a section on other parenting texts and how parents can seek additional professional help.

Harvey Parker has written *The ADD Hyperactivity Workbook* (1988). This paperback text is designed for parents, teachers and children. It includes brief but concise explanations as to causes, general treatment and medication for attention deficit. The text also provides guidelines for home and classroom behavior management and stories to be read to children to facilitate a common-sense understanding of attention problems. The text can be used as part of a parenting program by practitioners working with parents or by parents independently.

In *Families: Applications of Social Learning to Family Life* (1975), Gerald Patterson provides a text for the practitioner to be used as supplemental material for parent training programs. The primary goal of the text is to help parents learn child management skills based on social learning principles. The text is easy to follow and in some situations can be given to parents to read independently.

Patterson and Forgatch have authored a text specifically designed to assist in reducing conflict between parents and adolescents. In *Parents and Adolescents*

Living Together (1987), the authors have outlined basic social learning concepts and methods to help parents deal effectively with adolescents. The text is designed to assist parents to change the manner in which they relate to their adolescents.

The Art of Parenting (Wagonseller, Burnett, Salzberg & Burnett, 1977) is a multimedia program that includes text materials, audiocassettes, film strips and five parent review manuals covering the five sessions of the program. Sessions include communication, assertion training and behavioral management techniques, including motivation, specific methods and discipline. This program also devotes time to helping parents communicate and deal effectively with teachers.

Wagonseller and McDowell developed a five-session parent program titled Teaching Involved Parenting–TIP (1982). Their text, *You and Your Child: A Common Sense Approach To Successful Parenting* (1979) is meant to accompany TIP. This program deals with such issues as helping parents understand their role, dealing with expectations, communicating effectively, understanding behavior management principles and designing a behavior management program at home. The presenter's materials for this program include detailed suggestions for structuring each session, media materials and reproducible forms for parents.

SUMMARY

This chapter provided a model and philosophy to assist the practitioner in teaching parents to cope with and manage ADHD children. The model can be used in conjunction with a number of different parent training programs. The four steps of this model are:

1. Increase parental understanding.
2. Increase parental ability to differentiate incompetence from noncompliance.
3. Develop parental ability to provide positive direction to the child.
4. End interactions successfully.

It has been our experience that using this model has been of added benefit in both individual and group parent training. It is an essential component for effective parent training of ADHD children. Parents of ADHD children must be helped to understand the distinction between incompetent and noncompliant behavior. They must also be carefully coached to deal positively with their children and to understand the significant effects factors such as negative reinforcement and punishment can have upon the ADHD child. This chapter also presented a system for the application of a number of basic behavioral techniques as well as suggestions the practitioner can use to help parents deal with problematic behaviors and situations. The role of the practitioner as parent trainer must be both educational and supportive. Since ADHD children will present a chronic cluster of behavioral problems, the practitioner must be available on a long-term basis as needed. The chapter concluded with a review of parent training programs that, when used in conjunction with this model, provide a solid framework for the effective management and behavioral improvement of ADHD children in the home.

Concluding Remarks

In the future, researchers may unlock the mysteries of heredity and the intricacies of brain function. When that time arrives, medical, educational and mental health practitioners may gain an important understanding of many human behaviors, including those the scientific community labels attention-deficit hyperactivity disorder. With understanding may come a cure. Until that time, practitioners are faced with the responsibility of defining, observing, evaluating and managing these complex problems of childhood.

The definition of ADHD must serve the practitioner as a guideline for assessment and provide the families of these children with the means to understand the ADHD child's inability to meet the demands of the world we have designed. This is a disorder that for now is managed and not cured. Effective management requires understanding. It is essential that practitioners, families and the children themselves develop a common-sense understanding of ADHD problems. It is critical for the practitioner to recognize that the multiple behavioral problems comprising ADHD cause multiple and often varied problems for children. The practitioner must recognize the issue of incompetence versus noncompliance in the behavioral problems ADHD children present.

This is also a disorder that must be understood from a developmental perspective. Problems with attention span, overarousal, hyperactivity, impulsivity and difficulty with gratification have a varied impact on children of different ages. Although a group of ADHD children may share many similar skill deficits, any two children randomly compared within the group may be experiencing very different problems.

Because these are the most common problems of childhood, assessment must be conscientious: collecting and integrating medical, educational, psychological and behavioral data. The process of evaluation must consider alternative explanations for the problems the child is experiencing before deciding on the final explanation that this is an attention-disordered child. The practitioner must maintain perspective. Evaluation is incomplete if it only describes behavior and provides statistical analyses. Problems ADHD children experience must be placed within a real-life setting for each child, helping parents, teachers and others understand the powerful impact these behaviors are having on the child. It is up to the practitioner to help others see the world through the eyes of the ADHD child.

The multidisciplinary, multitreatment philosophy requires that each child's problems be addressed in a comprehensive fashion. A single treatment approach has not and will not prove effective in dealing with the myriad of problems ADHD children present. Education, behavior management, group and individual counseling, educational intervention and medication have proven to be an appropriate set of treatments for this disorder of childhood.

This text was conceived and written to comprehensively educate the practitioner about attention disorders in childhood. Effective evaluation and management of these problems in childhood is a reality, but requires time, effort, caring and understanding.

APPENDIX 1

Childhood History Form for
Attention Disorder

Child's Name _____

Birth Date _____ Age _____ Sex _____

Home Address _____
               Street   City

_____ Home Phone _____
State   Zip   Area Code

Child's School _____
             Name   Address

Grade _____ Special Placement (if any) _____

Child is presently living with:

___ Natural Mother ___ Natural Father ___ Stepmother ___ Stepfather
___ Adoptive Mother ___ Adoptive Father ___ Foster Mother
___ Foster Father ___ Other (Specify) _____

Non-residential adults involved with this child on a regular basis:
_____
_____

Source of Referral: Name _____
Address _____ Phone _____
Briefly state main problems of this child: _____
_____
_____
_____

PARENTS

Mother _____
Occupation _____ Bus. Phone _____

Age _____ Age at time of pregnancy with patient _____

School: Highest grade completed _____
        Learning problems _____
        Attention problems _____
        Behavior problems _____

Medical Problems _____

Have any of your blood relatives experienced problems similar to
those your child is experiencing? If so, describe _____
_____

From S. Goldstein and M. Goldstein. *The Multi-Disciplinary Evaluation and Treatment of Attention Disorders in Children: Symposium Handbook*. Copyright 1985 by Neurology, Learning and Behavior Center. Used with permission of the authors and publisher.

Parents (continued):

Father _____
Occupation _____ Bus. Phone _____

School: Highest grade completed _____
         Learning problems _____
         Attention problems_____
         Behavior problems _____

Medical Problems _____

Have any of your blood relatives experienced problems similar to
those your child is experiencing? If so, describe _____
_____

SIBLINGS

          Name   Age   Medical, social or school problems

1. _____
2. _____
3. _____
4. _____
5. _____
6. _____

PREGNANCY - Complications:
  Excessive vomiting _____ hospitalization required _____
  Excessive staining/blood loss _____ threatened miscarriage _____
  Infection(s) (specify) _____
  Toxemia _____ Operation(s) (specify) _____
  Other illness(es) (specify)_____
  Smoking during pregnancy _____ # cigarettes per day _____
  Alcoholic consumption during pregnancy _____ describe
    if beyond an occasional drink _____
  Medications taken during pregnancy _____
  X-ray studies during pregnancy _____
  Duration of pregnancy (weeks)_____

DELIVERY
  Type of labor: Spontaneous _____ Induced _____ Duration (hrs) _____
  Type of delivery: Normal _____ Breech _____ Caesarean _____
  Complications: Cord around neck _____ Hemorrhage _____
    Infant injured during delivery _____ Other _____
    Birth Weight _____

POST DELIVERY PERIOD
  Jaundice _____ Cyanosis (turned blue) _____ Incubator care _____
  Infection (specify) _____
  Number of days infant was in the hospital after delivery _____

INFANCY PERIOD

  Were any of the following present - to a significant degree -
  during the first few years of life? If so, describe.

     Did not enjoy cuddling _____
     Was not calmed by being held or stroked _____
     Difficult to comfort _____
     Colic _____ Excessive restlessness _____
     Excessively irritable _____
     Diminished sleep _____
     Frequent headbanging _____
     Difficulty nursing _____
     Constantly into everything _____

MEDICAL HISTORY

If your child's medical history includes any of the following,
please note the age when the incident or illness occurred and
any other pertinent information:

Childhood diseases (describe ages and any complications) ____

Operations _____
Hospitalizations for illness _____

Head injuries _____
Convulsions _____ with fever _____ without fever __
Coma _____ Persistent high fevers _____
Eye problems _____ Ear Problems _____
Allergies or Asthma _____
Poisoning _____
Sleep problems _____
Appetite _____

PRESENT MEDICAL STATUS

Height _____ Weight _____
Present illnesses for which the child is being treated _____
_____
Medications child is taking on ongoing basis _____
_____

DEVELOPMENTAL MILESTONES

If you can recall, record the age at which your child reached the
following developmental milestones. If you cannot recall exactly,
check item at right.

	Age	Early	Normal	Late
Smiled				
Sat without support				
Crawled				
Stood without support				
Walked without assistance				
Spoke first words				
Said phrases				
Said sentences				
Bladder trained, day				
Bladder trained, night				
Bowel trained, day				
Bowel trained, night				
Rode tricycle				
Rode bicycle (without training wheels)				
Buttoned clothing				
Tied shoelaces				
Named colors				
Named coins				
Said alphabet in order				
Began to read				

COORDINATION
Rate your child on the following skills:

	Good	Average	Poor
Walking			
Running			
Throwing			
Catching			
Shoelace tying			
Buttoning			
Writing			
Athletic abilities			
Exessive number of accidents compared to other children			

COMPREHENSION AND UNDERSTANDING

Do you consider your child to understand directions and situations as well as other children his or her age? If not, why not? _____
_____

How would you rate your child's overall level of intelligence compared to other children?

Below average _____   Above average _____   Average _____

SCHOOL

Were you concerned about your child's ability to succeed in kindergarten? If so, please explain _____
_____

Rate your child's school experiences related to **academic learning:**

	Good	Average	Poor
Nursery school			
Kindergarten			
Current grade			

To the best of your knowledge, at what grade level is your child functioning: reading _____ spelling _____ arithmetic _____

Has your child every had to repeat a grade? If so, when? _____

Present class placement: regular class ____ special class (if so specify) _____

Kinds of special counseling or remedial work your child is currently receiving _____

Describe briefly any academic school problems _____
_____
_____

Rate your child's school experiences related to **behavior:**

	Good	Average	Poor
Nursery school			
Kindergarten			
Current grade			

Does your child's teacher describe any of the following as significant classroom problems?

Doesn't sit still in his or her seat _____
Frequently gets up and walks around the classroom _____
Shouts out. Doesn't wait to be called on _____
Won't wait his or her turn _____
Doesn't cooperate well in group activities _____
Typically does better in a one to one relationship _____
Doesn't respect the rights of others _____
Doesn't pay attention during storytelling or show and tell _____
Describe briefly any other classroom behavioral problems _____
_____
_____

As best you can recall, please use the following space to provide a general description of your child's school progress in each grade. Use the back of this form if extra space is needed.
_____
_____
_____
_____
_____

PEER RELATIONSHIPS

Does your child seek friendships with peers? _____
Is your child sought by peers for friendship? _____
Does your child play with children primarily his or her own
  age? _____ younger? _____ older? _____
Describe briefly any problems your child may have with peers _____
_____
_____
_____

HOME BEHAVIOR

All children exhibit, to some degree, the behaviors listed below.
Check those that you believe your child exhibits to an excessive
or exaggerated degree when compared to other children his or her
own age.

Fidgets with hands, feet or squirms in seat _____
Has difficulty remaining seated when required to do so _____
Easily distracted by extraneous stimulation _____
Has difficulty awaiting turn in games or group situations _____
Blurts out answers to questions before they have been completed__
Has problems following through with instructions (usually not
  due to opposition or failure to comprehend) _____
Has difficulty paying attention during tasks or play activities__
Shifts from one uncompleted activity to another _____
Has difficulty playing quietly _____
Often talks excessively _____
Interrupts or intrudes on others (often not purposeful or planned
  but impulsive) _____
Does not appear to listen to what is being said _____
Loses things necessary for tasks or activities at home _____
Boundless energy and poor judgment _____
Impulsivity (poor self control) _____
Frustrates easily _____
History of temper tantrums _____
Temper outbursts _____
Frustrates easily _____
Sloppy table manners _____
Sudden outbursts of physical abuse of other children _____
Acts like he or she is driven by a motor _____
Wears out shoes more frequently than siblings _____
Excessive number of accidents _____
Doesn't seem to learn from experience _____
Poor memory _____
A "different child" _____

Does your child create more problems, either purposeful or nonpurposeful, within the home setting than his or her siblings? _____
_____

Does your child have difficulty benefiting from his experiences? __
_____

Types of discipline you use with your child _____
_____
_____

Is there a particular form of discipline that has proven effective?
_____

Have you participated in a parenting class or obtained other forms
of information concerning discipline and behavior management? _____
_____

INTERESTS AND ACCOMPLISHMENTS:

What are your child's main hobbies and interests? _____
_____

What are your child's areas of greatest accomplishment? _____
_____

What does your child enjoy doing most? _____
_____

What does your child dislike doing most? _____
_____

LIST NAMES AND ADDRESS OF ANY OTHER PROFESSIONALS CONSULTED:
(Including family physician or pediatrician)

1. _____
2. _____
3. _____
4. _____

ADDITIONAL REMARKS – Please write any additional remarks you may wish
to make regarding your child.

_____

_____

_____

_____

_____

_____

_____

_____

_____

_____

_____

_____

_____

_____

_____

_____

APPENDIX 2

Maternal Discipline Techniques—
Self Report Instrument

TYPICAL CHILD BEHAVIOR PROBLEMS

One of the things we're interested in is how you handle _____ when s/he misbehaves. I am going to describe some different ways in which children disobey their parents. I would like you to imagine your child in each situation and tell me how you would deal with him/her.

1. You need to take _____ out for an errand and you don't have much time. You call out for him, but he does not answer. After calling a few more times, you begin to look for him. Soon you become worried, but then find out that he has been hiding from you.

   First Method: What would you do?

   Second Method: What if he did it again the next day? What would you do then?

   Third Method: What would you probably do if he did it once again?

2. You're shopping in a store and _____ is with you. He sees something that he likes and asks you if he can have it. You tell him "NO," but he demands to have it and starts crying and screaming.

   First Method: What would you do?

   Second Method: What if she continues crying and screaming? What would you do?

   Third Method: What if she did it once again?

From A. K. Gardner, S. Scarr and C. Schwarz, in *Family Evaluation and Child Custody Litigation* by Richard A. Gardner. Copyright 1982 by Creative Therapeutics. Used with permission of the author and publisher.

3. You're busy cooking in the kitchen and you tell _____ to stay out for a while. Instead he climbs up on a table and knocks over a bowl, spilling all of the food on the floor.

First Method: What would you do?
Second Method: What if she came back into the kitchen and climbed back onto the table?
Third Method: What if she did it once again?

4. You and your family are in a strange area with lots of people and you tell _____ not to go too far away. However, he soon wanders off and you have to go looking all over the place for him.

First Method: What would you do when you found him?
Second Method: What if he wanders off again and you had to go looking for him again? What would you do when you found him?
Third Method: What if it happened again? What would you do when you found him?

5. _____ and a neighbor's child are playing together in your living room. _____ asks to play with a toy, but the other child refuses. _____ gets angry, hits his playmate, and takes the toy.

First Method: What would you do?
Second Method: What if she did it again?
Third Method: What if the next day, she did it again? What would you do?

6. After being told many times not to go into your closet, you come home to find that _____ has been playing there for a while and has made a big mess.

First Method: What would you do?
Second Method: What if later that same day you found him in your closet once again making a mess. What would you do?
Third Method: What if it happened again?

7. While playing in another room, _____ accidentally breaks a lamp, but does not come and tell you. You know that he has done it.

First Method: What would you do?
Second Method: What if the next time he broke something, he didn't tell you? What would you do?
Third Method: What if it happened again?

8. _____ is especially rude to one of the grandparents.

First Method: What would you do?

Second Method: What if later that day, it happened again? What would you do?

Third Method: What if it happened again the same day?

9. _____ "acts up" by running around and making a lot of noise while a neighbor or casual acquaintance is visiting and talking with you.

First Method: What would you do?

Second Method: What if he continues to distract the two of you by making lots of noise?

Third Method: What if it happened the next day? What would you do?

10. _____ has broken a very important possession of yours. When you ask him for an explanation, he denies having done it. You know he is lying.

First Method: What would you do?

Second Method: What if he continues to lie? What would you do?

Third Method: What if a similar thing happens the next day? What would you do? (Depending on the type of punishment described, could be replaced with: What if he still continues to lie?)

11. _____ refuses to go to bed when you tell him to.

First Method: What would you do?

Second Method: What if he still refuses to go to bed? What would you do then?

Third Method: What if the same thing happens the next night? What would you do?

12. Instead of eating his dinner, _____ plays with his food and then starts throwing it.

First Method: What would you do?

Second Method: What if he continues to throw his food? What would you do?

Third Method: What if he did the same thing at the next meal? What would you do?

13. You are busy in the kitchen and you ask him to do you a favor by answering the door. Instead of helping out, he just says "No."

First Method: What would you do?

Second Method: What if he still refused? What would you do then?

Third Method: What if later that same day, you asked him to do you another small favor, and he refused? What would you do?

14. You and your family are outside. When you are not looking he runs into a busy street, falls down and starts crying and calling for you. You pick him up and see that he doesn't seem to be hurt.

First Method: What would you do?

Second Method: What if later that day, it happens again? What would you do?

Third Method: What if the next day, it happens again? What would you do.

15. You're very tired and _____ has been pestering you. You have told him to stop, but he continues to bother you.

First Method: What would you do?

Second Method: What if he continues to pester you? What would you do?

Third Method: What if later that day, he began to bother you again? What would you do?

16. You are in a store. _____ reaches up on the counter, takes something, hides it in his pocket and walks away.

First Method: What would you do?

Second Method: What if he refused to give it back? What would you do?

Third Method: What if the next day, he did the same thing in a store? What would you do?

APPENDIX 3

Sources for Attention Assessment Instruments

Detroit Test of Auditory Attention Span for Unrelated Words
Detroit Test of Visual Attention Span for Objects
   from the Detroit Tests of Learning Aptitude
   Western Psychological Services
   12031 Wilshire Boulevard
   Los Angeles, CA 90025

WISC-R Digit Span Subtest
WISC-R Coding Subtest
WISC-R Auditory Arithmetic
WISC-R Mazes Subtest
   from the Wechsler Intelligence Scale for Children-Revised
   The Psychological Corporation
   P. O. Box 9954
   San Antonio, TX 78204-0954

Seashore Rhythm Test
Speech Sounds Perception Test
Trail Making Test
Progressive Figures Test
   Reitan Neuropsychology Laboratories, Inc.
   13387 East Edison Street
   Tucson, AZ 85719

Gordon Diagnostic System—Vigilance Task
Gordon Diagnostic System Delay Task
   Gordon Diagnostic System
   P. O. Box 746
   DeWitt, NY 13214

Cancellation of Rapidly Recurring Target Figures Test
  Journal of Brain and Language, **6**, 1978, pp. 52–62

Symbol Digit Modalities Test
  Western Psychological Services
  12031 Wilshire Boulevard
  Los Angeles, CA 90025

ITPA Visual Closure Subtest
  (from the Illinois Test of Psycholinguistic Abilities)
  University of Illinois Press
  University of Illinois
  Urbana, IL 61801

Gardner Steadiness Test
  Lafayette Instrument Company
  P. O. Box 1279
  Lafayette, IN 47902

Stroop Color Distraction Test
  Psychological Assessment Resources
  P.O. Box 998
  Odessa, FL 33556

Matching Familiar Figures Test
  Jerome Kagan, Ph.D.
  William James Hall
  Harvard University
  33 Kirkland Street
  Cambridge, MA 02138

APPENDIX 4

Software Manufacturers and Distributors

Academic Software
c/o Software City
22 East Quackenbush Avenue
Dumont, NJ 07628
1-201-837-8174

Activision, Inc.
P. O. Box 3047
Menlo Park, CA 94025
1-415-329-7699

Applesoft Basic
c/o Children's Television Workshop
One Lincoln Plaza
New York, NY 10023

Broderbund Software
17 Paul Drive
San Rafael, CA 94903-2101
1-415-492-3500

Cognitive Rehabilitation
NeuroScience Center
6555 Carrollton Avenue
Indianapolis, IN 46220
1-317-257-9672

Computer Courseware Services
300 York Avenue
Saint Paul, MN 55101

Davidson & Associates
3135 Kashwia Street
Torrance, CA 90505
1-213-534-4070

Designware, Inc.
185 Berry Street
San Francisco, CA 94107

DLM
One DLM Park
Allen, TX 75002-1302

Educational Resources
2354 Hassell Road, Suite B
Hoffman Estates, IL 60195

EPYX
600 Galveston Drive
Redwood City, CA 94063
1-415-366-0606

Fas Track Computer Products
4410 Westerville Road
Columbus, OH 43231
1-800-272-1600

Hartley Courseware, Inc.
133 Bridge Street
Diamondale, MI 48821
1-800-247-1380

Home Software Catalog
Scholastic Software
P. O. Box 7502
Jefferson City, MO 65102

Lambert Software Co.
P. O. Box 1257
Ramona, CA 92065
1-619-492-9721

Lambert Software Co.
10700 Northrup Way
Bellevue, WA 98004

The Learning Co.
545 Middlefield Road
Menlo Park, CA 94025

Life Science Associates
One Fenimore Road
Bayport, NY 11705

MECC
3490 Lexington Avenue N.
St. Paul, MN 55126
1-612-481-3500

Mindscape, Inc.
3444 Dundee Road
Northbrook, IL 60062
1-800-221-9884

Montezukma Micro
2544 W. Commerce Street
P. O. Box 224767
Dallas, TX 75222-4767
1-214-709-1986

Network Services
1915 Hugvenat Road
Richmond, VA 23235

Psychological Software Services Inc.
655 Carrollton Avenue
Indianapolis, IN 46220
1-317-257-9672

Random House Media
400 Hahn Road
Westminister, MD 21157
1-800-638-6460

Saint Lawrence Rehabilitation Center
1381 Lawrenceville Rd.
Lawrenceville, NJ 08648
1-609-896-9500

Scholastic Software, Inc.
P. O. Box 7502
2931 East McCarty Street
Jefferson City, MO 65102
1-800-541-5513

Soft Mart
217-A East Camp Wisdom Road
Suite #104
Duncanville, TX 75116
1-214-709-1986

Spinnaker Software Corp.
One Kendall Square
Cambridge, MA 02139
1-617-494-1225

Sunburst Communications
39 Washington Avenue
Pleasantville, NY 10570-9971
1-800-431-1934

Texas Instrument
P. O. Box 10508
Mail Station 5849
Lubbock, TX 79408

Wang Neuropsychological Laboratory
1720 LaLuna Court
San Luis Obispo, CA 93401
1-805-543-1552

Weekly Reader
10 Station Place
Norfolk, CT 06058
1-203-542-5553

References

Abikoff, H. (1985). Efficacy of cognitive training interventions in hyperactive children: A critical review. *Clinical Psychology Review* (Special issue. *Attention deficit disorder: Issues in assessment and intervention*), *5*, 479–512.

Abikoff, H. (1987). An evaluation of cognitive behavior therapy for hyperactive children. In B. B. Lahey and A. E. Kadzin (Eds.), *Advances in clinical child psychology* (Vol. 10, pp. 171–216). New York: Plenum Publishers Press.

Abikoff, H., Ganeles, G., Reiter, G., Blum, C., Foley, C., & Klein, R. G. (1988). Cognitive training in academically deficient ADDH boys receiving stimulant medication. *Journal of Abnormal Child Psychology, 16*, 411–432.

Abikoff, H., & Gittelman, R. (1985). Hyperactive children treated with stimulants: Is cognitive training a useful adjunct? *Archives of General Psychiatry, 42*, 953–961.

Abikoff, H., Gittelman-Klein, R., & Klein, D. F. (1977). Validation of a classroom observation code for hyperactive children. *Journal of Consulting and Clinical Psychology, 45*, 772–783.

Achenbach, T. M. (1975). Longitudinal study of relations between association of responding, I.Q. changes, and school performance from grades 3 to 12. *Developmental Psychology, 11*, 653-654.

Achenbach, T. M. (1978). The child behavior profile: I. Boys aged 6-11. *Journal of Consulting and Clinical Psychology, 46*, 478–488.

Achenbach, T. M. (1984). *Current status of the child behavior checklist and related materials.* Burlington, VT: University Associates in Psychiatry.

Achenbach, T. M., & Edelbrock, C. (1981). Behavioral problems and competencies reported by parents of normal and disturbed children aged 4 through 16. *Monographs of the Society for Research and Child Development, 46* (Serial No. 188).

Achenbach, T. M., & Edelbrock, C. (1983). *Manual for the child behavior checklist and revised child behavior profile.* Burlington, VT: Department of Psychiatry.

Ackerman, P. T., Dykman, R. A., & Oglesby, D. M. (1983). Sex and group differences in reading in attention disordered children with and without hyperkinesis. *Journal of Learning Disabilities, 16*, 407–414.

Ackerman, P. T., Dykman, R. A., & Peters, J. E. (1977). Teenage status of hyperactive and non-hyperactive learning disabled boys. *American Journal of Orthopsychiatry, 47*, 577–596.

Adams, M. J., Buschelia, J., DeSanchez, M., & Swets, J. A. (1986). *Odyssey: A curriculum for thinking—foundations of reasoning.* Watertown, MA: Mastery Education Corporation.

Aicardi, J. (1988). The Lennox-Gastaut Syndrome. *International Pediatrics, 3*, 152–157.

Aman, M. G., Mitchell, E. A., & Turbott, S. H. (1987). The effects of essential fatty acid supplementation by efamol in hyperactive children. *Journal of Abnormal Child Psychology, 15*, 75–90.

American Academy of Pediatrics. (1987). Committee on drugs report: Medication for children with an attention deficit disorder. *Pediatrics, 80,* 5.

American Psychiatric Association. (1968). *Diagnostic and statistical manual of mental disorders* (2nd ed.). Washington, DC: Author.

American Psychiatric Association. (1980). *Diagnostic and statistical manual of mental disorders* (3rd ed.). Washington, DC: Author.

American Psychiatric Association. (1987). *Diagnostic and statistical manual of mental disorders* (3rd ed., rev.). Washington, DC: Author.

Anderson, E. E., Clement, P. W., & Oettinger, L. (1981). Methylphenidate compared with behavioral self-control in attention deficit disorder. Preliminary report. *Developmental and Behavioral Pediatrics, 4,* 137–141.

Arnold, E., Molinoff, P., & Rutledge, C. (1977). The release of endogenous norepinephrine and dopamine from cerebral cortex by amphetamine. *Journal of Pharmacological Experimental Therapy, 202,* 544–557.

Asher, S. R., & Gottman, J. M. (1981). *The development of children's friendships.* New York: Cambridge University Press.

August, G. J., Stewart, M. A., & Holmes, C. S. (1983). Four year follow-up of hyperactive boys with and without conduct disorders. *British Journal of Psychiatry, 143,* 192–198.

Bachman, D. S. (1981). Pemoline-induced Tourette's disorder: A case report. *American Journal of Psychiatry, 138,* 1116–1117.

Bailey, D. P., Jr., & Simeonsson, R. J. (1985). A functional model of social competence. *Topics in Early Childhood, 4,* 20–31.

Baker, H. J., & Leland, B. (1967). *Detroit Tests of Learning Aptitude.* Indianapolis: Bobbs-Merrill.

Baker, L., & Cantwell, D. P. (1987). A prospective psychiatric follow-up of children with speech/language disorders. *Journal of the American Academy of Child Psychiatry, 26,* 546–553.

Bandura, A. (1977). *Social learning theory.* Englewood Cliffs, NJ: Prentice-Hall.

Barkley, R. A. (1976). Predicting the response of hyperkinetic children to stimulant drugs: A review. *Journal of Abnormal Child Psychology, 4,* 327–348.

Barkley, R. A. (1977). A review of stimulant drug research with hyperactive children. *Journal of Child Psychology and Psychiatry, 18,* 137–165.

Barkley, R. A. (1978). Recent developments in research on hyperactive children. *Journal of Pediatric Psychology, 3,* 158–163.

Barkley, R. A. (1981a). *Hyperactive children: A handbook for diagnosis and treatment.* New York: Guilford Press.

Barkley, R. A. (1981b). Hyperactivity. In E. Mash & L. Terdal (Eds.), *Behavioral assessment of childhood disorders.* New York: Guilford Press.

Barkley, R. A. (1987). *Defiant children: A clinician's manual for parent training.* New York: Guilford Press.

Barkley, R. A. (1988a). An alert to a national campaign of disinformation. *Clinical Child Psychology Newsletter,* (Section 1, Division 12), 3.

Barkley, R.A. (1988b). The effects of methylphenidate on the interactions of preschool ADHD children with their mothers. *Journal of American Academy of Child and Adolescent Psychiatry, 27,* 336–341.

Barkley, Russell (1989). Placebo "side effects" and Ritalin. *Clinical Child Psychology Newsletter, 3,* 2.

Barkley, R. A., Copeland, A. P., & Sivage, C. (1980). A self-controlled classroom for hyperactive children. *Journal of Autism and Developmental Disorders, 10,* 75–89.

Barkley, R. A., & Cunningham, C. E. (1979). The effects of methylphenidate on the mother-child interactions of hyperactive children. *Archives of General Psychiatry, 36,* 201–208.

Barkley, R. A., & Cunningham, C. E. (1980). The parent-child interactions of hyperactive children and their modification by stimulant drugs. In R. N. Knights and D. Bakker (Eds.), *Treatment of Hyperactive and Learning Disordered Children.* Baltimore: University Park Press.

Barkley, R. A., Karlsson, J., Strzelecki, E., & Murphy, J. V. (1984). Effects of age and Ritalin dosage on the mother-child interactions of hyperactive children. *Journal of Consulting and Clinical Psychology, 52,* 750–758.

Bash, M. S., & Camp, B. (1985). *Think aloud: Increasing social and cognitive skills—A problem-solving program for children.* Champaign, IL: Research Press.

Battle, E. S., & Lacey, B. (1972). A context for hyperactivity in children, over time. *Child Development, 43,* 757–773.

Beck, L., Langford, W. S., MacKay, M., & Sum, G. (1975). Childhood chemotherapy and later drug abuse and growth curve: A follow-up study of 30 adolescents. *American Journal of Psychiatry, 132,* 436–438.

Becker, W. C. (1971). *Parents are teachers: A child management program.* Champaign, IL: Research Press.

Behar, D., Rapoport, J. L., Adams, A. J., Berg, C. J., & Cornblath, M. (1984). Sugar challenge testing with children considered behaviorally "sugar reactive." *Journal of Nutrition and Behavior, 1,* 277–288.

Behar, D., Rapoport, J. L., Berg, C. J., Denckla, M. B., Mann, L., Cox, C., Fedio, P., Zahn, T., & Wolfman, M. G. (1984). Computerized tomography and neuropsychological test measures in adolescents with obsessive-compulsive disorder. *American Journal of Psychiatry, 141,* 363–369.

Behar, L. B. (1977). The Preschool Behavior Questionnaire. *Journal of Abnormal Child Psychology, 5,* 265–295.

Beitchman, J. H. (1987). Language delay and hyperactivity in preschoolers. *Canadian Journal of Psychiatry, 32,* 683–687.

Beitchman, J. H., Hood, J., Rochon, J., & Peterson, M. (1989). Empirical classification of speech/language impairment in children: II. Behavioral characteristics. *Journal of the American Academy of Child and Adolescent Psychiatry, 28,* 118–123.

Bellak, L. (Ed.). (1979). *Psychiatric aspects of minimal brain dysfunction in adults.* New York: Grune and Stratton.

Bellak, L., & Bellak, S. S. (1968). *Children's Apperception Test.* Los Angeles: Western Psychological Services.

Bender, L. (1942). Post encephalitic behavior disorders in children. In J. B. Neal (Ed.), *Encephalitis: A clinical study.* New York: Grune and Stratton.

Bender, L. (1956). *Psychopathology of children with organic brain disorders.* Springfield, IL: Charles C. Thomas.

Ben-Yishay, Y., Rattok, J., & Diller, L. (1979). *A clinical strategy for the systematic amelioration of attentional disturbances in severe head trauma patients* (Rehabilitation Monograph). New York: New York University Medical Center, Institute of Rehabilitation Medicine.

Bereiter, C., & Anderson, V. (1983). *Willy the wisher and other thinking stories: An Open Court thinking storybook.* LaSalle, IL: Open Court.

Berg, C., Hart, D., Quinn, P., & Rapoport, J. (1978). Newborn minor physical anomalies and prediction of infant behavior. *Journal of Autism and Childhood Schizophrenia, 8,* 427–439.

Berg, C., Quinn, P. O., & Rapoport, J. L. (1978). Clinical evaluation of one year old infants: Possible predictors of risk for the "hyperactive syndrome." *Journal of Pediatric Psychology, 3,* 164–167.

Berg, C., Rapoport, J. L., Barkley, L. S., Quinn, P. O., & Timmins, P. (1980). Newborn minor physical anomalies and problem behavior at age three. *Medical Journal of Psychiatry, 137,* 791–796.

Berry, C. A., Shaywitz, S. E., & Shaywitz, B. A. (1985). Girls with attention deficit disorder: A silent minority? A report on behavioral and cognitive characteristics. *Pediatrics, 76,* 801–809.

Berry, K., & Cook, V. J. (1980). Personality and behavior. In H. Rie & E. D. Rie (Eds.), *Handbook of minimal brain dysfunction.* New York: Wiley Interscience Press.

Birmaher, B., Quintana, H., & Greenhill, L. L. (1988). Methylphenidate treatment of hyperactive autistic children. *Journal of American Academy of Child and Adolescent Psychiatry, 27,* 248–251.

Blick, D. W., & Test, D. W. (1987). Effects of self-recording on high-school students' on-task behavior. *Learning Disability Quarterly, 10,* 203–213.

Block, G. H. (1977). Hyperactivity: A cultural perspective. *Journal of Learning Disabilities, 10,* 236–240.

Bloom, A. S., Russell, L. J., Weisskopf, B., & Blackerby, J. L. (1988). Methylphenidate-induced delusional disorder in a child with attention deficit disorder with hyperactivity. *Journal of American Academy of Child and Adolescent Psychiatry, 27,* 88–89.

Bloom, B. S. (1956). *Taxonomy of educational objectives.* New York: Longman.

Bond, E. P., & Partridge, C. E. (1926). Post encephalitic behavior disorders in boys and their management in the hospital. *American Journal of Psychiatry, 6,* 103.

Borden, K. A., Brown, R. T., Jenkins, P., & Clingerman, S. R. (1987). Achievement attributions and depressive symptoms in attention-deficit disordered and normal children. *Journal of School Psychology, 25,* 399–404.

Borland, B. L., & Hechtman, H. K. (1976). Hyperactive boys and their brothers: A 25-year follow-up study. *Archives of General Psychiatry, 33,* 669–675.

Bornstein, P., & Quevillon, R. (1976). The effects of a self-instructional package on overactive preschool boys. *Journal of Applied Behavior Analysis, 9,* 179–188.

Bradley, C. (1937). The behavior of children receiving benzedrine. *American Journal of Psychiatry, 94,* 577–585.

Breen, M. J. (1986). Normative data on the Home Situations and School Situations Questionnaires. *ADD/Hyperactivity Newsletter, 3,* 6.

Broden, M., Hall, R. V., & Mitts, B. (1971). The effect of self-recording on the classroom behavior of two eighth-grade students. *Journal of Applied Behavior Analysis, 4,* 191–199.

Brown, G. L., Hunt, R. D., Ebert, M. H., Bunney, W. E., & Kopin, I. J. (1979). Plasma levels of d-amphetamine in hyperactive children. *Psychopharmacology, 62,* 133–140.

Brown, L., Sherbenou, R. J., & Dollar, S. J. (1983). *Test of Non-Verbal Intelligence.* Austin, TX: Pro-Ed.

Brown, R. P., Ingber, P. S., & Tross, S. (1983). Pemoline and lithium in a patient with attention deficit disorder. *Journal of Clinical Psychiatry, 44,* 146–148.

Brown, R. T. (1980). Impulsivity and psychoeducational intervention in hyperactive children. *Journal of Learning Disabilities, 13*, 249–254.

Brown, R. T. (1985). The validity of teacher ratings and differentiating between two sub-groups of attention deficit disordered children with or without hyperactivity. *Educational and Psychological Measurement, 45*, 661–669.

Brown, R. T., Borden, K. A., Wynne, M. E., Schleser, R., & Clingerman, S. R. (1986). Methylphenidate and cognitive therapy with ADD children: A methodological consideration. *Journal of Abnormal Child Psychology, 14*, 481–497.

Brown, R. T., Borden, K. A., Wynne, M. E., Spunt, A. L., & Clingerman, S. R. (1987). Compliance with pharmacological and cognitive treatments for attention deficit disorder. *American Academy of Child and Adolescent Psychiatry, 26*, 521–526.

Brown, R. T., Wynne, M. E., & Medenis, A. (1985). Methylphenidate in cognitive therapy: A comparison of treatment approaches with hyperactive boys. *Journal of Abnormal Child Psychology, 13*, 69–87.

Brunquell, P., Russman, B. S., & Lerer, T. (1988, September). The mental status examination by pediatric neurologists in children with learning problems. Presentation made at the seventeenth national meeting of the Child Neurology Society, Halifax, Canada.

Bryant, L. E., & Budd, K. S. (1984). Teaching behaviorally handicapped preschool children to share. *Journal of Applied Behavioral Analysis, 17*, 45–56.

Buckley, N. K., & Walker, H. M. (1970). *Modifying classroom behavior*. Champaign, IL: Research Press.

Bugental, D. B., Collins, S., Collins, L., & Chaney, L. F. (1978). Attributional and behavioral changes following two behavior management interventions with hyperactive boys: A follow-up study. *Child Development, 49*, 247–250.

Bunney, B. S., & Aghajanian, C. K. (1976). d-Amphetamine-induced inhibition of central dopaminergic neurons: Mediation by striatonigral feedback pathway. *Science, 192*, 391.

Burd, L., & Fisher, W. (1986). Central auditory processing disorder or attention deficit disorder? *Developmental and Behavioral Pediatrics, 7*, 215.

Burns, B. J. (1972). The effect of self-directed verbal commands in arithmetic performance and activity level of urban hyperactive children. Unpublished doctoral dissertation. Cited in D. M. Ross and S. A. Ross (1982). *Hyperactivity: Current issues, research and theory* (2nd ed.). New York: John Wiley & Sons.

Bushell, D. (1973). *Classroom behavior*. Englewood Cliffs, NJ: Prentice-Hall.

Byers, R. K. (1959). Lead poisoning: Review and report of 45 cases. *Pediatrics, 23*, 585.

Call, J. D. (1985). Psychological and behavioral development of infants and children. In V. C. Kelley (Ed.), *Practice of Pediatrics*. Philadelphia: Harper & Row.

Cameron, M. I., & Robinson, V. M. (1980). Effects of cognitive training on academic and on-task behavior of hyperactive children. *Journal of Abnormal Child Psychology, 8*, 405–419.

Camp, B. W., & Bash, M. S. (1981). *Think aloud–increasing social and cognitive skills: A problem-solving program for children*. Champaign, IL: Research Press.

Campbell, S. B. (1975). Mother-child interaction: A comparison of hyperactive, learning-disabled, and normal boys. *American Journal of Orthopsychiatry, 45*, 51–57.

Campbell, S. B. (1985). Hyperactivity in preschoolers: Correlates and prognostic implications. *Clinical Psychology Review, 5*, 405–428.

Campbell, S. B., & Cluss, P. (1982). Peer relationships of young children with behavior problems. In K. H. Rubin and H. S. Ross (Eds.), *Peer relationships and social skills in childhood*. New York: Springer-Verlag.

Campbell, S. B., Endman, M. W., & Bernfeld, G. (1977). A three-year follow-up of hyperactive preschoolers into elementary school. *Journal of Child Psychology and Psychiatry, 18*, 239–249.

Campbell, S. B., & Paulauskas, S. (1979). Peer relations in hyperactive children. *Journal of Child Psychology and Psychiatry, 20*, 233–246.

Campbell, S. B., Szumowski, E. K., Ewing, L. J., Gluck, D. S., & Breaux, A.M. (1982). A multi-dimensional assessment of parent-identified behavior problem toddlers. *Journal of Abnormal Child Psychology, 10*, 569–591.

Cantwell, D. P. (1972). Psychiatric illness in the families of hyperactive children. *Archives of General Psychiatry, 27*, 414–417.

Cantwell, D. P. (1975). Genetics of hyperactivity. *Journal of Child Psychology and Psychiatry, 16*, 261–264.

Cantwell, D. P. (1979). The "hyperactive" child. *Hospital Practice,14*, 65–73.

Cantwell, D. P., & Baker, L. (1977). Psychiatric disorder in children with speech and language retardation. *Archives of General Psychiatry, 34*, 583–591.

Cantwell, D. P., & Baker, L. (1985). Psychiatric and learning disorders in children with speech and language disorders: A descriptive analysis. *Advances in Learning and Behavioral Disabilities, 4*, 29–47.

Cantwell, D. P., & Baker, L. (1987). Differential diagnosis of hyperactivity/Response to commentary. *Journal of Developmental Behavioral Pediatrics, 8*, 159–165, 169–170.

Cantwell, D. P., & Baker, L. (1988). Issues in classification of child and adolescent psychopathology. *Journal of the American Academy of Child and Adolescent Psychiatry, 27*, 521–533.

Cantwell, D. P., Baker, L., & Mattison, R. (1981). Prevalence, type and correlates of psychiatric disorder in 200 children with communication disorder. *Journal of Developmental and Behavioral Pediatrics, 2*, 131–136.

Cantwell, D. P., & Carlson, G. A. (1978). Stimulants. In J. S. Werry (Ed.), *Pediatric psychopharmacology: The use of behavior modifying drugs in children*. New York: Brunner/Mazel.

Cantwell, D. P., & Satterfield, J. H. (1978). The prevalence of academic underachievement in hyperactive children. *Journal of Pediatric Psychology, 3*, 168–171.

Caresia, L., Pugnetti, L., Besana, R., Barteselli, F., Cazzullo, A. G., Musetti, L., & Scarone, S. (1984). EEG and clinical findings during pemoline treatment in children and adults with attention deficit disorder. *Neuropsychobiology, 11*, 158–167.

Carey, W. B. (1970). A simplified method for measuring infant temperament. *Journal of Pediatrics, 77*, 188–194.

Carlson, C. L., Lahey, B. B., Frame, C. L., & Walker, J. (1987). Sociometric status of clinic-referred children with attention deficit disorders with and without hyperactivity. *Journal of Abnormal Child Psychology, 15*, 537–547.

Carlson, C. L., Lahey, B. B., & Neeper, R. (1986). Direct assessment of the cognitive correlates of attention deficit disorders with and without hyperactivity. *Journal of Psychopathology and Behavioral Assessment, 8*, 69–86.

Carter, E. N., and Reynolds, J. N. (1976). Imitation in the treatment of a hyperactive child. *Psychotherapy: Theory, Research and Practice, 13*, 160–161.

Cartledge, G., & Milburn, J. F. (1980). *Teaching social skills to children*. New York: Pergamon Press.

Casat, C. D., Pleasants, D. Z., & Van Wyck Fleet, J. (1987). A double-blind trial of bupropion in children with attention deficit disorder. *Psychopharmacology Bulletin, 23,* 120–122..

Ceaser, L. D. (1986). *Comprehension capers: Main ideas and inferences.* Belmont, CA: David S. Lake.

Charles, L., Schain, R. J., & Zelniker, T. (1981). Optimal dosages of methylphenidate for improving the learning and behavior of hyperactive children. *Behavioral Pediatrics, 2,* 78–81.

Chase, S. N., & Clement, P. W. (1985). Effects of self-reinforcement and stimulants on academic performance in children with attention deficit disorder. *Journal of Clinical Child Psychology, 14,* 323–333.

Chelune, G. J., Ferguson, W., Koon, R., & Dickey, T. O. (1986). Frontal lobe disinhibition in attention deficit disorder. *Child Psychiatry and Human Development, 16,* 221–232.)

Christie, D. J., Hiss, M., & Lozanoff, B. (1984). Modification of inattentive classroom behavior: Hyperactive children's use of self-recording with teacher guidance. *Behavior Modification, 8,* 391–406.

CIBA Pharmaceuticals. (1974). *NBD compendium* (Vol. 1, pp.1–12). Summit, NJ: Author.

Clark, L. (1986). *SOS: Help for parents.* Bowling Green, KY: Parent's Press.

Clark, L., & Elliott, S. (1988). The influence of treatment strength information on knowledgable teachers' pretreatment evaluations of social skills training methods. *Professional School Psychology, 3,* 241–251.

Clark, M. L., Cheyne, J. A., Cunningham, C. E., & Siegel, L. S. (1988). Dyadic peer interaction and task orientation in attention deficit disordered children. *Journal of Abnormal Child Psychology, 16,* 1–15.

Clement, P. W., Anderson, E. E., Arnold, J. H., Butman, R. E., Fantuzzo, J. W., & Mays, R. (1978). Self-observation and self-reinforcement as sources of self-control in children. *Biofeedback Self-Regulation, 3,* 247–267.

Clements, S. D., & Peters, J. E. (1962). Minimal brain dysfunctions in the school-aged child. *Archives of General Psychiatry, 6,* 185–197.

Cohen, N. J., Davine, M., & Meloche-Kelly, M. (1989). Prevalence of unsuspected language disorders in a child psychiatric population. *Journal of the American Academy of Child and Adolescent Psychiatry, 28,* 107–111.

Cohen, N. J., Sullivan, S., Minde, K. K., Novak, C., & Helwig, C. (1981). Evaluation of the relative effectiveness of methylphenidate and cognitive behavior modification in the treatment of kindergarten-aged hyperactive children. *Journal of Abnormal Child Psychology, 9,* 43–54.

Cohen, N. J., Weiss, G., & Minde, K. (1972). Cognitive styles in adolescents previously diagnosed as hyperactive. *Journal of Child Psychology and Psychiatry, 13,* 203–209.

Coie, J. D., & Kuperschmidt, J. B. (1983). A behavioral analysis of emerging social status in boys' groups. *Child Development, 54,* 1400–1416.

Coleman, W. S. (1988). *Attention deficit disorders, hyperactivity and associated disorders: A handbook for parents and professionals* (5th Ed.). Madison, WI: Calliope Books.

Collier, C. P., Soldin, S. J., Swanson, J. M., MacLeod, S. M., Weinberg, F., & Rochefort, J. G. (1985). Pemoline pharmacokinetics and long-term therapy in children with attention deficit disorder and hyperactivity. *Clinical Pharmacokinetics, 10,* 269–278.

Collins, B. E., Whalen, C. K., & Henker, B. (1980). Ecological and pharmacological influences on behaviors in the classroom. The hyperkinetic behavioral syndrome. In S. Salzinger, J. Antrobus, & J. Glick (Eds.), *The ecosystem of the "sick" child.* New York: Academic Press.

Comalli, P. E., Wapner, S., & Werner, H. (1962). Interference effects of Stroop Color-Wood Test in childhood, adulthood and aging. *Journal of Genetic Psychology, 100*, 47–52.

Conners, C. K. (1969). A teacher rating scale for use with drug studies with children. *American Journal of Psychiatry, 126,* 885–888.

Conners, C. K. (1970). Symptom patterns in hyperkinetic, neurotic and normal children. *Child Development, 41*, 667–682.

Conners, C. K. (1972). Symposium: Behavior modification of drugs: II. Psychological effects of stimulant drugs in children with minimal brain dysfunction. *Pediatrics, 49*, 702–708.

Conners, C. K. (1973). Rating scales for use in drug studies with children. *Psychopharmacology Bulletin* (Special Issue: *Pharmacotherapy with Children)*, 24–84.

Conners, C. K. (1975a). Minimal brain dysfunction and psychopathology in children. In A. Davids (Ed.), *Child personality and psychopathology: Volume 2. Current topics.* New York: Wiley Interscience Press.

Conners, C. K. (1975b). Control trial of methylphenidate in preschool children with minimal brain dysfunction. *International Journal of Mental Health, 4*, 61–74.

Conners, C. K. (1980). *Food additives and hyperactive children.* New York: Plenum Press.

Conners, C. K. (1982). Parent and teacher rating forms for the assessment of hyperkinesis in children. In P. A. Keller & L. G. Ritt (Eds.), *Innovations in clinical practice: A source book* (Vol. I). Sarasota, FL: Professional Resource Exchange.

Conners, C. K. (1987). How is the Teacher Rating Scale used in the diagnosis of attention deficit disorder? In J. Loney (Ed.), *The young hyperactive child: Answers to questions about diagnosis, prognosis and treatment* (p.142). New York: Halworth Press.

Conners, C. K., (1989a). *Connors' Teacher Rating Scales.* Toronto: Multi-Health Systems.

Conners, C. K., (1989b). *Connors' Parent Rating Scales.* Toronto: Multi-Health Systems.

Conners, C. K., Eisenberg, L., & Sharpe, L. (1964). Effects of methylphenidate (Ritalin) on paired-associate learning and Porteus Maze performance in emotionally disturbed children. *Journal of Consulting and Clinical Psychology, 28*, 14–22.

Conners, C. K., & Taylor, E. (1980). Pemoline, methylphenidate and placebo in children with minimal brain dysfunction. *Archives of General Psychiatry, 37*, 922–930.

Conners, C. K., Taylor, E., Meo, G., Kurtz, M. A., & Fournier, M. (1972). Magnesium pemoline and dextroamphetamine: A controlled study in children with minimal brain dysfunction. *Psychopharmocologia, 26*, 321–336.

Conners, C. K., & Wells, K. C. (1985). ADD-H Adolescent Self-Report Scale. *Psychopharmacology Bulletin, 21*, 921–922.

Conners, C. K., & Wells, K. C. (1986). *Hyperkinetic children: A neuropsychosocial approach.* Beverly Hills, CA: Sage.

Conners, C. K., & Werry, J. S. (1979). *Psychopathological disorders of childhood* (2nd ed.), New York: John Wiley & Sons.

Connoloy, A. J., Nachtman, W., & Pritchett, E. M. (1976). *Key Math Diagnostic Arithmetic Test.* Circle Pines, MN: American Guidance Service.

Copeland, A. P. (1979). Types of private speech produced by hyperactive and non-hyperactive boys. *Journal of Abnormal Child Psychology, 7*, 169–177.

Copeland, L., Wolraich, M., Lindgren, S., Milich, R., & Woolson, R. (1987). Pediatricans' reported practices in the assessment and treatment of attention deficit disorders. *Journal of Developmental and Behavioral Pediatrics, 8*, 191–197.

Cowart, V. S. (1988a). Reply to behavior disorders and the Ritalin controversy. *Journal of the American Medical Association, 260,* 2219.

Cowart, V. S. (1988b). The Ritalin controversy: What's made this drug's opponents hyperactive? *Journal of the American Medical Association, 259,* 2521–2523.

Cowen, E., Pederson, A., Babigan, H., Izzo, L., & Trost, M. (1973). Long-term follow-up of early detected vulnerable children. *Journal of Consulting and Clinical Psychology, 41,* 438–446.

Cox, R. D., & Gunn, W. B. (1980). Interpersonal skills in the schools: Assessment and curriculum development. In D. P. Rathjen and J. P. Foreyt (Eds.), *Social competence: Interventions for children and adults.* New York: Pergamon Press.

Cunningham, C. E., & Barkley, R. A. (1978a). The role of academic failure in hyperactive behavior. *Journal of Learning Disabilities, 11,* 15–21.

Cunningham, C. E., & Barkley, R. A. (1978b). The effects of methylphenidate on the mother-child interaction of hyperactive identical twins. *Developmental Medicine and Child Neurology, 20,* 634–642.

Cutler, M., Little, J. W., & Strauss, A. A. (1940). The effect of benzedrine on mentally deficient children. *American Journal of Mental Deficiency, 45,* 59–65.

Dainer, K. B., Klorman, R., Salzman, L. F., Hess, D. W., Davidson, P. W., & Michael, R. L. (1981). Learning-disordered children's evoked potentials during sustained attention. *Journal of Abnormal Child Psychology, 9,* 79–94.

Davids, A. (1971). An objective instrument for assessing hyperkinesis in children. *Journal of Learning Disabilities, 4,* 499–501.

DeBrueys, M. T. (Project Coordinator). (1986). *125 ways to be a better student: A program for study skill success.* Moline, IL: LinguiSystems.

de la Burde, B., & Choate, M. S. (1975). Early asymptomatic lead exposure and development at school age. *Behavioral Pediatrics, 4,* 638–642.

Delaney-Black, V., Camp, B. W., Lubchenco, L. O., Swanson, C., Roberts, L., Gaherty, P., & Swanson, B. (1989). Neonatal hyperviscosity association with lower achievement and I.Q. scores at school age. *Pediatrics, 83,* 662–667.

DeMarco, S., Sunder, T., Batts, C., Fruitiger, A. D., & Levey, B. (1988, September). The incidence of a developmental right-hemisphere deficit syndrome in dyseidetic children. Presentation made at the seventeenth national meeting of the Child Neurology Society, Halifax, Canada.

Denckla, M. B. (1985). Revised neurological examination for subtle signs. *Psychopharmacology Bulletin, 21,* 773–789.

Denckla, M. B., Bemporad, J. R., & MacKay, M. C. (1976). Tics following methylphenidate administration. *Journal of American Medical Association, 235,* 1349–1351.

Denckla, M. B., LeMay, M., & Chapman, C. A. (1985). Few CT scan abnormalities found even in neurologically impaired learning disabled children. *Journal of Learning Disabilities, 18,* 132–135.

Denckla, M. B., & Rudel, R. G. (1978). Anomalies of motor development in hyperactive boys. *Annals of Neurology, 3,* 231–233.

Denckla, M. B., Rudel, R. G., Chapman, C., & Krieger, J. (1985). Motor proficiency in dyslexic children with and without attentional disorders. *Archives of Neurology, 42,* 228–231.

Denhoff, E., Davids, A., & Hawkins, R. (1971). Effects of dexedrine on hyperkinetic children: A controlled double-blind study. *Journal of Learning Disabilities, 4,* 27–34.

Denman, S. B. (1984). *Denman Neuropsychology Memory Scale.* Charleston, SC: Author.

Deno, S. L. (1980). Direct observation approach to measuring classroom behavior. *Exceptional Children, 46*, 396–399.

Dinkmeyer, D., & McKay, G. D. (1982). *Systematic training for effective parenting: The parent's handbook.* Circle Pines, MN: American Guidance Service.

Dodge, K. A., McCluskey, C. L., & Feldman, E. (1985). Situational approach to the assessment of social competence in children. *Journal of Consulting and Clinical Psychology, 53*, 344–353.

Dougherty, P. M., & Redomski, N. V. (1987). *The cognitive rehabilitation workbook.* Rockville, MD: Aspen.

Douglas, V. I. (1972). Stop, look and listen: The problem of sustained attention and impulse control in hyperactive and normal children. *Canadian Journal of Behavioral Science, 4*, 259–282.

Douglas, V. I. (1974). Sustained attention and impulse control: Implications for the handicapped child. In J. A. Swets & L. L. Elliott (Eds.), *Psychology and the handicapped child* (DHEW Pub. No. (OE) 73-05000). Washington, DC: U.S. Department of Health, Education and Welfare.

Douglas, V. I. (1980). Treatment and training approaches to hyperactivity: Establishing internal or external control. In C. K. Whalen and B. Henker (Eds.), *Hyperactive children: The social ecology of identification and treatment.* New York: Academic Press.

Douglas, V. I. (1985). The response of ADD children to reinforcement: Theoretical and clinical implications. In L. N. Bloomingdale (Ed.), *Attention deficit disorder: Identification, course and rationale.* Jamaica, NY: Spectrum.

Douglas, V. I., Barr, R. G., O'Neil, M. E., & Britton, B. G. (1986). Short-term effects of methylphenidate on the cognitive, learning, and academic performance of children with attention deficit disorder in the laboratory and classroom. *Journal of Child Psychology and Psychiatry, 27*, 191–211.

Douglas, V. I., Parry, P., Martin, P., & Garson, C. (1976). Assessment of a cognitive training program for hyperactive children. *Journal of Abnormal Child Psychology, 4*, 389–410.

Douglas, V. I., & Peters, K. G. (1979). Toward a clearer definition of the attentional deficit of hyperactive children. In G. A. Hale and M. Lewis (Eds.), *Attention and the development of cognitive skills.* New York: Plenum Press.

Drabman, R. S., Spitalnik, R., & O'Leary, K. D. (1973). Teaching self-control to disruptive children. *Journal of Abnormal Psychology, 82*, 10–16.

Duffy, F. H., Denckla, M. B., Bartels, P. H., Sandini, G., & Kiessling, L. S. (1980a). Dyslexia: Regional differences in brain electrical activity by topographic mapping. *Annals of Neurology, 7*, 412–420.

Duffy, F. H., Denckla, M. B., Bartels, P. H., Sandini, G., & Kiessling, L. S. (1980b). Dyslexia: Automated diagnosis by computerized classification of brain electrical activity. *Annals of Neurology, 7*, 421–428.

Dunn, L. M., & Markwardt, F. C. (1970). *Peabody Individual Achievement Test.* Circle Pines, MN: American Guidance Service.

Dweck, C. S. (1975). The role of expectations and attributions in the alleviation of learned helplessness. *Journal of Personality and Social Psychology, 31*, 674–685.

Dykman, R. A., Ackerman, P. T., Clements, S. D., & Peters, J. E. (1971). Specific learning disabilities: An attentional deficit syndrome. In H. R. Myklebust (Ed.), *Progress in learning disabilities* (Vol. 2, pp. 56–93). New York: Grune and Stratton.

Dykman, R. A., McGrew, J., & Ackerman, P. T. (1974). A double-blind clinical study of pemoline on MBD children: Comments on the psychological test results. In C. K. Conners, (Ed.), *Clinical use of stimulant drugs in children*, *Excerpta Medica*, 125–129.

Dykman, R. A., McGrew, J., Harris, T. S., Peters, J. E. & Ackerman, P. T. (1976). Two blinded studies of the effects of stimulant drugs on children: Pemoline, methylphenidate and placebo. In R. T. Anderson and C. G. Halcomb (Eds.), *Learning disability/minimal brain dysfunction syndrome* (pp. 217-235). Springfield, IL: Thomas.

Ebaugh, F. G. (1923). Neuropsychiatric sequelae of acute epidemic encephalitis in children. *American Journal of Diseases of Children, 25,* 89–97.

Edelbrock, C., & Achenbach, T. (1984). The teacher version of the Child Behavior Profile: I. Boys age 6–11. *Journal of Consulting and Clinical Psychology, 52,* 207–217.

Edelbrock, C., Costello, A.J., & Kessler, M.D. (1984). Empirical corroboration of attention deficit disorder. *Journal of the American Academy of Child Psychiatry, 23,* 285–290.

Egeland, B., & Weinberg, R. A. (1976). The Matching Familiar Figures Test: A look at psychometric credibility. *Child Development, 47,* 483–491.

Egger, J., Carter, C. M., Graham, P. J., Gumley, D., & Soothill, J. F. (1985). Controlled trial of oligoantigenic treatment in the hyperkinetic syndrome. *Lancet*, March 9, 540–545.

Elardo, P., & Cooper, M. (1977). *AWARE: Activities for social development*. Menlo Park, CA: Addision-Wesley.

Ellis, A., & Harper, R. (1975). *A new guide to rational living*. New York: Wilshire Book Company.

Epstein, L. C., Lasgna, L., Conners, C. K., & Rodriguez, A. (1968). Correlation of dextroamphetamine excretion and drug response in hyperactive children. *Journal of Nervous and Mental Disease, 146*(2), 136–146.

Erenberg, G., Cruse, R. P., and Rothmer, A. D. (1985). Gilles de la Tourette's syndrome: Effect of stimulant drugs. *Neurology, 35,* 1346–1348.

Farnett, C., Forte, I., & Loss, B. (1976). *Special kid's stuff*. Nashville, TN: Incentive Publications.

Feehrer, C. E., & Adams, M. J. (1986). *Odyssey: A curriculum for thinking—decision making*. Watertown, MA: Mastery Education Corporation.

Feingold, B. F. (1974). *Why your child is hyperactive*. New York: Random House.

Feldman, M. J., & Drasgow, J. (1981). *The Visual-Verbal Test*. Los Angeles: Western Psychological Services.

Finch, A. J., Saylor, C. F., & Edwards, G. L. (1985). Children's Depression Inventory: Sex and grade norms for normal children. *Journal of Consulting and Clinical Psychology, 53,* 424–425.

Fleischman, M. J., Horne, A. M., & Arthur, J. L. (1983). *Troubled families: A treatment program*. Champaign, IL: Research Press.

Freidling, C., & O'Leary, S. G. (1979). Effects of self-instructional training on second and third grade hyperactive children: A failure to replicate. *Journal of Applied Behavior Analysis, 12,* 211–219.

Friedman, J. T., Carr, R., Elders, J., Ringdahal, I., & Roache, A. (1981). Effect on growth in pemoline treated children with attention deficit disorder. *Medical Journal Dis. Child, 135,* 329–332.

Friedman, R. J. (1988). Attention-deficit Hyperactivity Disorder. *A video tape*. St. Clair Shores, MI.

Friedman, R. J., & Doyal, G. T. (1987). *Attention deficit disorder and hyperactivity* (2nd ed.). Danville, IL: Interstate Printers & Publishers, Inc.

Fromm-Auch, D., & Yeudall, L. T. (1983). Normative data for the Halstead-Reitan Neuropsychological Test. *Journal of Clinical Neuropsychology, 5*, 221–232.

Funk, J. B., & Ruppert, E. S. (1984). Language disorders and behavioral problems in preschool children. *Developmental and Behavioral Pediatrics, 5*, 357–360.

Gajar, A. H., Schloss, P. J., Schloss, C. N., & Thompson, C. K. (1984). Effects of feedback and self-monitoring on head trauma youths' conversational skills. *Journal of Applied Behavioral Analysis, 17*, 353–358.

Gardner, R. A. (1978). *The Talking, Feeling and Doing Game.* Cresskill, NJ: Creative Therapeutics.

Gardner, R. A. (1979). *The objective diagnosis of minimal brain dysfunction.* Cresskill, NJ: Creative Therapeutics.

Gardner, R. A. (1982a). *Psychostimulant medication assessment battery.* Unpublished.

Gardner, R. A. (1982b). *Family evaluation and child custody litigation.* Cresskill, NJ: Creative Therapeutics.

Gardner, R. A., Gardner, A. K., Caemmerer, A., & Broman, M. (1979). An instrument for measuring hyperactivity and other signs of minimal brain dysfunction. *Journal of Clinical Child Psychology, 8*, 173–179.

Garfinkel, B. D. (1989, June). Recent advances in Attention Deficit Disorder. Presentation made at the First National Conference on Attention Deficit Disorders, Orlando, FL.

Garfinkel, B. G., & Klee, S. H. (1983). A computerized assessment battery for attention deficits. *Psychiatric Hospitalization, 14*, 163–166.

Garfinkel, B. G., Wender, P. H., Sloman, L., & O'Neill, I. (1983). Tricyclic antidepressant and methylphenidate treatment of attention deficit disorder in children. *Journal of the American Academy of Child Psychiatry, 22*, 343–348.

Gascon, G. G., Johnson, R., & Burd, L. (1986). Central auditory processing and attention deficit disorders. *Journal of Child Neurology, 1*, 27–33.

Gittelman, R. (1985). Self-Evaluation (teenagers) Self-Report. *Psychopharmacology Bulletin, 21*, 925–926.

Gittelman, R., Klein, D. F., & Feingold, I. (1983). Children with reading disorders. Two effects of methylphenidate in combination with reading remediation. *Journal of Child Psychology and Psychiatry, 24*, 193–212.

Gittelman, R., Mannuzza, S., Shenker, R., & Bonagura, N. (1985). Hyperactive boys almost grown up: I. Psychiatric status. *Archives of General Psychiatry, 42*, 937–947.

Gittelman-Klein, R., Abikoff, H., Pollack, E., Klein, D. F., Katz, S., & Mattes, J. (1980) A controlled trial of behavior modification and methylphenidate in hyperactive children. In C. K. Whalen and B. Henker (Eds.), *Hyperactive Children: The social ecology of identification and treatment.* New York: Academic Press.

Gittelman-Klein, R., Klein, D. F., Katz, S., Saraf, K., & Pollack, E. (1976). Comparative effects of methylphenidate and thioridazine in hyperkinetic children: I. Clinical results. *Archives of General Psychiatry, 33*, 1217–1231.

Glow, R. A., & Glow, P. H. (1980). Peer and self-rating: Children's perception of behavior relevant to hyperkinetic impulse disorder. *Journal of Abnormal Psychology, 8*, 471–490.

Goldberg, J. O., & Konstantareas, M. M. (1981). Vigilance in hyperactive and normal children on a self-paced operant task. *Journal of Child Psychology and Psychiatry, 22*, 55–63.

Golden, G. S. (1977). Tourette's Syndrome: The pediatric perspective. *American Medical Journal of Diseases in Children, 131*, 531–534.

Goldstein, A. P. (1988). *The Prepare curriculum: Teaching prosocial competencies.* Champaign, IL: Research Press.

Goldstein, A. P., & McGinnis, E. (1988). *The skill streaming video.* Champaign, IL: Research Press.

Goldstein, A. P., Sprafkin, R. P., Gershaw, N. J., & Klein, P. (1980). *Skill-streaming the adolescent: A structured learning approach to teaching prosocial skills.* Champaign, IL: Research Press.

Goldstein, K. (1942). *After-effects of brain injuries in war.* New York: Grune and Stratton.

Goldstein, S. (1987a). *Adolescent School Situations Questionnaire.* Salt Lake City, UT: Neurology, Learning and Behavior Center.

Goldstein, S. (1987b). *Incomplete Sentences Form.* Salt Lake City, UT: Neurology, Learning and Behavior Center.

Goldstein, S. (1988a). *Social Skills Assessment Questionnaire.* Salt Lake City, UT: Neurology, Learning and Behavior Center.

Goldstein, S. (1988b). *Teacher Observation Checklist.* Salt Lake City, UT: Neurology, Learning and Behavior Center.

Goldstein, S. (1989a). *ADHD Diagnostic Checklist.* Salt Lake City, UT: Neurology, Learning and Behavior Center.

Goldstein, S. (1989b). *Why won't my child pay attention? A video guide for parents.* Salt Lake City, UT: Neurology, Learning and Behavior Center.

Goldstein, S., & Goldstein, M. (1985). *The multi-disciplinary evaluation and treatment of attention deficit disorders in children: Symposium handbook.* Salt Lake City, UT: Neurology, Learning and Behavior Center.

Goldstein, S., & Goldstein, M. (1986). *A parent's guide: attention deficit disorders in children.* Salt Lake City, UT: Neurology, Learning and Behavior Center.

Goldstein, S., & Goldstein, M. (1987). *A teachers guide: attention deficit disorders in children.* Salt Lake City, UT: Neurology, Learning and Behavior Center.

Goldstein, S., & Hinerman, P. (1988). *Language and behavior problems in children.* Salt Lake City, UT: Neurology, Learning and Behavior Center.

Goldstein, S., & Pollock, E. (1988a). *Problem solving skills training for attention deficit children.* Salt Lake City, UT: Neurology, Learning and Behavior Center.

Goldstein, S., & Pollock, E. (1988b). *Social skills training for attention deficit children.* Salt Lake City, UT: Neurology, Learning and Behavior Center.

Goodman, L. S., & Gilman, A. (Eds.). (1975). *The pharmacological basis of therapeutics* (5th ed.). New York: Macmillan.

Goodwin, S. E., & Mahoney, M. J. (1975). Modification of aggression through modeling: An experimental probe. *Journal of Behavior Therapy and Experimental Psychiatry, 6,* 200–202.

Gordon, M. (1979). The assessment of impulsivity and mediating behaviors in hyperactive and non-hyperactive boys. *Journal of Abnormal Child Psychology, 7,* 317–326.

Gordon, M. (1983). *The Gordon Diagnostic System.* Dewitt, NY: Gordon Systems.

Gordon, M., Mammen, O., DiNiro, D., & Mettelman, B. (1988). Source-dependent subtypes of ADHD. *ADHD-Hyperactivity Newsletter, 10,* 2–4.

Gordon, M., & McClure, F. D. (1983, August). *The objective assessment of attention deficit disorders.* Paper presented at the 91st annual convention of the American Psychological Association, Anaheim, CA.

Gordon, M., & Mettelman, B. B. (1987). *Technical guide to the Gordon Diagnostic System.* Syracuse, NY: Gordon Systems.

Gorenstein, E. E., & Newman, J. P. (1980). Disinhibitory psychopathology: A new perspective and model for research. *Psychology Review, 87*, 301–315.

Goulden, K. J., & Shinnar, S. (1988, September). Epilepsy and behavior disturbance in children with multiple developmental disabilities. Presentation made at the seventeenth national meeting of the Child Neurology Society, Halifax, Canada.

Goyer, P. F., Davis, G. C., & Rapoport, J. L. (1979). Abuse of prescribed stimulant medication by a 13-year-old hyperactive boy. *Journal of the American Academy of Child Psychiatry, 18*, 170–175.

Goyette, C. H., Conners, C. K., & Ulrich, R. F. (1978). Normative data on the revised Conners Parent and Teacher Rating Scales. *Journal of Abnormal Child Psychology, 6*, 221–236.

Gray, W. S. (1967). *Gray Oral Reading Test*. New York: Bobbs-Merrill.

Graziano, A. M. (1983). Behavioral approaches to child and family systems. *Counseling Psychologist, 11*, 47–56.

Greenhill, L., Cooper, T., Solomon, M., Fried, J., & Cornblatt, B. (1987). Methylphenidate saliva levels in children. *Psychopharmacology Bulletin, 23*, 115–119.

Greenhill, L. L., Rieder, R. O., & Wender, P. H. (1973). Lithium carbonate in the treatment of hyperactive children. *Archives of General Psychiatry, 28*, 636–645.

Gregorich, B., & Armstrong, B. (1985). *Logical logic*. Santa Barbara, CA: The Learning Works.

Gresham, F. (1986). Conceptual issues in the assessment of social competence in children. In P. Strain, M. Guralnick, & H. M. Walker (Eds.), *Children's social behavior: Development, assessment and modification*. New York: Academic Press.

Gresham, F., & Elliott, S. (1984). Assessment and classification of children's social skills: A review of methods and issues. *School Psychology Review, 13*, 292–300.

Grignetti, M. C. (1986). *Odyssey: A curriculum for thinking—Problem solving*. Watertown, MA: Mastery Education Corporation.

Gross, M. D. (1976). Growth of hyperkinetic children taking methylphenidate, dextroamphetamine or imipramine/desipramine. *Pediatrics, 58*, 423–431.

Gualtieri, C. T., & Hicks, R. E. (1985). Neuropharmacology of methylphenidate and a neural substitute for childhood hyperactivity. *Psychiatric Clinics of North America, 8*, 875–892.

Gualtieri, C. T., Hicks, R. E., Patrick, K., Schroeder, S. R., & Breese, G. R. (1984). Clinical correlates of methylphenidate blood levels. *Therapeutic Drug Monitoring, 6*, 379–392.

Guy, W. (1976). *ECDEU Assessment Manual for Psychopharmacology*. Rockville, MD: National Institute of Mental Health, 383–406.

Haenlein, M., & Caul, W. F. (1987). Attention deficit disorder with hyperactivity: A specific hypothesis of reward dysfunction. *Journal of the American Academy of Child and Adolescent Psychiatry, 26*, 356–362.

Hagerman, R. J., & Falkenstein, A. R. (1987). An association between recurrent otitis media in infancy and later hyperactivity. *Clinical Pediatrics, 5*, 253–257.

Hagerman, R. J., Kemper, M., & Hudson, M. (1985). Learning disabilities and attentional problems in boys with Fragile-x Syndrome. *American Journal of Diseases of Children, 139*, 674–678.

Hallahan, D. P., Marshall, K. J., & Lloyd, J. W. (1981). Self-recording during group instruction: Effects on attention to task. *Learning Disability Quarterly, 4*, 407–413.

Hallahan, D. P., & Sapona, R. (1983). Self-monitoring of attention with learning-disabled children: Past research and current issues. *Journal of Learning Disabilities, 16*, 616–620.

Halperin, J. M., & Gittelman, R. (1986). Do hyperactive children and their siblings differ in I.Q. and academic achievement? *Psychiatry Research, 6*, 253–258.

Halperin, J. M., Gittelman, R., Katz, S., & Struve, F. A. (1986). Relationship between stimulant effect, electroencephalogram, and clinical neurological findings in hyperactive children. *Journal of the American Academy of Child Psychiatry, 25*, 820–825.

Halperin, J. M., Gittelman, R., Klein, D. F., & Rudel, R. G. (1984). Reading-disabled hyperactive children: A distinct subgroup of attention deficit disorder with hyperactivity? *Journal of Abnormal Child Psychology, 12*, 1–14.

Hammill, D. D. (1985). *Detroit Tests of Learning Aptitude−2*. Austin, TX: Pro-Ed.

Hanf, C. (1978). *Parent training for behaviorally disordered children*. Workshop presented for the psychology staff in Granite School District, Salt Lake City, UT.

Harcherik, D. F., Cohen, D. J., Ort, S., Paul, R., Shaywitz, B. A., Volkmar, F. R., Rothman, S. L. G., & Leckman, J. F. (1985). Computed tomographic brain scanning in four neuropsychiatric disorders of childhood. *Medical Journal of Psychiatry, 142*, 731–734.

Harris, K. R. (1986). Self-monitoring of attentional behavior versus self-monitoring of productivity: Effects on-task behavior. An academic response rate among learning disabled children. *Journal of Applied Behavior Analysis, 19*, 417–423.

Hartsough, C. S., & Lambert, N. M. (1985). Medical factors in hyperactive and normal children. *American Journal of Orthopsychiatry, 55*, 190–201.

Hayes, S. C., & Nelson, R. O. (1983). Similar reactivity produced by external cues and self-monitoring. *Behavior Modification, 7*, 193–196.

Hazel, J. S., Bragg Schumaker, J. , Sherman, J. A., & Sheldon-Wildgen, J. (1981). *Asset: A social skills program for adolescents*. Champaign, IL: Research Press.

Hechtman, L., Weiss, G., & Perlman, T. (1980). Hyperactives as young adults: Self-esteem and social skills. *Canadian Journal of Psychiatry, 25*, 478–483.

Hechtman, L., Weiss, G., & Perlman, T. (1984). Young adult outcome of hyperactive children who received long-term stimulant treatment. *Journal of American Academy of Child Psychiatry, 23*, 261–269.

Heins, E. D., Lloyd, J. W., & Hallahan, D.P. (1986). Cued and non-cued self-recording of attention to task. *Behavior Modification, 10*, 235–254.

Helsel, W. J., Hersen, M., & Lubetsky, M. J. (1989). Stimulant medication and the retarded. *Journal of the American Academy of Child and Adolescent Psychiatry, 28*, 138–139.

Henker, B., & Whalen, C. K. (1980). The changing faces of hyperactivity: Retrospect and prospect. In C. K. Whalen & B. Henker (Eds.), *Hyperactive children: The social ecology of identification and treatment*. New York: Academic Press.

Henker, B., Whalen, C., & Hinshaw, S. (1980). The attributional contexts of cognitive motivational strategies. *Exceptional Educational Quarterly, 1*, 17–30.

Hier, D., LeMay, M., Rosenberger, P., & Perlo, V. (1978). Developmental dyslexia: evidence for a subgroup with reversal of cerebral asymmetry. *Archives of Neurology, 35*, 90–92.

Hinshaw, S. P. (1987). On the distinction between attention deficits/hyperactivity and conduct problems/aggression in child psychopathology. *Psychological Bulletin, 101*, 443–463.

Hinshaw, S. P., Henker, B., & Whalen, C. K. (1984a). Self-control in hyperactive boys and anger-inducing situations: Effects of cognitive-behavioral training and of methylphenidate. *Journal of Abnormal Child Psychology, 12*, 55–78.

Hinshaw, S. P., Henker, B., & Whalen, C. K. (1984b). Cognitive-behavioral and pharmacologic interventions for hyperactive boys: Comparative and combined effects. *Journal of Consulting and Clinical Psychology, 52*, 739–749.

Hodges, K., Kline, J., Stern, L., Cytryn, L., & McKnew, D. (1982). The development of a child assessment interview for research and clinical use. *Journal of Abnormal Child Psychology, 10*, 173–189.

Hohman, L. B. (1922). Post-encephalitic behavior disorder in children. *Johns Hopkins Hospital Bulletin, 33*, 372–375.

Holborow, P. L., & Berry, P. S. (1986). Hyperactivity and learning difficulties. *Journal of Learning Disabilities, 19*, 426–431.

Horn, W. (1988). *Parent training program*. Unpublished manuscript.

Horn, W. F., Chatoor, I., & Conners, C. K. (1983). Additive effects of dexedrine and self-control training: A multiple assessment. *Behavior Modification, 7*, 383–402.

Horn, W. F., & Ialongo, N. (1988) Multi-modal treatment of attention deficit hyperactivity disorder in children. In H. Fitzgerald, B. Lester, & M. Yogman (Eds.), *Theory and research in behavioral pediatrics* (Vol. 4). New York: Plenum Press.

Horn, W. F., Ialongo, N., Popovich, S., & Peradotto, D. (1987). Behavioral parent training and cognitive-behavioral self-control therapy with ADD-H children: Comparative and combined effects. *Journal of Clinical Child Psychology, 16*, 57–68.

Hoy, E., Weiss, G., Minde, K., & Cohen, N. (1978). The hyperactive child at adolescence: Cognitive, emotional and social functioning. *Journal of Abnormal Child Psychology, 6*, 311–324.

Huang, Y. H., & Maas, J. W. (1981). d-Amphetamine at low doses suppresses noradrenergic functions. *European Journal of Pharmacology, 75*, 187.

Huessy, H.R. (1988). Behavior disorders and the Ritalin controversy. *Journal of the American Medical Association, 260*, 2219.

Huessy, H. R., & Wright, A. I. (1970). The use of imipramine in children's behavior disorders. *ACTA Paedopsychiatrica, 37*, 194–199.

Humphrey, L. L. (1982). Children's and teachers' perspectives on children's self-control: The development of two rating scales. *Journal of Consulting and Clinical Psychology, 50*, 624–633.

Humphries, T., Kinsbourne, M., & Swanson, J. (1978). Stimulant effects on cooperation and social interaction between hyperactive children and their mothers. *Journal of Psychology and Psychiatry, 19*, 13–22.

Hunt, R. D. (1987). Treatment effects of oral and transdermal clonidine in relation to methylphenidate: An open pilot study in ADD-H. *Psychopharmacology Bulletin, 23*, 111–114.

Hunt, R. D., Minderra, R., & Cohen, D. J. (1985). Clonidine benefits children with attention deficit disorder and hyperactivity: Report of a double-blind placebo cross over therapeutic trial. *Journal of the American Academy of Child Adolescent Psychiatry, 24*, 617–629.

Jackson, D. A., & Monroe, C. (1983). *Getting along with others: Teaching social effectiveness to children*. Champaign, IL: Research Press.

Jaffe, S. L. (1989). Pemoline and liver function. *Journal of the American Academy of Child and Adolescent Psychiatry, 28*, 457–458.

James, W. (1890). *The principles of psychology*. New York: Holt.

Jastak, J. F., Bijou, S. W., & Jastak, S. (1978). *Wide Range Achievement Test*. Wilmington, DE: Jastak Associates.

Jastak, S., & Wilkinson, G. S. (1984). *Wide Range Achievement Test:. Administration manual.* Wilmington, DE: Jastak Associates.

Jensen, J. B., Burke, N., & Garfinkel, B. D. (1988). Depression and symptoms of attention deficit disorder with hyperactivity. *Journal of the American Academy of Child and Adolescent Psychiatry, 27,* 742–747.

Jensen, W. (1982). *Children's behavior therapy unit parenting program.* Unpublished manuscript.

Johnson, S. M., & White, G. (1971). Self-observation as an agent of behavioral change. *Behavior Therapy, 2,* 488–497.

Kagan, J. (1964). *The Matching Familiar Figures Test.* Unpublished. Harvard University, Cambridge.

Kagan, J., Rosman, B. L., Day, D., Albert, J., & Phillips, W. (1964). Information processing in the child: Significance of analytic and reflective attitudes. *Psychological Monographs, 78.* (1, Whole No. 578).

Kalachnik, J. E., Sprague, R. L., Sleator, E. K., Cohen, M. N., & Ullmann, R. K. (1982). Effect of methylphenidate hydrochloride on stature of hyperactive children. *Developmental Medicine Child Neurology, 24,* 586–595.

Kanfer, F. H. (1970). Self-regulation: Research, issues, and speculations. In C. Neuringer and J. L. Michel (Eds.), *Behavior modification in clinical psychology.* New York: Appleton-Century-Crofts.

Kaplan, B. J., McNicol, J., Conte, R. A., & Moghadam, H. K. (1989). Dietary replacement in preschool-aged hyperactive boys. *Pediatrics, 83,* 7–17.

Kaplan, H. K., Wamboldt, F., & Barnhardt, R. D. (1986). Behavioral effects of dietary sucrose in disturbed children. *American Journal of Psychology, 7,* 143.

Karp, S. A., & Konstadt, N. (1971). *Children's Embedded Figures Test.* Palo Alto, CA: Consulting Psychologist Press.

Kashani, J., Chapel, J., & Ellis, J. (1979). Hyperactive girls. *Journal of Operational Psychiatry, 10,* 145–149.

Kaufman, A. S. (1979). *Intelligence testing with the WISC-R.* New York: John Wiley & Sons.

Kaufman, K. F., & O'Leary, K. D. (1972). Reward, cost and self-evaluation procedures for disruptive adolescents in a psychiatric hospital school. *Journal of Applied Behavior Analysis, 5,* 293–309.

Kazdin, A. E. (1975). Recent advances in token economy research. In M. Hersen, R. M. Eisler, and P. M. Miller (Eds.), *Progress in behavior modification* (Vol. 1). New York: Academic Press.

Kazdin, A. E., & Matson, J. L. (1981). Social validation and mental retardation. *Applied Research in Mental Retardation, 2,* 39–53.

Kelly, J. A., & Drabman, R. S. (1977). The modification of socially detrimental behavior. *Journal of Behavioral Therapy and Experimental Psychiatry, 8,* 101–104.

Kelly, L. M., Sonis, W., Fialkov, J., Kazdin, A., & Matson, J. (1986). Behavioral assessment of methylphenidate in a child with frontal lobe damage. *Journal of Psychopathology and Behavioral Assessment, 8,* 47–54.

Kelly, P. C., Cohen, M. L., Walker, W. O., Caskey, O. L., & Atkinson, A. W. (1989). Self-esteem in children medically managed for Attention Deficit Disorder. *Pediatrics, 83,* 211–217.

Kendall, P. C. (1988). *Stop and think workbook.* Marion Station, PA.

Kendall, P. C., & Brasswell, L. (1982). Cognitive-behavioral self-control therapy for children. A component analysis. *Journal of Consulting and Clinical Psychology, 50,* 672–689.

Kendall, P. C., & Brasswell, L. (1985). *Cognitive-behavioral therapy for impulsive children.* New York: The Guilford Press.

Kendall, P. C., & Wilcox, L. E. (1979). Self-control in children: Development of a rating scale. *Journal of Consulting and Clinical Psychology, 47,* 1020–1029.

Keough, B. K., & Barkett, C. J. (1980). An educational analysis of hyperactive children's achievement problems. In C. K. Whalen and B. Henker (Eds.), *Hyperactive children: The social ecology of identification and treatment.* New York: Academic Press.

King, C., & Young, R. D. (1982). Attentional deficits with and without hyperactivity: Teacher and peer perceptions. *Journal of Abnormal Child Psychology, 10,* 483–495.

Kirby, E. A., & Grimley, L. K. (1986). *Understanding and treating attention deficit disorder.* New York: Pergamon Press.

Kirby, E. A., & Horne, A. (1986). A comparison of hyperactive and aggressive children. In E. A. Kirby & L. K. Grimley (Eds.), *Understanding and treating attention deficit disorder.* New York: Pergamon Press.

Kirby, F., & Shields, F. (1972). Modification of arithmetic response rate and attending behavior in a seventh-grade student. *Journal of Applied Behavior Analysis, 5,* 79–84.

Kirk, S. A., McCarthy, J. J., and Kirk, W. D. (1968). *The Illinois Test of Psycholinguistic Abilities* (rev. ed.). Urbana, IL: University of Illinois Press.

Klein, A. R., & Young, R. D. (1979). Hyperactive boys in their classroom: Assessment of teacher and peer perceptions, interactions and classroom behaviors. *Journal of Abnormal Child Psychology, 7,* 425–442.

Klein, R. D. (1979). Modifying academic performance in the grade school classroom. In M. Hersen, R. M. Eisler, & P. M. Miller (Eds.), *Progress in behavior modification* (Vol. 8, pp. 293–321). New York: Academic Press.

Klorman, R. M., Salzman, L., Borgstedt, A., & Dainer, K. (1981). Normalizing effects of methylphenidate on hyperactive children's vigilance, performance and evoked potentials. *Psychopharmacology, 6,* 665–667.

Klorman, R. M., Salzman, L. F., Pass, H. L., Borgstedt, A. D., & Dainer, K. B. (1979). Effects of methylphenidate on hyperactive children's evoked responses during passive and active attention. *Psychophysiology, 16,* 23–29.

Kneedler, R. D., & Hallahan, D. P. (1981). Self-monitoring of on-task behavior with learning-disabled children: Current study and directions. *Exceptional Education Quarterly, 2,* 73–82.

Knights, R. N. (1966). *Normative data on tests for evaluating brain damage in children from five to fourteen years of age* (Research Bulletin #20). London, Canada: University of Western Ontario.

Knobel, M., Walman, M. B., & Mason, E. (1959). Hyperkinesis and organicity in children. *Archives of General Psychiatry, 1,* 310–321.

Knobolc, H., & Pasamanick, B. (1959). The syndrome of minimal cerebral damage in infancy. *Journal of the American Medical Association, 70,* 1384–1386.

Konstantareas, M. M., & Hermatidis, S. (1983). Effectiveness of cognitive mediation and behavior modification with hospitalized hyperactives. *Canadian Journal of Psychiatry, 28,* 462–470.

Kounin, J. S. (1970). *Discipline and group management in classrooms.* Melbourne, FL: Krieger.

Kovacs, M. (1983). *The Children's Depression Inventory: A self-rated depression scale for school-aged youngsters.* Unpublished manuscript. University of Pittsburgh.

Kramer, J. R. (1987). What are hyperactive children like as young adults? In J. Loney (Ed.), *The young hyperactive child: Answers to question about diagnosis, prognosis and treatment.* New York: Haworth Press.

Kramer, J. R., & Loney, J. (1982). Childhood hyperactivity and substance abuse: A review of the literature. In A. D. Gadow and I. Bailer (Eds.), *Advances in learning and behavioral disabilities* (Vol. 1). Greenwich, CT: JAI Press.

Kuehne, C. (1985). *A discriminant analysis of behavioral and psychometric measures of attention in children with attention deficit disorder and specific learning disabilities.* Unpublished doctoral dissertation. University of Utah.

Kupietz, S., Winsberg, B., Richardson, E., Maitinsky, S., & Mendell, N. (1988). Effects of methylphenidate dosage on hyperactive reading-disabled children: I. Behavior and cognitive performance effects. *Journal of the American Academy of Child and Adolescent Psychiatry, 27,* 70–77.

L'Abate, L., & Milan, M. (1985). *Handbook of social skills training and research.* New York: John Wiley & Sons.

Lahey, B. B., Pelham, W. E., Schaughency, E. A., Atkins, M. S., Murphy, H. A., Hynd, G., Russo, M., Hartdagen, S., & Lorys-Vernon, A. (1988). Dimensions in types of attention deficit disorder. *Journal of American Academy of Child and Adolescent Psychiatry, 27,* 330–335.

Lahey, B. B., Schaughency, E. A., Frame, C. L., & Strauss, C. C. (1985). Teacher ratings of attention problems in children experimentally classified as exhibiting attention deficit disorders with and without hyperactivity. *Journal of the American Academy of Child and Adolescent Psychiatry, 24,* 613–616.

Lahey, B. B., Schaughency, E. A., Hynd, G. W., Carlson, C. L., & Nieves, N. (1987). Attention deficit disorder with and without hyperactivity: See comparison of behavioral characteristics of clinic-referred children. *Journal of the American Academy of Child and Adolescent Child Psychiatry, 26,* 718–723.

Lahey, B. B., Schaughency, E. A., Strauss, C. C., & Frame, C. L. (1984). Are attention deficit disorders with and without hyperactivity similar or dissimilar disorders? *Journal of the American Academy of Child and Adolescent Psychiatry, 23,* 302–309.

Lambert, N. M., & Sandoval, J. (1980). The prevalence of learning disabilities and a sample of children considered hyperactive. *Journal of Abnormal Child Psychology, 8,* 33–50.

Lambert, N. M., Sandoval, J., & Sassone, D. (1978). Prevalence of hyperactivity in elementary school children as a function of social system definers. *American Journal of Orthopsychiatry, 48,* 446–463.

Landau, S., & Milich, R. (1988). Social communication patterns of attention-deficit-disordered boys. *Journal of Abnormal Child Psychology, 16,* 69–81.

Landau, S., Milich, R., & Whitten, P. (1984). A comparison of teacher and peer assessment of social status. *Journal of Clinical Child Psychology, 13,* 44–99.

Landrigan, P. J., Whitworth, R. H., Baloh, R. W., Staehling, N. W., Barthel, W. F., & Rosenbloom, B. F. (1975). Neuropsychological dysfunction in children with chronic low-level lead absorption. *Lancet,* March 29, 708–712.

Langhorne, J. E., & Loney, J. (1979). A 4-fold model for subgrouping the hyperkinetic/MBD syndrome. *Child Psychiatry and Human Development, 9,* 153–159.

Lapouse, R., & Monk, M. (1958). An epidemiological study of behavior characteristics in children. *American Journal of Public Health, 48,* 1134–1144.

Larsen, V. (1964). Physical characteristics of disturbed adolescents. *Archives of General Psychiatry, 10,* 55.

Lasley, T. J. (1986). Issues in teacher education, Volume II: Background papers from the national commission for excellence in teacher education. Washington, DC: American Association of Colleges for Teacher Education. Teacher education monograph #6.

Laufer, M. W., & Denhoff, E. (1957). Hyperkinetic behavior syndrome in children. *Journal of Pediatrics, 50,* 463–474.

Leimbach, J. (1986). *Primarily logic.* San Luis Obispo, CA: Dandilion Publications.

Lester, M. L., & Fishbein, D. H. (1988). Nutrition and childhood neuropsychological disorders. In R. E. Tarter, D. H. Van Thiel & K. L. Edwards (Eds.), *Medical neuropsychology* (pp. 291–325). New York: Plenum Press.

Levine, M. D. (1987) Attention deficit: The diversive effects of weak control systems in childhood. *Pediatric Annals, 16,* 117–130.

Lezak, M. D. (1983). *Neuropsychological assessment (2nd ed.).* New York: Oxford University Press.

Licht, B. G., Kistner, J. A., Ozkaragoz, T., Shapiro, S., & Clausen, L. (1985). Causal attributions of learning disabled children: Individual differences and their implications for persistence. *Journal of Educational Psychology, 77,* 208–216.

Linn, R. T., & Hodge, G. K. (1982). Locus of control in childhood hyperactivity. *Journal of Consulting and Clinical Psychology, 50,* 592–593.

Loeber, R., & Dishion, T. (1983). Early predictors of male delinquency: A review. *Psychological Bulletin, 94,* 68–99.

Logan, W. J., Farrell, J. E., Malone, M. A., & Taylor, M. J. (1988, September). Effect of stimulant medications on cerebral event-related potentials. Presentation made at the seventeenth national meeting of the Child Neurology Society. Halifax, Canada.

Loney, J. (1974). The intellectual functioning of hyperactive elementary school boys: A cross sectional investigation. *American Journal of Orthopsychiatry, 44,* 754–762.

Loney, J. (1980a). Hyperkinesis comes of age: What do we know and where should we go? *American Journal of Orthopsychiatry, 50,* 28–42.

Loney, J. (1980b). The Iowa theory of substance abuse among hyperactive adolescents. In D. J. Lettieri, M. Sayers, & H. W. Pearson (Eds.), *Theories on drug abuse: Selective contemporary perspectives (NIDA Research Monograph 30,* March).

Loney, J. (1986). Hyperactivity and aggression in the diagnosis of Attention Deficit Disorder. In B. B. Lahey and A. E. Kazdin (Eds.), *Advances in Clinical Child Psychology.* New York: State University Press.

Loney, J. (Ed.). (1987). *The young hyperactive child: Answers to questions about diagnosis, prognosis and treatment.* New York: Haworth Press.

Loney, J., Kramer, J., & Milich, R. (1981). The hyperkinetic child grows up: Predictors of symptoms, delinquency and achievement at follow-up. In K. D. Gadow & J. Loney (Eds.), *Psychosocial aspects of drug treatment for hyperactivity.* Boulder, CO: Westview Press.

Loney, J., & Milich, R. S. (1981). Hyperactivity, inattention, and aggression in clinical practice. In M. Wolraich & D. K. Routh (Eds.), *Advances in behavioral pediatrics* (Vol. 2). Greenwich, CT: JAI Press.

Lou, H. C., Henriksen, L., & Bruhn, P. (1984). Focal cerebral hypoperfusion in children with dysphasia and/or attention deficit disorder. *Archives of Neurology, 41,* 825–829.

Love, A. J., & Thompson, M. G. G. (1988). Language disorders and attention deficit disorders in young children referred for psychiatric services: Analysis of prevalence and a conceptual synthesis. *American Journal of Orthopsychiatry, 58,* 52–64.

Lovitt, T. C. (1973). Self-management projects with children with behavioral disorders. *Journal of Learning Disabilities, 6,* 138–150.

Lovitt, T. C., & Curtiss, K. A. (1969). Academic response rate as a function of teacher- and self-imposed contingencies. *Journal of Applied Behavior Analysis, 2,* 49–53.

Lovrich, D., & Stamm, J. S. (1983). Event-related potential and behavioral correlates of attention in reading retardation. *Journal of Clinical Neuropsychology, 5,* 13–37.

Lowe, T. L., Cohen, D. J., Detlor, J., Kremenitzer, M. W., & Shaywitz, B. A. (1982). Stimulant medications precipitate Tourette's Syndrome. *Journal of the American Medical Association, 247,* 1729–1731.

Luisada, P. V. (1969). REM deprivation and hyperactivity in children. *The Chicago Medical School Quarterly, 28,* 97–108.

Luria, A. R. (1959). The directive function of speech in development. *Word, 15,* 341–352.

Luria, A. R. (1961). *The role of speech and the regulation of normal and abnormal behaviors.* New York: Liveright.

Mahoney, M. J. (1977). Some applied issues in self-monitoring. In J. D. Cone and R. P. Hawkins (Eds.), *Behavioral assessment: New direction in clinical psychology* (pp. 245–254). New York: Brunner/Mazel.

Mainville, F., & Friedman, R. J. (1976). Peer relations of hyperactive children. *Ontario Psychologist, 8,* 17–20.

Mash, E. J., & Johnston, C. (1983). Sibling interactions of hyperactive and normal children and their relationship to reports of maternal stress and self-esteem. *Journal of Clinical Child Psychology, 12,* 91–99.

Massman, P. J., Nussbaum, N.L., & Bigler, E. D. (1988). The mediating effect of age on the relationship between child behavior checklist hyperactivity scores and neuropsychological test performance. *Journal of Abnormal Child Psychology, 16,* 89–95.

Mattes, J. A. (1980). The role of frontal lobe dysfunction in childhood hyperkinesis. *Comprehensive Psychiatry, 21,* 358–369.

McConnell, S., & Odom, S. (1986). Sociometrics: Peer referenced measures and the assessment of social competence. In P. Strain, M. Guralnick, & H. M. Walker (Eds.). *Children's social behavior: Development, assessment and modification.* New York: Academic Press.

McDaniel, K. D. (1986). Pharmacologic treatment of psychiatric and neurodevelopmental disorders in children and adolescents (Part 2). *Clinical Pediatrics, 25,* 143–146.

McGee, R., & Share, D. L. (1988). Attention deficit disorder hyperactivity and academic failure: Which comes first and what should be treated? *Journal of the American Academy of Child and Adolescent Psychiatry, 27,* 318–325.

McGee, R., Williams, S., & Silva, P. A. (1987). A comparison of girls and boys with teacher-identified problems of attention. *Journal of the American Academy of Child and Adolescent Psychiatry, 26,* 711–716.

McGinnis, E., Goldstein, A. P., Sprafkin, R. P., & Gershaw, N. J. (1984). *Skill-streaming the elementary school child: A guide for teaching prosocial skills.* Champaign, IL: Research Press.

McMahon, S. A., & Greenberg, L. M. (1977). Serial neurologic examination of hyperactive children. *Pediatrics, 59,* 584–587.

McNamara, J. J. (1972). Hyperactivity in the apartment bound child. *Clinical Pediatrics, 11*, 371–372.

McNutt, B., Ballard, J. E., & Boileau, R. (1976). The effects of long-term stimulant medication on growth and body composition of hyperactive children. *Psychopharmocology Bulletin, 12*, 13–14.

Meichenbaum, D. (1975). Self-instructional methods. In F. H. Kanfer and A. P. Goldstein (Eds.), *Helping people change*. New York: Pergamon Press.

Meichenbaum, D. (1976). Cognitive-behavior modification. In J. T. Spence, R. C. Carson, & J. W. Thibaut (Eds.), *Behavioral approaches to therapy*. Morristown, NJ: General Learning Press.

Meichenbaum, D. (1977). *Cognitive-behavior modification*. New York: Plenum Press.

Meichenbaum, D., & Goodman, J. (1969). Reflection-impulsivity and verbal control of motor behavior. *Child Development, 40*, 785–797.

Meichenbaum, D. H., & Goodman, J. (1971). Training impulsive children to talk to themselves: A means of developing self-control. *Journal of Abnormal Psychology, 77*, 115–126.

Messer, S. B. (1976). Reflection-impulsivity. A review. *Psychological Bulletin, 83*, 1026–1052.

Mesulam, M. M. (1985). *Principals of behavioral neurology*. Philadelphia: F. A. Davis.

Mikkelsen, E. J., Brown, G. L., Minichiello, M. D., Millican, F. K., & Rapoport, J. L. (1982). Neurologic status in hyperactive, enuretic, encopretic and normal boys. *Journal of American Academy of Child Psychiatry, 21*, 75–81.

Milich, R. S., & Landau, S. (1981). Socialization and peer relations in the hyperactive child. In K. D. Gadow & I. Bailer (Eds.), *Advances in learning and behavior disabilities* (Vol. 1). Greenwich, CT: JAI Press.

Milich, R. S., Landau, S., Kilby, G., & Whitten, P. (1982). Preschool peer perceptions of the behavior of hyperactive and aggressive children. *Journal of Abnormal Child Psychology, 10*, 497–510.

Milich, R. S., & Loney, J. (1979). The role of hyperactive and aggressive symptomatology in predicting adolescent outcome among hyperactive children. *Journal of Pediatric Psychology, 4*, 93–112.

Milich, R. S., & Pelham, W. E. (1986). Effects of sugar ingestion on the classroom and playgroup behavior of attention deficit disordered boys. *Journal of Consulting and Clinical Psychology, 54*, 714–718.

Milich, R., Whidiger, T. A., & Laundau, S. (1987). Differential diagnosis of attention deficit and conduct disorders using conditional probabilities. *Journal of Consulting and Clinical Psychology, 55*, 762–767.

Miller, P., & Bigi, L. (1979). The development of children's understanding and attention. *Merrill-Palmer Quarterly, 25*, 235–250.

Millon, T., Green, C. J., & Meagher, R. B. (1982). *Millon Adolescent Personality Inventory*. Minneapolis: National Computer Systems.

Minde, K. K., Lewin, D., Weiss, G., Lavigueur, H., Douglas, V., & Sykes, E. (1971). The hyperactive child in elementary school: A five-year controlled follow-up. *Exceptional Children, 38*, 215–221.

Mischel, W., Shoda, Y., & Rodriguez, M. L. (1989). Delay of gratification in children. *Science, 244*, 933–938.

Mitchell, E., & Matthews, K. L. (1980) Gilles de la Tourette's disorder associated with pemoline. *American Journal of Psychiatry, 137*, 1618–1619.

Mitchell, W. G., Chavez, J. M., Zhou, Y., & Guzman, B. L. (1988, September). Relationship of antiepileptic drugs to reaction time, impulsivity, and attention in children with epilepsy. Presentation made at the seventeenth national meeting of the Child Neurology Society. Halifax, Canada.

Molitch, M., & Eccles, A. K. (1937). Effects of benzedrine sulphate on intelligence scores of children. *American Journal of Psychiatry, 94*, 587–590.

Moreland, J. R., Schwebel, A. I., Beck, S., & Wells, R. T. (1982). Parents as therapists: A review of the behavior therapy parent training literature, 1975–1981. *Behavior Modification, 6*, 250–276.

Morgan, C. D., & Murray, H. A. (1935). A method for investigating fantasies: The Thematic Apperception Test. *Archives of Neurology and Psychiatry, 34*, 289–307.

Morrison, J., & Stewart, M. (1971). A family study of hyperactive child syndrome. *Biological Psychiatry, 3*, 189–195.

Morrison, J., & Stewart, M. (1973). The psychiatric status of legal families of adopted hyperactive children. *Archives of General Psychiatry, 28*, 888–891.

Mostovsky, D. I. (1970). *Attention: Contemporary theory and analysis.* New York: Appleton-Century Crofts.

Murray, J. B. (1987). Psychophysiological effects of methylphenidate (Ritalin). *Psychological Reports, 61*, 315–336.

Needleman, H. L., Gunnoe, C., Leviton, A., Reed, R., Peresie, H., Maher, C., & Barrett, P. (1979). Deficits in psychologic and classroom performance of children with elevated dentine lead levels. *New England Journal of Medicine, 300*, 689–695.

Nelson, K. B., & Ellenberg, J. H. (1979a). Apgar scores and long-term neurological handicap. *Annals of Neurology, 6*, 1982 (Abstract).

Nelson, K. B., & Ellenberg, J. H. (1979b). Neonatal signs as predictors of cerebral palsy. *Pediatrics, 64*, 225–232.

Netter, F. H. (1986.) *The CIBA Collection of Medical Illustrations. Nervous System: Part II. Neurologic and Neuromuscular Disorders.* West Caldwell, NJ: CIBA.

Nichamin, S. J. (1972). Recognizing minimum cerebral dysfunction in the infant and toddler. *Clinical Pediatrics, 11*, 255–257.

Nicholi, A. M., Jr. (1978). The adolescent. In A. M. Nicholi, Jr. (Ed.), *The Harvard guide to modern psychiatry.* London: Belnap.

Nickerson, R. S. (1986). *Odyssey: A curriculum for thinking—Verbal reasoning.* Watertown, MA: Mastery Education Corporation.

Norman, D. A. (1969). *Memory and attention.* New York: John Wiley & Sons.

Olweus, D. (1979). Stability of aggressive reaction patterns in males: A review. *Psychological Bulletin, 86*, 852–875.

Ostrom, N. N., & Jensen, W. R. (1988). Assessment of attention deficits in children. *Professional School Psychology, 3*, 253–269.

Ottinger, D., Halpin, B., Miller, M., Durmain, L., & Hanneman, R. (1985). Evaluating drug effectiveness in an office setting for children with attention deficit disorders. *Clinical Pediatrics, 24*, 245–251.

Ozawa, J. P., & Michael, W. B. (1983). The concurrent validity of a behavioral rating scale for assessing attention deficit disorder (DSM-III) in learning disabled children. *Educational and Psychological Measurement, 43*, 623–632.

Page, J. G., Bernstein, J. E., Janicki, R. S., & Michelli, F. A. (1974). A multi-clinical trial of pemoline in childhood hyperkinesis. *Excerpta Medica, 48*, 99–124.

Paine, S. C., Ridicchi, J., Rosellini, L. C., Deutchman, L., & Darch, C. B. (1983). *Structuring your classroom for academic success*. Champaign, IL: Research Press.

Palkes, H. S., & Stewart, M. A. (1972). Intellectual ability and performance of hyperactive children. *American Journal of Orthopsychiatry, 42*, 35–39.

Palkes, H. S., Stewart, M. A., & Freedman, J. (1971). Improvement in maze performance of hyperactive boys as a function of verbal-training procedures. *Journal of Special Education, 5*, 337–342.

Palkes, H. S., Stewart, M. A., & Kahana, B. (1968). Porteus Maze. Performance of hyperactive boys after training in self-directed verbal commands. *Child Development, 39*, 817–826.

Parker, H. C. (1988). *The ADD hyperactivity workbook*. Plantation, FL: Impact Publications.

Parker, V. S., & TenBrooek, N. L. (1987). *Problem solving, planning and organizational tasks: Strategies for retraining*. Tuscon, AZ: Communication Skill Builders.

Paternite, C. E., & Loney, J. (1980). Childhood hyperkinesis: Relationships between symptomatology and home environment. In C. K. Whalen and B. Henker (Eds.), *Hyperactive children: The social ecology of identification and treatment*. New York: Academic Press.

Paternite, C. E., Loney, J., & Langhorne, J. E. (1976). Relationships between symptomatology and SES-related factors in hyperkinetic/MBD boys. *American Journal of Orthopsychiatry, 46*, 291–301.

Patterson, G. R. (1974). Interventions for boys with conduct problems: Multiple settings, treatments, and criteria. *Journal of Consulting and Clinical Psychology, 42*, 471–481.

Patterson, G. R. (1975). *Families: Applications of social learning to family life*. Champaign, IL: Research Press.

Patterson, G. R. (1976). *Living with children: New methods for parents and teachers*. Eugene, OR: Castialia.

Patterson, G. R., & Forgatch, M. S. (1987). *Parents and adolescents living together. Part 1: The basics. Part 2: Family problem solving*. Eugene, OR: Castialia.

Pearson, D. E., Teicher, M. H., Shaywitz, B. A., Cohen, D. J., Young, J. G., & Anderson, G. M. (1980). Environmental influences on body weight and behavior in developing rats after neonatal 6-hydroxydopamine science. *Science, 209*, 715–717.

Pelham, W. E. (1987). What do we know about the use and effects of CNS stimulants in ADD? In J. Loney (Ed.), *The young hyperactive child: Answers to questions about diagnosis, prognosis and treatment*. New York: Haworth Press.

Pelham, W. E., Atkins, M.S., Murphy, H.A., & White, K.S. (1981a). Attention deficit disorder with and without hyperactivity: Definitional issues and correlates. In W. Pelham (Ed.), *DSM-III category of attention deficit disorders: Rationale, operationalization and correlates*. Los Angeles: American Psychological Association.

Pelham, W. E., Atkins, M.S., Murphy, H.A., & White, K.S. (1981b). Operationalization and validation of attention deficit disorder. Paper presented at the annual meeting of the Association for Advancement of Behavioral Therapy, Toronto, Canada.

Pelham, W. E., & Bender, M. E. (1982). Peer relationships and hyperactive children: Description and treatment. In K. Gadow & I. Bailer (Eds.), *Advances in learning and bevhavioral disabilities (Vol. 1)*. Greenwich, CT: JAI Press.

Pelham, W. E., Bender, M. E., Caddel;, J., Booth, S., & Moorer, S. H. (1985a). Methylphenidate and children with Attention Deficit Disorder: Dose effects on classroom, academic and social behavior. *Archives of General Psychiatry, 42*, 948–952.

Pelham, W. E., Bender, M. E., Caddell, J., Booth, S., & Moorer, S. H. (1985b). Medication effect on arithmetic learning. *Archives of General Psychiatry, 42,* 948–951.

Pelham, W. E., & Milich, R. (1984). Peer relations of children with hyperactivity/attention deficit disorder. *Journal of Learning Disabilities, 17,* 560–568.

Pelham, W. E., Schnedler, R. W., Bologna, N., & Contreras, J. A. (1980). Behavioral and stimulant treatment of hyperactive children: A therapy study with methylphenidate probes in a within-subject design. *Journal of Applied Behavior Analysis, 13,* 221–236.

Pelham, W. E., Schnedler, R. W., Miller, J., Ronnei, M., Paluchowski, C., Budrow, M., Marx, D., Nilsson, D. , & Bender, M. E. (1986). The combination of behavior therapy and psychostimulant medication in the treatment of hyperactive children: A therapy outcome study. In L. Bloomingdale (Ed.), *Attention deficit disorders.* New York: Spectrum Books.

Pelham, W. E., Sturges, J., Hoza, J., Schmidt, C., Bijlsma, J. J., Milich, R., & Moorer, S. (1987) Sustained release and standard methylphenidate effects on cognitive and social behavior in children with attention deficit disorder. *Pediatrics, 4,* 1987. 491–501.

Pelham, W. E., Swanson, J., Bender, M., & Wilson, J. (1980, August). *Effects of pemoline on hyperactivity: Laboratory and classroom measures.* Read before the annual meeting of the American Psychological Association, Montreal.

Pellock, J. M., Culbert, J. P., Garnett, W. R., Crumrine, P. K., Kaplan, A. M., O'Hara, K. A., Driscoll, S. M., Frost, M. M., Alvin, R., Hamer, R. M., Handen, B., Horowitz, I. W. , & Nichols, C. (1988, September). *Significant differences of cognitive and behavioral effects of antiepileptic drugs in children.* Presentation made at the seventeenth national meeting of the Child Neurology Society, Halifax, Canada.

Perkins, D. N., & Laserna, C. (1986). *Odyssey: A curriculum for thinking—Inventive thinking.* Watertown, MA: Mastery Education Corporation.

Persson-Blennow, I., & McNeil, T. F. (1988). Frequencies and stability of temperament types in childhood. *Journal of the American Academy of Child and Adolescent Psychiatry, 27,* 619–622.

Phillips, J. S. , & Ray, R. S. (1980). Behavioral approaches to childhood disorders: Review and critique. *Behavior Modification, 4,* 3–34.

Physician's Desk Reference. (1989). Oradell, NJ: Medical Economics Company.

Piers, E. V., & Harris, D. B. (1984). *Piers-Harris Children's Self-Concept Scale.* Los Angeles: Western Psychological Services.

Pleak, R., Birmaher, B., Gavrilescu, A., Abichandini, A., & Williams, D. (1988). Mania and neuropsychiatric excitation following carbamazepine. *Journal of the American Academy of Child and Adolescent Psychiatry, 27,* 500–503.

Plenk, A. (1975). *Plenk Storytelling Test.* Salt Lake City, UT: The Children's Center.

Pliszka, S. R. (1987). Tricyclic antidepressants in the treatment of children with attention deficit disorder. *Journal of the American Academy of Child and Adolescent Psychiatry, 26,* 127–132.

Polirstok, S. R. (1987). Training handicapped students in the mainstream to use self-evaluation techniques. *Techniques: A Journal for Remedial Education and Counseling, 3,* 9–18.

Pollard, S., Ward, E. N., & Barkley, R. A. (1983). The effects of parent training and Ritalin on the parent-child interactions of hyperactive boys. *Child and Family Behavior Therapy, 5,* 51–69.

Pomeroy, J. C., Sprafkin, J., & Gadow, K. D. (1988). Minor physical anomalies as a biologic marker for behavior disorders. *Journal of the American Academy of Child and Adolescent Psychiatry, 27,* 466–473.

Popkin, M. (1986). *Active parenting*. Atlanta, GA: Author.

Porrino, L. J., Lucignani, G., Dow-Edwards, D., & Sokoloff, L. (1984). Dose dependent effects and acute amphetamine administration on functional brain metabolism in rats. *Brain Research, 307*, 311–320.

Porrino, L. J., Rapoport, J. L., Behar, D., Sceery, W., Ismond, D.R., & Bunney, W. E. (1983). A naturalistic assessment of the motor activity of hyperactive boys: I. Comparison with normal controls. *Archives of General Psychiatry, 40*, 681–687.

Posner, N. I. (1987). Selective attention in head injury. In H. S. Levin, J. Grafman, & H. M. Eisenberg (Eds.), *Neurobehavioral recovery from head injury*. New York: Oxford University Press.

Posner, N. I., & Snyder, C. R. (1975). Attention and cognitive control. In R. Solso (Ed.), *Information processing and cognition: The Loyola symposium*. Hillsdale, NJ: Earlbaum Press.

Preskorn, S. H., Bupp, S. J., Weller, E. B., & Weller, R.A. (1989). Plasma levels of imipramine and metabolites in 68 hospitalized children. *Journal of the American Academy of Child and Adolescent Psychiatry, 28*, 373–375.

Prichep, A., Sutton, S., & Hakerm, G. (1976). Evoked potentials in hyperkinetic and normal children under certainty and uncertainty: A placebo and methylphenidate study. *Psychophysiology, 13*, 419–428.

Prinz, R. J., Connor, P. A., & Wilson, C. C. (1981). Hyperactive and aggressive behaviors in childhood: Intertwined dimensions. *Journal of Abnormal Psychology, 9*, 191–192.

Prinz, R. J., & Loney, J. (1974). Teacher-rated hyperactive elementary school girls: An exploratory developmental study. *Child Psychiatry in Human Development, 4*, 246–257.

Quinn, P. O., & Rapoport, M. D. (1974). Minor physical anomalies and neurologic status in hyperactive boys. *Pediatrics, 53*, 742–747.

Rapoport, M. D. (1987). *The Attention Training System*. DeWitt, NY: The Gordon Systems.

Rapoport, M. D. (1988). Hyperactivity and attention deficits. In Hersen and V. B. Van Hesselt (Eds.), *Behavior therapy with children and Adolescents*. New York: John Wiley & Sons.

Rapoport, M. D., DuPaul, G. J., Stoner, G., Birmingham, B. K., & Massey, G. (1985). Attention deficit disorder with hyperactivity. Differential effects of methylphenidate on impulsivity. *Pediatrics, 76*, 938–943.

Rapoport, M. D., DuPaul, G. J., Stoner, G., & Jones, T. J. (1986). Comparing classroom and clinic measures of attention deficit disorder: Differential, idiosyncratic and dose-response effects of methylphenidate. *Journal of Consulting and Clinical Psychology, 54*, 334–341.

Rapoport, M. D., Murphy, H. A., & Bailey, J. S. (1982). Ritalin vs. response cost in the control of hyperactive children: A within-subject comparison. *Journal of Applied Behavior Analysis., 15*, 205–216.

Rapoport, M. D., Stoner, G., DuPaul, G. J., Birmingham, B. K. & Tucker, S. (1985). Methylphenidate in hyperactive children: Differential effects of dose on academic learning and social behavior. *Journal of Abnormal Child Psychology, 13*, 227–244.

Rapoport, M. D., Stoner, G., DuPaul, G., Kelly, K. L., Tucker, S. B., & Schoeler, T. (1988). Attention deficit disorder and methylphenidate: A multilevel analysis of dose-response effects on children's impulsivity across settings. *American Academy of Child and Adolescent Psychiatry, 27*, 60–69.

Raskin, L. A., Shaywitz, S. E., Shaywitz, B. A., Anderson, G. M., & Cohen, D. J. (1984). Neurochemical correlates of attention deficit disorder. *Pediatric Clinics of North America, 54*, 714–718.

Reeves, J. C., & Werry, J. S. (1987). Soft signs in hyperactivity. In David E. Tupper (Ed.), *Soft neurological signs*. Troy, NY: Grune and Stratton.

Reid, M. K., & Borkowski, J. G. (1987). Causal attributions of hyperactive children: Implications for teaching strategies and self-control. *Journal of Educational Psychology, 79*, 296–307.

Reitan, R. M. (1958). Validity of the Trail-Making Test as an indication of organic brain damage. *Perceptual Motor Skills, 8*, 271–276.

Reitan, R. M. (1987). *Neuropsychological evaluation of children* (Workshop training manual). Tuscon, AZ: Neuropsychology Press.

Reitan, R. M., & Wolfson, D. (1985). *The Halstead-Reitan Neuropsychological Test Battery: Theory and clinical interpretation*. Tuscon, AZ: Neuropsychology Press.

Reynolds, W. M. (1987). *Reynolds' Adolescent Depression Scale*. Odessa, FL: Psychological Assessment Resoursces, Inc.

Rhode, G., Morgan, D. P., & Young, K. R. (1983). Generalization and maintenance of treatment gains of behaviorally handicapped students from resource rooms to regular classrooms using self-evaluation procedures. *Journal of Applied Behavioral Analysis, 16*, 171–188.

Richardson, E., Kupietz, S., & Maitinsky, S. (1987). What is the role of academic intervention in the treatment of hyperactive children with reading disorders? In J. Loney (Ed.), *The young hyperactive child: Answers to questions about diagnosis, prognosis and treatment*. New York: Haworth Press.

Richardson, E., Kupietz, S. S., Winsberg, B. G., Maitinsky, S., & Mendell, N. (1988). Effects of methylphenidate dosage in hyperactive reading-disabled children: II. Reading achievement. *Journal of American Academy of Child and Adolescent Psychiatry, 27*, 78–87.

Riddle, K. D., & Rapoport, J. L. (1976). A 2-year follow-up of 72 hyperactive boys. Classroom behavior and peer acceptance. *The Journal of Nervous and Mental Disease, 162*, 126–134.

Rie, H. E. (1980). Definitional problems. In H. E. Rie and E. D. Rie (Eds.), *Handbook of minimal brain dysfunctions: A critical view*. New York: Wiley Interscience Press.

Roberts, G. E. (1982). *Robert's Apperception Test for children*. Los Angeles: Western Psychological Services.

Robin, A. L. (1979). Problem-solving communication training: A behavioral approach to the treatment of parent-adolescent conflict. *American Journal of Family Therapy, 7*, 69–82.

Robin, A. L., & Foster, S. L. (1989). *Negotiating parent-adolescent conflict*. New York: Guilford Press.

Robins, L. N. (1979). Follow-up studies. In H. C. Quay and J. S. Werry (Eds.), *Psychopathological disorders of childhood*. New York: John Wiley & Sons.

Rodriguez, M. L., Shoda, Y., Mischel, W., & Wright, J. (1989, March). *Delay of gratification in children's social behavior in natural settings*. Paper presented at a meeting of the Eastern Psychological Association, Boston.

Rooney, K. J., Hallahan, D. P., & Lloyd, J. W. (1984). Self-recording of attention by learning-disabled students in the regular classroom. *Journal of Learning Disabilities, 17*, 360–364.

Rosenbaum, M., & Baker, E. (1984). Self-control behavior in hyperactive and non-hyperactive children. *Journal of Abnormal Child Psychology, 12*, 303–331.

Rosenbaum, M. S., & Drabman, R. S. (1979). Self-control training in the classroom: A review and critique. *Journal of Applied Behavior Analysis, 12*, 467–485.

Rosenthal, R. H., & Allen, T. W. (1978). An examination of attention, arousal and learning dysfunctions of hyperkinetic children. *Psychological Bulletin, 85*, 689–715.

Ross, D. M., & Ross, S. A. (1976). *Hyperactivity: Research, theory and action*. New York: John Wiley & Sons.

Ross, D. M., & Ross, S. A. (1982). *Hyperactivity: Current issues, research and theory* (2nd ed.). New York: John Wiley & Sons.

Rosse, R. B., & Licamele, W. L. (1984). Slow release methylphenidate problems when children chew tablets. *Journal of Clinical Psychiatry, 45*, 525.

Rosvold, H. E., Mirsky, A. F., Sarason, I., Bransome, E. D., & Beck, L. H. (1956). A continuous performance test of brain damage. *Journal of Consulting Psychology, 20*, 343–350.

Rotter, J. B. (1950). *Incomplete Sentences Blank—High School Form*. New York: The Psychological Corporation.

Routh, D. K. (1978). Hyperactivity. In P. R. Magrab (Ed.), *Psychological management of pediatric problems* (Vol. 2). Baltimore: University Park Press.

Routh, D. K., Schroeder, C. S., & O'Tauma, L. (1974). Development of activity level in children. *Developmental Psychology, 10*, 163–168.

Rudel, R. G., Denckla, M. B., & Broman, N. (1978). Rapid silent response to repeated target symbols by dyslexic and non-dyslexic children. *Brain and Language, 6*, 52–62.

Rutter, M. (1988). DSM-III-R: A postscript. In M. Rutter, A. H. Tuma, & I. S. Lann (Eds.), *Assessment and diagnosis in child psychopathology* (pp. 453–464). New York: Guilford Press.

Safer, D. J., Allen, R. P. (1973). Factors influencing the suppressant effects of two stimulant drugs on the growth of hyperactive children. *Pediatrics, 51*, 660–667.

Safer, D. J., & Allen, R. P. (1976). *Hyperactive children: Diagnosis and management*. Baltimore: University Park Press.

Safer, D. J., Allen, R. P., & Barr, E. (1972). Depression of growth in hyperactive children on stimulant drugs. *New England Journal of Medicine, 287*, 217–220.

Safer, D. J., & Krager, J. M. (1983). Trends in medication treatment of hyperactive children. *Clinical Pediatrics, 22*, 500–504.

Safer, D. J., & Krager, J. M. (1988). A survey of medication treatment for hyperactive/inattentive students. *Journal of the American Medical Association, 260*, 2256–2258.

Sallee, F., Stiller, R., Perel, J. & Bates, T. (1985). Oral pemoline, kinetics and hyperactive children. *Clinical Pharmacology Therapy., 37*, 606–609.

Sandberg, S. T., Rutter, M., & Taylor, E. (1978). Hyperkinetic disorder in psychiatric clinic attenders. *Developmental Medicine in Child Neurology, 20*, 279–299.

Santostefano, S., & Paley, E. (1964). Development of cognitive controls in children. *Journal of Clinical Psychology, 20*, 213–218.

Sarasone, S. B. (1949). *Psychological problems in mental deficiency*. New York: Harper and Row.

Sassone, D., Lambert, N. M., & Sandoval, J. (1982). The adolescent status of boys previously identified as hyperactive. In D. M. Ross and S. A. Ross (Eds.), *Hyperactivity: Current issues, research and theory* (2nd ed.). New York: John Wiley & Sons.

Satin, M. S., Winsberg, B. G., Monetti, C. H., Sverd, J., & Ross, D. A. (1985). A general population screen for attention deficit disorder with hyperactivity. *Journal of the American Academy of Child Psychiatry, 24*, 756–764.

Satterfield, B. (1988, February). *Multi-modal therapy in treating ADDH conduct disorder.* Presented at the Taboroff Child and Adolescent Child Psychiatry Conference on Conduct Disorders, Snowbird, UT.

Satterfield, J. H., & Bradley, B. W. (1977). Evoked potentials in brain maturation in hyperactive children. *Electroencephalography and Clinical Neurophysiology, 43*, 43–51.

Satterfield, J. H., Cantwell, D., & Satterfield, B. (1974). Pathophysiology of the hyperactive child syndrome. *Archives of General Psychiatry, 31*, 839–844.

Satterfield, J. H., Cantwell, D. P., & Satterfield, B. T. (1979). Multi-modality treatment. *Archives of General Psychiatry, 36*, 965–974.

Satterfield, J. H., Cantwell, D. P., Saul, R. E., Lesser, L. I., & Podosin, R. L. (1973). Response to stimulant drug treatment in hyperactive children: Prediction from EEG and neurological findings. *Autism Childhood Schizophrenia, 3*, 36–48.

Satterfield, J. H., & Dawson, M. E. (1971). Electrodermal correlates of hyperactivity in children. *Psychophysiology, 8*, 191–197.

Satterfield, J. H., Hoppe, C. M., & Schell, A. M. (1982). A perspective study of delinquency in 110 adolescent boys with attention deficit disorder and 88 normal adolescent boys. *American Journal of Psychiatry, 139*, 795–798.

Satterfield, J. H., Satterfield, B. T., & Cantwell, D. P. (1981). Three-year multi-modality treatment study of 100 hyperactive boys. *Journal of Pediatrics, 98*, 650–655.

Satterfield, J. H., Schell, A. M., & Backs, R. W. (1987). Longitudinal study of AERPs in hyperactive and normal children: Relationship to antisocial behavior. *Electroencephalography and Clinical Neurophysiology, 67*, 531–536.

Schachar, R., Taylor, E., Wieselberg, M. B., Thorley, G., & Rutter, M. (1987). Changes in family function and relationships in children who respond to methylphenidate. *Journal of the American Academy of Child and Adolescent Psychiatry, 26*, 728–732.

Schleifer, M., Weiss, G., Cohen, N. J., Elman, M., Cvejic, H., & Kruger, E. (1975). Hyperactivity in preschoolers and the effect of methylphenidate. *American Journal of Orthopsychiatry, 45*, 35–50.

Schloss, P. J., Schloss, C. N., Wood, C. E., & Kiehl, W. S. (1986). A critical review of social skills research with behaviorally disordered students. *Behavioral Disorders, 12*, 1–14.

Schneider, M. (1978). Turtle technique in the classroom. Described in M. Herbert, *Conduct disorders of childhood and adolescents* (p. 119). New York: John Wiley & Sons.

Schoenfield, M., & Rosenblatt, J. (1985). *Adventures with logic.* Belmont, CA: David S. Lake.

Seashore, C. E., Lewis, D., & Saetveit, D. L. (1960). *Seashore Measures of Musical Talents* (rev. ed.). New York: Psychological Corporation.

Sebrechts, M. M., Shaywitz, S. E., Shaywitz, B. A., Jatlow, P., Anderson, G. M., & Cohen, D. J. (1986). Components of attention, methylphenidate dosage, and blood levels in children with attention deficit disorder. *Pediatrics, 77*, 222–228.

Senf, G. M. (1988). Neurometric brain mapping in the diagnosis and rehabilitation of cognitive dysfunction. *Cognitive Rehabilitation, 6*, 20–37.

Shaffer, D., & Schonfeld, I. (1984). A critical note on the value of attention deficit as a basis for a clinical syndrome. In L. M. Bloomingdale (Ed.), *Attention deficit disorders: Diagnostic, cognitive, and therapeutic understanding.* Long Island, NY: Spectrum.

Shapiro, E. A. K. (1981). Tic disorders. *Journal of the American Medical Association, 245*, 1583–1585.

Shapiro, S. K., & Garfinkel, B. D. (1986). The occurrence of behavior disorders in children: The interdependence of attention deficit disorder and conduct disorder. *Journal of the American Academy of Child Psychiatry, 25*, 809–819.

Shaywitz, B. A., Cohen, D. J., & Bowers, M. B. (1977). CSF monoamine metabolites in children with minimal brain dysfunction: Evidence for alteration of brain dopamine. *Journal of Pediatrics, 1*, 67–71.

Shaywitz, B. A., Gordon, J. W., Klopper, J. H., & Zelterman, D. (1977). The effect of 6-hydroxydopamine of habituation and activity in the developing rat pup. *Pharmacology, Biochemistry and Behavior, 6*, 391–396.

Shaywitz, B. A., Klopper, J. H., & Gordon, J. W. (1978). Methylphenidate in 6-hydroxydopamine-treated developing rat pups. *Archives of Neurology, 35*, 463–469.

Shaywitz, B. A., & Pearson, D. E. (1978). Effects of phenobarbital on activity and learning in 6-hydroxydopamine-treated rat pups. *Pharmacology, Biochemistry and Behavior, 9*, 173–179.

Shaywitz, B. A., Shaywitz, S. E., Anderson, G. M., Jatlow, P., Gillespie, S. M., Sullivan, B. M., Riddle, M. A., Leckman, J. F., & Cohen, D. J. (1988, September). D-Amphetamine Affects Central Noradrenergic Mechanisms in Children with Attention Deficit Hyperactivity Disorder. *Presentation made at the seventeenth national meeting of the Child Neurology Society, Halifax, Canada.*

Shaywitz, B. A., Yager, R. D., & Klopper, J. H. (1976). Selective brain dopamine depletion in developing rats: An experimental model of minimal brain dysfunction. *Science, 191*, 305-307.

Shaywitz, S. E. (1986). Prevalence of attentional deficits and an epidemiologic sample of school children (unpublished raw data). In J. F. Kavanaugh and T. J. Truss (Eds.), *Learning Disabilities: Proceedings of the national conference, 1988* (p. 457) Parkton, MD: York Press.

Shaywitz, S. E., Hunt, R. D., Jatlow, P., Cohen, D. J., Young, J. G., Pierce, R. N., Anderson, G. M., & Shaywitz, B. A. (1982). Psychopharmacology of attention deficit disorder: Pharmacokinetic neuroendocrine and behavioral measures following acute and chronic treatment with methylphenidate. *Pediatrics, 69*, 688–694.

Shaywitz, S. E., & Shaywitz, B. A. (1986). Attention Deficit Disorder: Current perspectives. In J. F. Kavanaugh and T. J. Truss (Eds.), *Learning Disabilities: Proceedings of the national conference, 1988* (369–523). Parkton, MD: York Press.

Shaywitz, S. E., & Shaywitz, B. A. (1988). Increased medication use in attention deficit hyperactivity disorder: Regressive or appropriate? (Editorial). *Journal of the American Medical Association, 260*, 2270–2272.

Shekim, W. O., Dekirmenjian, H., & Chapel, J. L. (1977). Urinary catecholamine metabolites in hyperkinetic boys treated with d-amphetamine. *American Journal of Psychiatry, 11*, 1276–1279.

Shekim, W. O., Dekirmenjian, H., Chapel, J. L., Javaid, J. and Davis, J. M. (1979). Norepinephrine metabolism and clinical response to dextroamphetamine in hyperactive boys. *Journal of Pediatrics, 95*, 389–394.

Shekim, W. O., Sinclair, E., Glaser, R., Horwitz, E., Javaid, J., & Bylund, D. (1987). Norepinephrine and dopamine metabolites and educational variables in boys with attention deficit disorder and hyperactivity. *Journal of Child Neurology, 2*, 50–56.

Shelley, E. M., & Riester, A. (1972). Syndrome of minimal brain damage in young adults. *Diseases of the Nervous System, 33*, 335–338.

Shetty, T., & Chase, T. N. (1976) Central monoamines and hyperkinesis of childhood. *Neurology, 26,* 1000–1002.

Shure, M. B. (1981). Social competence as a problem-solving skill. In J. D. Wine and M. D. Smye (Eds.), *Social competence.* New York: Guilford Press.

Shure, M. B. & Spivack, G. (1978). *Problem-solving techniques in child rearing.* San Francisco: Josey-Bass.

Silver, L. B. (1980a). *Attention deficit disorders: Booklet for parents.* Summit, NJ: CIBA.

Silver, L. B. (1980b). *Attention deficit disorders: Booklet for the classroom teacher.* Summit, NJ: CIBA.

Silver, L. B. (1981). The relationship between learning disabilities, hyperactivity, distractability and behavioral problems. A clinical analysis. *Journal of the American Academy of Child Psychiatry, 20,* 385–397.

Sleator, E. K. (1982). Office diagnosis of hyperactivity by the physician. In K. D. Gadow and I. Bialer (Eds.), *Advances in Learning and Behavioral Disabilities* (Vol. 1). Greenwich, CT: JAI.

Sleator, E. K., Ullmann, R. K., & von Neumann, A. (1982). How do hyperactive children feel about taking stimulants and will they tell their doctor? *Clinical Pediatrics, 21,* 474–479.

Smith, A. (1973). *Symbol Digit Modalities Test Manual.* Los Angeles: Western Psychological Services.

Smith, H. F. (1986). The elephant on the fence: Approaches to the psychotherapy of attention deficit disorder children. *American Journal of Psychotherapy, 40,* 252–264.

Snyder, S. H., & Meyerhoff, J. L. (1973). How amphetamine acts in minimal brain dysfunction. *Annals New York Academy of Sciences, 205,* 310–319.

Speltz, M. L., Varley, C. K., Peterson, K., & Beilke, R. L. (1988). Effects of dextroamphetamine and contingency management on a preschooler with ADHD and oppositional defiant disorder. *Journal of American Academy of Child Adolescent Psychiatry, 27,* 175–178.

Spivack, G., & Shure, M. B. (1974). *Social adjustment of young children: A cognitive approach to solving real-life problems.* San Francisco: Josey-Bass.

Sprague, R. L., & Sleator, E. K. (1977). Methylphenidate in hyperkinetic children: Differences in dose effects on learning and social behavior. *Science, 198,* 1274–1276.

Spring, C., Blunden, D., Greenberg, L. M., & Yellin, A. M. (1977). Validity and norms of a hyperactivity rating scale. *Exceptional Children, 11,* 313–321.

Spring, C., Yellin, A. M., & Greenberg, L. M. (1976). Effects of imipramine and methylphenidate on perceptual-motor performance of hyperactive children. *Perceptual and Motor Skills, 43,* 459–470.

Stanton, R. D., & Brumback, R. A. (1981). Non-specificity of motor hyperactivity as a diagnostic criterion. *Perceptual Motor Skills, 52,* 323–332.

Starke, K., & Montel, H. (1973). Involvement of a-receptors in clonidine-induced inhibition of transmitter release from central monoamine neurons. *Neuropharmacology, 12,* 1073–1080.

Stedman, J. M., Lawlis, G. F., Cortner, R. H., & Achterberg, G. (1978). Relationships between WISC-R factors, Wide-Range Achievement Test scores, and visual-motor maturation in children referred for psychological evaluation. *Journal of Consulting and Clinical Psychology, 46,* 869–872.

Steinberg, G. G., Troshinsky, C., & Steinberg, H. R. (1971). Dextroamphetamine responsive behavior disorder in school children. *American Journal of Psychiatry, 128,* 174–179.

Sternbach, H. (1981). Pemoline induced mania. *Biological Psychiatry, 16*, 987–989.

Stevenson, R. S., Pelham, W., & Skinner, R. (1984). Dependent and main effects of methylphenidate and pemoline on paired associate learning and spelling in hyperactive children. *Journal of Counseling and Clinical Psychology, 52*, 104–113.

Stewart, M. A. (1980). Genetic, perinatal, and constitutional factors in minimal brain dysfunction. In H. E. Rie and E. D. Rie (Eds.), *Handbook of minimal brain dysfunctions*. New York: Wiley Interscience Press.

Stewart, M. A., DeBlois, C. S., & Cummings, C. (1980). Psychiatric disorders in parents of hyperactive boys and those with conduct disorder. *Journal of Child Psychology and Psychiatry, 21*, 283–292.

Stewart, M. A., & Olds, S. W. (1973). *Raising a hyperactive child*. New York: Harper and Row.

Stewart, M. A., Thatch, B. T., & Freidin, M. R. (1970). Accidental poisoning in the hyperactive child syndrome. *Diseases of the Nervous System, 31*, 403–407.

Still, G. F. (1902). The Coulstonian Lectures on some abnormal physical conditions in children. *Lancet, 1*, 1008–1012.

Stokes, T. R., & Baer, D. M. (1977). An implicit technology of generalization. *Journal of Applied Behavior Analysis, 10*, 349–367.

Strain, P., Guralnick, M., & Walker, H. M. (1986). *Children's social behavior*. New York: Academic Press.

Strauss, A. A., & Kephart, N. C. (1955). *Psychopathology and education of the brain-injured child: Vol. 2. Progress in theory and clinic*. New York: Grune and Stratton.

Strauss, A. A., & Lehtinen, L. E. (1947). *Psychopathology and education of the brain-injured child*. New York: Grune and Stratton.

Strayhorn, J. M., Rapp, N., Donina, W., & Strain, P. S. (1988). Randomized trial of methylphenidate for an autistic child. *Journal of American Academy of Child and Adolescent Psychiatry, 27*, 244–247.

Stroop, J. R. (1935). Studies of interference in serial verbal reactions. *Journal of Experimental Psychology, 18*, 643–661.

Strub, R. L., & Black, F. W. (1977). *The mental status examination in neurology*. Philadelphia: F.A. Davis.

Sulzer-Azaroff, B., & Mayer, G. R. (1977). *Applying behavior-analysis procedures with children and youth*. New York: Holt, Rinehart & Winston.

Sunder, T. R., DeMarco, S., Fruitiger, A. D., & Levey, B. (1988, September). A developmental right hemisphere deficit syndrome in childhood. Presentation made at the seventeenth national meeting, of the Child Neurology Society, Halifax, Canada.

Swanson, J. M. (1988). Discussion. In J. F. Kavanaugh and T. J. Truss (Eds.), *Learning disabilities: Proceedings of the national conference, 1988*. (pp. 542–546). Parkton, Maryland: York Press, 542–546.

Swanson, J., & Kinsbourne, M. (1980). Food dyes impair performance of hyperactive children on a laboratory learning test. *Science, 207*, 1485–1487.

Swanson, J., Kinsbourne, M., Roberts, W., & Zucker, K. (1978). Time-response analysis of the effect of stimulant medication on the learning ability of children referred for hyperactivity. *Pediatrics, 61*, 21–29.

Tarnowski, K. J., Prinz, R. J., & Ney, S. M. (1986). Comparative analysis of attentional deficits in hyperactive and learning disabled children. *Journal of Abnormal Psychology, 95*, 341–345.

Tawney, J. W., & Gast, D. L. (1984). *Applied behavior analysis for teachers*. Columbus, OH: Charles R. Merrill.

Taylor, E. (1980). Development of attention. In M. Rutter (Ed.), *Scientific foundations of developmental psychiatry*. London: Heineman Medical Books.

Terestman, N. (1980). Mood quality and intensity in nursery school children as predictors of behavior disorder. *American Journal of Orthopsychiatry, 50*, 125–138.

Thomas, A., & Chess, S. (1977). *Temperament and development*. New York: Brunner/-Mazel.

Thompson, J., Ross, R., & Horwitz, S. (1980). The role of computed tomography in the study of children with minimal brain dysfunction. *Journal of Learning Disabilities, 13*, 48–51.

Thorndike, R. L., Hagen, E. P., & Satler, J. M. (1986). *Revised Stanford Binet Intelligence Scale*. Boston: Houghton Mifflin.

Tofte-Tipps, S., Mendonca, P., & Peach, R. V. (1982). Training and generalization of social skills: A study with two developmentally handicapped, socially isolated children. *Behavior Modification, 6*, 45–71.

Trenerry, M. R., Crosson, B., DeBoe, J. & Leber, W. R. (1989). *The Stroop Neuropsychological Screening Test*. Odessa, FL: Psychological Assessment Resources.

Trites, R. (1979). Prevalence in hyperactivity in Ottawa, Canada. In R. Trites (Ed.), *Hyperactivity in children*. Baltimore: University Park Press.

Trites, R. L., Blouin, A. G. A., & Laprade, K. (1982). Factor analysis of the Conners Teacher Rating Scale based on a large normative sample. *Journal of Consulting and Clinical Psychology, 50*, 615–623.

Trommer, B. L., Bernstein, L. P., Rosenberg, R. S., & Armstrong, K. J. (1988, September). Topographic mapping of P300 in attention deficit disorder. Presentation made at the seventeenth national meeting of the 1988 Child Neurology Society, Halifax, Canada.

Ullmann, R. K., & Sleator, E. (1985). Attention deficit disorder. Children with or without hyperactivity. Which behaviors are helped by stimulants? *Clinical Pediatrics, 24*, 547–551.

Ullmann, R. K., & Sleator, E. (1986). Responders, nonresponders, and placebo responders among children with attention deficit disorder. Importance of blinded placebo evaluation. *Clinical Pediatrics, 25*, 594–599.

Ullmann, R. K., Sleator, E. K., & Sprague, R. K. (1985a). *Add-H: Comprehensive teacher's rating scale*. Champaign, IL: MetriTech.

Ullmann, R. K., Sleator, E. K., & Sprague, R. K. (1985b). Introduction to the use of ACTeRs. *Psychopharmacology Bulletin, 21*, 915–920.

Urion, D. K. (1988, September). Attention deficit hyperactivity disorder: Pharmacological response predicted by neurological subtype. Presentation made at the seventeenth national meeting of the Child Neurology Society, Halifax, Canada.

Van Zomeren, A. H. (1981). *Reaction time and attention after closed head injury*. Lisse, Switzerland: Swets & Zeitinger.

Van Zomeren, A. H., & Brouwer, W. H. (1987). Head injury and concepts of attention. In H. S. Levin, J. Grafman, & H. M. Eisenberg (Eds.), *Neurobehavioral recovery from head injury*. New York: Oxford University Press.

Varni, J. W., & Henker, B. (1979). A self-regulation approach to the treatment of three hyperactive boys. *Child Behavior Therapy, 1*, 171–191.

Vaughn, V. (1969). Growth and development. In W. Nelson (Ed.), *Textbook of pediatrics* (9th ed.). Philadelphia: W.B. Saunders.

Voelker, S., Lachar, D., & Gadowski, C. L. (1983). The Personality Inventory for Children and response to methylphenidate: Preliminary evidence for predictive utility. *Journal of Pediatric Psychology, 8*, 161–169.

Voeller, K. K. S., & Heilman, K. M. (1988, September). Motor impersistence in children with attention deficit hyperactivity disorder: Evidence for right-hemisphere dysfunction. Presentation made at the seventeenth national meeting of the Child Neurology Society, Halifax, Canada.

Vygotsky, L. (1962). *Thought and language*. New York: John Wiley & Sons.

Waddell, K. J. (1984). The self-concept and social adaptation of hyperactive children and adolescents. *Journal of Clinical Child Psychology, 13*, 50–55.

Wagonseller, B. R., Burnett, M., Salzberg, B., & Burnett, J. (1977). *The art of parenting: A complete training guide*. Champaign, IL: Research Press.

Wagonseller, B. R., & McDowell, R.L. (1979). *You and your child: A common sense approach to successful parenting*. Champaign, IL: Research Press.

Wagonseller, B. R., & McDowell, R. L. (1982). *Teaching involved parenting*. Champaign, IL: Research Press.

Walker, H. M., Todis, B., Holmes, D., & Horton, G. (1988). *The Walker social skills curriculum: The ACCESS Program*. Austin, TX: Pro-Ed.

Wallander, J. L., Schroeder, S. R., Michelli, J. A., & Gualitieri, C. T. (1987). Classroom social interactions of attention deficit disorder with hyperactivity children as a function of stimulant medication. *Journal of Pediatric Psychology, 12*, 61–76.

Webb, T. E., & Oski, F. A. (1973). Iron deficiency anemia may affect scholastic achievement in young adolescents. *Journal of Pediatrics, 82*, 827–829.

Webb, T. E., & Oski, F. A. (1974). Behavioral status of young adolescents with iron deficiency anemia. *Journal of Special Education, 2*, 153–156.

Wechsler, D. (1974). *Wechsler Intelligence Scale For Children—Revised*. New York: Psychological Corporation.

Wehrli, K. (1971). *A self-instruction workbook for visual accuracy*. Worthington, OH: Ann Arbor.

Weiner, B. (1979). A theory of motivation for some classroom experiences. *Journal of Educational Psychology, 71*, 3–25.

Weiss, G., & Hechtman, L. (1979). The hyperactive child syndrome. *Science, 205*, 1348–1354.

Weiss, G., & Hechtman, L. T. (1986). *Hyperactive children grown up*. New York: Guilford Press.

Weiss, G., Hechtman, L., & Perlman, T. (1978). Hyperactives as young adults: Social, employer and self-rating scales obtained during ten-year follow-up evaluation. *American Journal of Orthopsychiatry, 48*, 438–445.

Weiss, G., Kurger, E., Danielson, U., & Elman, M. (1975). Effect of long-term treatment of hyperactive children with methylphenidate. *CMA Journal, 112*, 159–163.

Weiss, G., Minde, K., Werry, J. S., Douglas, V. I., & Nemeth, E. (1971). Studies on the hyperactive child: VII Five-year follow-up. *Archives of General Psychiatry, 24*, 409–414.

Wender, E. H. (1986). The food additive-free diet in the treatment of behavior disorders: A review. *Developmental and Behavioral Pediatrics, 7*, 35–42.

Wender, P. H. (1971). *Minimal brain dysfunction in children*. New York: John Wiley & Sons.

Wender, P. (1972). The minimal brain dysfunction syndrome in children. *Journal of Nervous and Mental Disease, 155*, 55–71.

Wender, P. H. (1975). The minimal brain dysfunction syndrome. *Annual Review of Medicine, 26*, 45–62.

Wender, P. H. (1979). The concept of adult minimal brain dysfunction. In L. Bellak (Ed.), *Psychiatric aspects of minimal brain dysfunction in adults.* New York: Grune and Stratton.

Wender, P. H. (1987). Differential diagnosis of hyperactivity. *Developmental and Behavioral Pediatrics, 8,* 166–167.

Werner, E. E., Bierman, J. M., French, F. E., Simonian, K., Connor, A., Smith, R. S. & Campbell, M. (1968). Reproductive and environmental casualties: A report on the 10-year follow up of the children of the Kauai pregnancy study. *Pediatrics, 42,* 112-127.

Werner, E. E., & Smith, R. S. (1977). *Kauai's children come of age.* Honolulu: University of Hawaii Press.

Werry, J. S. (1968). Developmental hyperactivity. *Pediatric Clinics of North America, 15,* 581–599.

Werry, J. S. (1978). Measures in pediatric psychopharmacology. In J. S. Werry (Ed.), *Pediatric psychopharmacology: The use of behavior modifying drugs in children.* New York: Brunner/Mazel.

Werry, J. S. (1988). In memoriam—DSM-III [Letter to the editor]. *Journal of the American Academy of Child and Adolescent Psychiatry, 27,* pp. 138–139.

Werry, J. S., Aman, M. G., & Lampen, E. (1975). Halperidol and methylphenidate in hyperactive children. *ACTA Paedopsychiatrica, 42,* 26–40.

Werry, J. S., Minde, K., Guzman, A., Weiss, G., Dogan, K., & Hoy, E. (1972). Studies on the hyperactive child: VII. Neurological status compared with neurotic and normal children. *American Journal of Orthopsychiatry, 42,* 441–449.

Whalen, C. K., Collins, B. E., Henker, B., Alkus, S. R., Adams, D., & Stapp, S. (1978). Behavior observations of hyperactive children and methylphenidate (Ritalin) effects in systematically structured classroom environments: Now you see them, now you don't. *Journal of Pediatric Psychology, 3,* 177–184.

Whalen, C. K., & Henker, B. (1976). Psychostimulants and children: A review and analysis. *Psychological Bulletin, 83,* 1113–1130.

Whalen, C. K., & Henker, B. (1980). The social ecology of psychostimulant treatment: A model for conceptual and empirical analysis. In C. K. Whalen and B. Henker (Eds.), *Hyperactive children: The social ecology of identification and treatment.* New York: Academic Press.

Whalen, C. K., & Henker, B. (1985). The social worlds of hyperactive (ADDH) children. *Clinical Psychology Review, 5,* 447–478.

Whalen, C. K., Henker, B., Castro, J., & Granger, D. (1987). Peer perceptions of hyperactivity and medication effects. *Child Development, 58,* 816–828.

Whalen, C. K., Henker, B., Collins, B. E., Finck, D., & Dotemoto, S. (1979). A social ecology of hyperactive boys: Medication effects in structured classroom environments. *Journal of Applied Behavior Analysis, 12,* 65–81.

Whalen, C. K., Henker, B., Collins, B., McAuliffe, S., & Vaux, A. (1979). Peer interaction in a structured communication task: Comparisons of normal and hyperactive boys and of methylphenidate (Ritalin) and placebo effects. *Child Development 50,* 388–401.

Whalen, C. K., Henker, B., & Dotemoto, S. (1981). Teacher response to methylphenidate (Ritalin) versus placebo status of hyperactive boys in the classroom. *Child Development, 52,* 1005–1014.

Whalen, C. K., Henker, B., & Hinshaw, S. P. (1985). Cognitive-behavioral therapies for hyperactive children: Premises, problems and prospects. *Journal of Abnormal Child Psychology, 13,* 391–410.

Whalen, C. K., Henker, B., Swanson, J. M., Granger, D., Kliewer, W., & Spencer, J. (1987). Natural social behaviors in hyperactive children: Dose effects of methylphenidate. Journal of *Consulting and Clinical Psychology, 55,* 187–193.

Whimbey, A., & Lochhead, J. (1986). *Problem solving and comprehension.* Hillsdale, NJ: Lawrence Erlbaum Associates.

White, M. (1975). Natural rates of teacher approval and disapproval in the classroom. *Journal of Applied Behavior Analysis, 8,* 367–372.

Whitehead, P. L., & Clark, L. D. (1970). Effect of lithium carbonate, placebo and thyridizine on hyperactive children. *Medical Journal of Psychiatry, 127,* 824–825.

Whitehill, M. B., Hersen, M., & Bellack, A. S. (1980). Conversational skills training for socially isolated children. *Behavior Research Therapy, 12,* 217–225.

Whitehouse, D., Shah, U., & Palmer, F. B. (1980). Comparison of sustained release and standard methylphenidate in the treatment of minimal brain dysfunction. *Journal of Clinical Psychiatry, 41,* 282–285.

Willerman, L. (1973). Activity level and hyperactivity in twins. *Child Development, 44,* 288–293.

Winnicott, D. W. (1974). *Pediatrics through psychoanalysis: The collective papers of D.W. Winnicott.* New York: Basic Books.

Winsberg, B. G., Camp-Bruno, J. A., Vink, J., Timmer, C. J., & Sverd, J. (1987). Mianserin pharmacokinetics and behavior in hyperkinetic children. *Journal of Clinical Psychopharmacology, 7,* 143–147.

Winsberg, B., Maitinsky, S., Kupietz, S., & Richardson, E. (1987). Is there dose dependent tolerance associated with chronic methylphenidate therapy in hyperactive children: Oral dose of plasmic concentrations. *Psychopharmacology Bulletin, 23,* 107–110.

Winsberg, B. G., Maitinsky, S., Richardson, E., & Kupietz, S. S. (1988). Effects of methylphenidate on achievement in hyperactive children with reading disorders. *Psychopharmacology Bulletin, 24,* 238–241.

Winsberg, D. J., Kupietz, S. S., Sverd, J., Hungdung, B. L., & Young, N. L. (1982). Methylphenidate oral dose plasma concentrations and behavioral response in children. *Psychopharmacology, 76,* 329–332.

Wirt, R. D., Lacher, D., Klinedinst, J. K., & Seat, P. D. (1977). *Multi-dimensional description of child personality: A manual for the Personality Inventory for Children.* Los Angeles: Western Psychological Services.

Wolff, P. H. (1969). The natural history of crying and other vocalizations in early infancy. In B. M. Foss (Ed.), *Determinants of infant behavior* (Vol. 4). London: Methuen.

Wolraich, M., Drummond, T., Salomon, M., O'Brien, M., & Sivage, C. (1978). Effects of methylphenidate alone and in combination with behavior management of hyperactive children. *Journal of Abnormal Child Psychology, 6,* 149–161.

Wolraich, M., Milich, R., Stumbo, P., & Schultz, F. (1985). Effects of sucrose ingestion on the behavior of hyperactive boys. *Journal of Pediatrics, 106,* 675–682.

Womack, R. L. (1985). *Creating line designs: Books 1-4.* Bothell, WA: Golden Educational Center.

Woodcock, R. W. (1973). *Woodcock Reading Mastery Tests.* Circle Pines, MN: American Guidance Service.

Woodcock, R. W., & Johnson, M. B. (1977). *Woodcock-Johnson Psycho-Educational Battery*. Hingham, MA: Teaching Resources.

Woodcock, R. W. (1989). *Woodcock-Johnson Psychoeducational Battery - Revised*. Allen, Texas: Teaching Resources.

Woodside, D. B., Brownstone, D., & Fisman, S. (1987). The Dexamethasone Suppression Test and the Children's Depression Inventory in psychiatric disorders in children. *Canadian Journal of Psychiatry, 32*, 2–4.

Wyngaarden, J. B. (1988). Adverse effects of low-level lead exposure on infant development. *Journal of the American Medical Association, 259*, 2524.

Yanow, M. (1973). Report on the use of behavior modification drugs on elementary school children. In M. Yanow (Ed.), *Observations from the treadmill*. New York: Viking Press.

Zachman, L., Husingh, R., & Barrett, M. (1988). *Blooming: Language arts*. Moline, IL: LinguiSystems.

Zachman, L., Jorgenson, C., Barrett, M., Husingh, R. & Snedden, M. K. (1982). *Manual of exercises for expressive reasoning*. Moline, IL: LinguiSystems.

Zagar, R., Arbit, J., Hughes, J. R., Busell, R. E., & Busch, K. (1989). Developmental and disruptive behavior disorders among delinquents. *Journal of the American Academy of Child and Adolescent Psychiatry, 28*, 437–440.

Zametkin, A. J., Karoum, F., & Rapoport, J. L. (1987). Treatment of hyperactive children with d-phenylalanine. *American Journal of Psychiatry, 144*, 792–794.

Zametkin, A. J., & Rapoport, J. L. (1987). Neurobiology of attention deficit disorder with hyperactivity: Where have we come in 50 years? *Journal of American Academy of Child and Adolescent Psychiatry, 26*, 676–686.

Zametkin, A., Reeves, J. C., Webster, L., & Werry, J. C. (1986). Promethazine treatment of children with attention deficit disorder and hyperactivity—ineffective and unpleasant. *Journal of the American Academy of Child Psychiatry, 25*, 854–856.

Author Index

Lacher, D., 13, 113, 114
Lahey, B. B., 6, 10, 37, 336
Lambert, N. M., 4, 6, 16, 17, 21, 23, 24, 29
Lampen, E., 254
Landau, S., 26, 161, 329, 334, 336
Landrigan, P. J., 33
Langford, W. S., 230
Langhorne, J. E., 26, 76
Lapouse, R., 5
Laprade, K., 73
Larsen, V., 63
Laserna, C., 294
Lasgna, L., 56
Lasley, T. J., 326
Laufer, M. W., 5
Lavigeuer, H., 21
Lawlis, G. F., 127
Leber, W. R., 141
Leckman, J. F., 60
Lehtinen, L. E., 5, 314
Leimbach, J., 292
Leland, B., 131
LeMay, M., 60
Lerer, T., 51
Lesser, L. I., 56
Lester, M. L., 32
Levey, B., 40
Levine, M. D., 41
Leviton, A., 33
Lewin, D., 21
Lewis, D., 133
Lezak, M. D., 131, 133
Licamele, W. L., 264
Licht, B. G., 267, 280
Lindgren, S., 222
Linn, R. T., 280
Little, J. W., 231
Lloyd, J. W., 267, 270, 272
Lochhead, J., 295
Loeber, R., 330
Logan, W. J., 58
Loney, J., 21, 23, 24, 25, 26, 27, 76, 230, 238, 313, 330
Lorys-Vernon, A., 37
Loss, B., 294
Lou, H. C., 29
Love, A. J., 19
Lovitt, T. C., 268, 272
Lovrich, D., 58

Lowe, T. L., 215
Lozanoff, B., 267, 270, 273
Lubchenco, L. O., 29
Lubetsky, M. J., 231
Luisada, P. V., 16
Luria, A. R., 217, 267

Maas, J. W., 39
MacKay, M., 230
MacKay, M. C., 227
MacLeod, S. M., 251
Maher, C., 33
Mahoney, M. J., 273, 274
Mainville, F., 334
Maitinsky, S., 236, 237, 238, 242
Malone, M. A., 58
Mammen, O., 14
Mann, L., 61
Mannuzza, S., 2, 3, 24, 25, 230
Markwardt, F. C., 96, 145
Marshall, K. J., 267
Martin, P., 275
Marx, D., 217
Mash, E. J., 18, 336
Massman, P. J., 127
Matson, J. L., 232, 332
Mattes, J., 216, 217
Matthews, K. L., 227, 251
Mattison, R., 19
Mayer, G. R., 320, 323
Mays, R., 282
McAuliffe, S., 330
McCarthy, J. J., 138, 139
McClure, F. D., 7, 135
McCluskey, C. L., 333
McConnell, S., 332
McDaniel, K. D., 227
McDowell, R. L., 366
McGee, R., 3, 6, 36
McGinnis, E., 331, 333, 334, 339, 340
McGrew, J., 249, 251
McKay, G. D., 365
McKnew, D., 110
McMahon, S. A., 63, 64
McNamara, J. J., 4
McNeil, T. F., 15
McNicol, J., 32
McNutt, B., 229
Meagher, R. B., 146
Medenis, A., 234

Subject Index